Baillière's
CLINICAL
ENDOCRINOLOGY
AND
METABOLISM
INTERNATIONAL PRACTICE AND RESEARCH

Baillière's

CLINICAL ENDOCRINOLOGY AND METABOLISM

INTERNATIONAL PRACTICE AND RESEARCH

Volume 2/Number 2
May 1988

Non-insulin-dependent Diabetes

M. NATTRASS BSc, MBChB, PhD, FRCP
P. J. HALE MA, DM, MRCP
Guest Editors

Baillière Tindall
London Philadelphia Sydney Tokyo Toronto

Baillière Tindall   24–28 Oval Road
W.B. Saunders   London NW1 7DX, UK

The Curtis Center, Independence Square West,
Philadelphia, PA 19106–3399, USA

1 Goldthorne Avenue
Toronto, Ontario M8Z 5T9, Canada

Harcourt Brace Jovanovich Group (Australia) Pty Ltd,
32–52 Smidmore Street, Marrickville, NSW 2204, Australia

Exclusive Agent in Japan:
Maruzen Co. Ltd. (Journals Division)
3–10 Nihonbashi 2-chome, Chuo-ku, Tokyo 103, Japan

ISSN 0950–351X

ISBN 0–7020–1294–7 (single copy)

Baillière's Clinical Endocrinology and Metabolism is published four times each year by
Baillière Tindall. Annual subscription prices are:

TERRITORY	ANNUAL SUBSCRIPTION	SINGLE ISSUE
1. UK & Republic of Ireland	£35.00 post free	£15.00 post free
2. USA & Canada	US$68.00 post free	US$25.00 post free
3. All other countries	£45.00 post free	£18.50 post free

The editor of this publication is Katharine Hinton, Baillière Tindall,
24–28 Oval Road, London NW1 7DX, UK.

Baillière's Clinical Endocrinology and Metabolism was published from 1972 to 1986 as
Clinics in Endocrinology and Metabolism.

Typeset by Phoenix Photosetting, Chatham.
Printed and bound in Great Britain by Mackays of Chatham PLC, Chatham, Kent.

Contributors to this issue

CLIFFORD J. BAILEY BSc, PhD, Senior Tutor, Biology Division, Department of Pharmaceutical Sciences, Aston University, Birmingham B4 7ET, UK.

JOHN C. BROWN PhD, DSC, FRSC, Professor of Physiology, University of British Columbia, 2146 Health Sciences Mall, Vancouver, BC V6T 1W5, Canada.

ANNE CLARK BSc, PhD, Research Fellow, Diabetes Research Laboratories, Radcliffe Infirmary, Woodstock Road, Oxford OX2 6HE, UK.

P. L. DRURY, Consultant Physician, Department of Diabetes, King's College Hospital, Denmark Hill, London SE5 9RS, UK.

STEWART MAXWELL DUNN, BA, MAPsS, PhD, Research Fellow, Department of Medicine, University of Sydney, NSW 2006, Australia; Consultant Psychologist, Royal Prince Alfred Hospital, Missenden Road, Camperdown, NSW 2050, Australia.

MICHAEL G. FITZGERALD MD, FRCP, Consultant Physician, General Hospital, Steelhouse Lane, Birmingham B4 6NH, UK.

WENDY GATLING DM, MRCP, MBChB, Senior Registrar, Poole General Hospital, Longfleet Road, Poole, Dorset, UK.

JOHN E. GERICH MD, Professor of Medicine and Physiology, University of Pittsburgh School of Medicine, Clinical Research Center, 3488 Presbyterian University Hospital, 230 Lothrop Street, Pittsburgh, PA 15261, USA.

PETER JOHN HALE MA, DM, MRCP, Senior Registrar in Medicine, General Hospital, Steelhouse Lane, Birmingham B4 6NH, UK.

LENE HEICKENDORFF MD, Department of Clinical Chemistry, Kommunehospitalet, University of Århus, DK-8000 Århus C, Denmark.

ROBERT J, HEINE MD, Senior Lecturer, Department of Internal Medicine, Free University Hospital, De Boelelaan 1117, 1081 HV Amsterdam, The Netherlands.

RONALD DAVID HILL FRCP, Consultant Physician, Poole General Hospital, Longfleet Road, Poole, Dorset, UK.

HILARY KING MD, MSc, MFCM, Consultant, Division of Noncommunicable Diseases, World Health Organization, CH-1211 Geneva 27, Switzerland.

THOMAS LEDET MD, PhD, Senior Lecturer, Institute of Experimental Clinical Research, University Institute of Pathology, Kommunehospitalet, DK-8000 Århus C, Denmark.

J. LEVY MA, MBBS, MRCP, Honorary Senior Registrar, Diabetes Research Laboratories, Radcliffe Infirmary, Woodstock Road, Oxford OX2 6HE, UK.

DAVID RICHARD MATTHEWS MA, DPhil, BM, BCH, MRCP, Honorary Consultant Physician, Diabetes Research Laboratories, Radcliffe Infirmary, Woodstock Road, Oxford OX2 6HE, UK.

ARNE MELANDER, MD, PhD, Professor and Head, Division of Clinical Pharmacology, Department of Research in Primary Health Care, Lund University Health Sciences Centre, S-24010 Dalby, Sweden.

MALCOLM NATTRASS BSc, MBChB, PhD, FRCP, Consultant Physician, General Hospital, Steelhouse Lane, Birmingham B4 6NH, UK.

STEPHEN O'RAHILLY MD, MRCP, Registrar in Endocrinology, Radcliffe Infirmary, Woodstock Road, Oxford OX2 6HE, UK.

GILLIAN C. PEARSON, BSc, MPhil, Senior Lecturer in Nutrition and Dietetics, Leeds Polytechnic, Department of Applied Science, Calverley Street, Leeds LS1 3HE, UK.

LARS MELHOLT RASMUSSEN MD, Research Fellow, University Institute of Pathology, Kommunehospitalet, DK-8000 Århus C, Denmark.

DOUGLAS ANDREW ROBERTSON MA, BM, BCh, MRCP, Research Registrar, Diabetic Clinic, General Hospital, Steelhouse Lane, Birmingham B4 6NH, UK.

A. S. RUDENSKI, Registrar in Clinical Biochemistry, John Radcliffe Hospital, Oxford OX3 7DU, UK.

J. D. RUTTER BSc, FIA, Actuary, Wesleyan and General Assurance Company Limited, Maple House, 150 Corporation Street, Birmingham B4 6AR, UK.

BALDEV M. SINGH MBBS, MRCP, Registrar in General Medicine/Diabetes Mellitus, General Hospital, Steelhouse Lane, Birmingham B4 6NH, UK.

ROBERT CHARLES TURNER MD, FRCP, Clinical Reader, Nuffield Department of Clinical Medicine, Diabetes Research Laboratories, Radcliffe Infirmary, Woodstock Road, Oxford OX2 6HE, UK.

JOHN K. WALES MD, FRCP, Senior Lecturer and Honorary Consultant Physician, University Department of Medicine, General Infirmary, Leeds LS1 3EX, UK.

Table of contents

Foreword

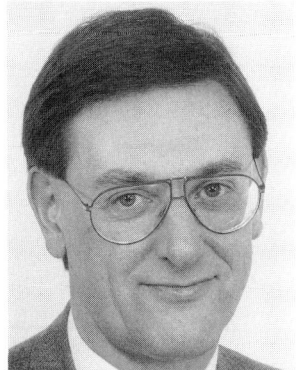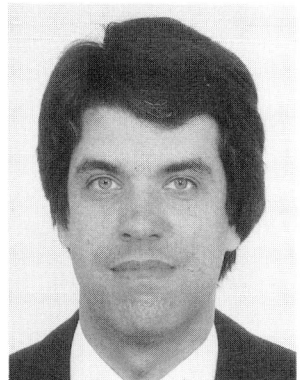

Despite the considerably greater prevalence of non-insulin-dependent diabetes and the terrible costs in patient mortality and morbidity it remains a poor relation of insulin-dependent diabetes. The aetiology and pathogenesis continue to be shrouded in mystery, while treatment and management have developed little in the 30 years since the introduction of the first oral hypoglycaemic agent. Contrast this with progress in insulin chemistry giving pure human insulin preparations, newer methods of insulin delivery, and major attempts at intervention in the early stages of insulin-dependent diabetes based on a surer knowledge of causation.

Yet if recent advances cannot be chronicled there is still reason enough why an issue of *Baillière's Clinical Endocrinology and Metabolism* devoted to non-insulin-dependent diabetes is timely. There is ample scope for reminder and reiteration while presenting the modest advances that have been made.

In the first three chapters the accent is upon updating the aetiology and pathogenesis with King, Gerich, and Turner and his colleagues presenting rather different points of view. Aetiology, of course, determines prevalence which is a matter of great concern to all involved in the care of these patients while it is a firm belief that rational treatment must be based in knowledge of the pathogenesis.

If a reminder be needed of the shocking costs of non-insulin-dependent diabetes these are set out in the chapter by Singh, Rutter and FitzGerald. This serves as a prelude to an examination of current knowledge of the role of the major destructive agent atherosclerosis. The natural history of a disease such as diabetes must, of necessity, be that of the treated disorder and it is therefore a matter of some sadness that it can be written about as unchanging over the last 20 or more years reflecting the paucity of progress. Nowhere is our ignorance more exposed than in the 'hyperinsulinaemia' hypothesis, first mooted nearly 20 years ago, referred to by almost every contributor to the volume, and yet still awaiting confirmation or refutation.

To the reiteration of those trusty options of treatment—diet, updated by Pearson and Wales, and tablets—there is increasing consideration being given to insulin treatment of this group of patients as outlined by Heine. There is added the relatively new supporting role for education, which has yet to be given the same degree of attention both in terms of evaluation and management. In his contribution, Dunn introduces a cautionary note imploring us to approach the topic with scientific principles intact. Yet this contribution widens the view of treatment to include a more comprehensive approach to management. This point is further taken up by Gatling and Hill in their chapter on the organization of care.

Underlying all the contributions is a genuine concern for patients with non-insulin-dependent diabetes and a realization that major challenges still exist if the outlook is to be improved for these people. It will do no harm for us to be reminded of this.

M. NATTRASS
P. J. HALE

1

Aetiology

HILARY KING

Major advances in our understanding of the aetiology of diabetes mellitus became possible with the recognition of the heterogeneity of the disorder, and the clear distinction between insulin-dependent (Type 1) diabetes mellitus (IDDM), non-insulin-dependent (Type 2) diabetes mellitus (NIDDM) and various other forms of the disease (National Diabetes Data Group, 1979; World Health Organization, 1980; 1985).

While many insights into the aetiology of NIDDM stem originally from astute clinical observations, aetiological hypotheses are generally tested by epidemiological study and it is to the epidemiological literature that one must turn for many of the important contributions to this field.

There is general agreement today that the aetiology of NIDDM should be considered on the one hand in terms of underlying genetic susceptibility and on the other with respect to precipitants, which have been traditionally described under the somewhat confusing heading of 'environmental risk factors'. Such thinking mirrors modern aetiological theory regarding a number of other chronic disorders including cardiovascular disease and cancer.

As knowledge of environmental influences on disease patterns has grown, it has become increasingly necessary to refine and expand the concept of environmental risk, as will be discussed later. However, it is convenient to consider first the evidence of genetic influence in the aetiology of NIDDM.

GENETICS OF NIDDM

Assisted by rapid technological advances, genetic research into human diseases has grown steadily as practical implications of such work have become widely appreciated. For NIDDM, as for other conditions, these not only include genetic counselling but also selective intervention with a view to prevention of the disease, both in high risk individuals and in entire high risk communities.

The present evidence of genetic influence in NIDDM may be conveniently considered under three headings: family studies; genetic markers; and ethnicity and genetic admixture.

Family studies

An increase in prevalence or positive family history of diabetes in family members of NIDDM patients, as compared with non-diabetic subjects, was observed some time ago. Studies include a nation-wide survey in Canada (Simpson, 1968) and the Whitehall Survey in Great Britain (Reid et al, 1974). Although such findings are suggestive of genetic influence, they must be treated with caution. Firstly, biases such as differential ascertainment (family members of diabetic subjects may be more likely to be tested for diabetes) and enhanced recall, as well as influence of family size and age factors, are difficult to control. Secondly, family members share not only genetic factors but also a variable degree of environmental influence. Both Kobberling (1971) and Baird (1973) attempted to overcome these problems with more complex study designs. While not conclusive, their results lend weight to the genetic hypothesis by demonstrating greater familiality in non-obese, as compared to obese, probands. The reasoning here is that obese probands may have a greater environmental component to their disease, however their non-obese counterparts may be suffering from a more genetically penetrant form. These results also give some insight into the potential heterogeneity of the disease.

More persuasive than general family studies are those of twins. Since monozygous twins share genes and (usually) early environment, concordance may suggest genetic determination, whereas discordance is strongly suggestive of environmental effects. The well-known work of the King's College Hospital group in London (Barnett et al, 1981) confirmed earlier studies performed before the present classification for diabetes was adopted, by showing that of 53 identical twin pairs all but five were concordant for NIDDM. The likelihood of genetic influence, given such high concordance, was considered high, although the study design was subject to some criticism on the basis of ascertainment bias.

Recently, a study based on military records in the USA (Newman et al, 1987) excluded ascertainment bias and overestimation of concordance by investigating male twin pairs recruited without regard to the diabetic status of either twin. The authors confirmed marked concordance in monozygotic twin pairs (58% versus an expected figure of 10%). They also found that only one of 15 originally NIDDM-discordant monozygotic twin pairs remained discordant for the disease at second examination 10 years later, and that 65% of non-diabetic monozygotic co-twins of subjects with NIDDM had elevated blood glucose concentrations. They concluded that there was a strong genetic predisposition to NIDDM, but that lack of complete concordance and variation in the age of onset between twins indicated a non-genetic component in the aetiology of the disease. Evidence suggesting the importance of shared environmental effects came from the finding that disease-concordant twins were more likely to be in current weekly contact with one another than were other twin pairs.

Genetic markers

Unlike IDDM, in which substantial risk associated with the possession of certain human leukocyte antigens (HLA) has been demonstrated, specific markers that have been found to be associated with NIDDM are relatively weak and inconsistent. This is all the more surprising in view of the higher degree of twin concordance for NIDDM than for IDDM.

The positive reports of HLA associations with NIDDM all come from non-Caucasian populations suspected of having enhanced risk of NIDDM. HLA–A2 has shown a weak association with NIDDM in the Xhosa blacks of South Africa (Briggs et al, 1980) and the Pima Indians in North America (Williams et al, 1981). Another reported association is with HLA–BW61 in Asian Indians in both South Africa (Hammond and Asmal, 1980) and Fiji (Serjeantson et al, 1981). HLA–BW22 has been demonstrated with increased frequency in Polynesians (Serjeantson et al, 1982).

In Caucasian populations, attention was drawn to a possible association between polymorphism of the insulin gene and NIDDM (Owerbach and Nerup, 1982; Rotwein et al, 1983). However, subsequent support for this association has not been forthcoming (Owerbach et al, 1983).

Mention should also be made, in passing, of another possible genetic marker for NIDDM which received widespread attention in the late 1970s—the chlorpropamide-alcohol flush. Also from the investigations of the King's College Hospital group, it was reported that, following chlor-propamide treatment, more NIDDM patients experienced facial flushing after ingestion of alcohol when compared with control subjects and, more-over, that flushing was also related to positive first degree family history of diabetes in NIDDM patients (Leslie and Pyke, 1978). Unfortunately, a number of sources of bias were identified in this study and other workers failed to reproduce the findings.

While the weak nature of the genetic associations that have been described to date might lead one to suppose that the inheritance of NIDDM is probably determined by multiple genes, pedigree analyses in two populations severely affected by NIDDM, the Pima Indians (Yamashita et al, 1984) and the Nauruans (Serjeantson and Zimmet, 1984) both suggest a major gene determination with a dominant mode of inheritance. If sup-ported by further study, this finding could have important implications for the prevention of NIDDM. However, major gene determination of NIDDM may yet prove to apply only to a small number of unusual, high-risk communities.

Ethnicity and genetic admixture

High-risk populations, particularly the Pima Indians (Knowler et al, 1978) and the Nauruans (Zimmet et al, 1984), have provided a continuing spur to the investigation of the genetics of NIDDM. In both of these groups, approximately one-third of the adult population suffer from NIDDM and, as in the case of identical twin concordance, it has generally been acknowl-edged that such a high frequency of the disease is unlikely to be due to environmental factors alone.

One approach in such studies has been to determine the occurrence of NIDDM in relation to proportional genetic admixture from 'high risk' (i.e. indigenous) and other (generally Caucasian) sources. Brosseau et al (1979) demonstrated a fivefold excess in full-blooded American Indians in North

Dakota as compared with those with one-half Indian inheritance. In Nauruans, data of Serjeantson et al (1983) also suggested that foreign genetic admixture was protective against NIDDM. A threefold excess in prevalence of diabetes in Nauruans, as compared with their nearest Micronesian neighbours, was also demonstrated after controlling for various confounding factors, including age and obesity (King et al, 1984a).

Comparable findings have been reported in Mexican Americans in Texas (Stern et al, 1983; Gardner et al, 1984) and, most recently, in Australian Aborigines (Williams et al, 1987). An interesting relationship between mean two-hour plasma glucose concentration and degree of Austronesian genetic admixture (which is thought to confer susceptibility to NIDDM) has been described for six Pacific populations (King et al, 1984b) (Figure 1). A similar association has also been demonstrated for Mexican Americans (Chakraborty et al, 1986).

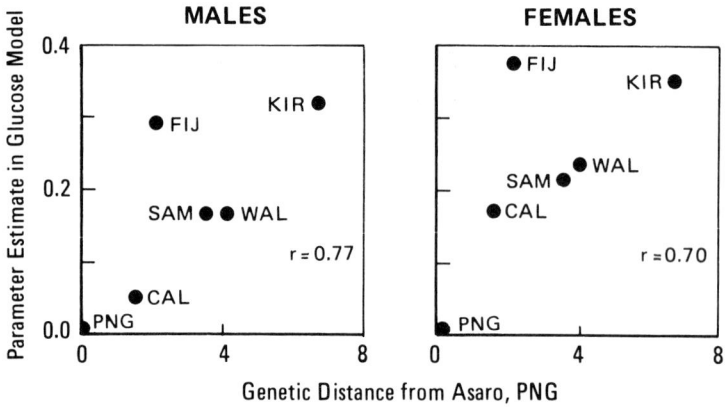

Figure 1. The relationship between the parameter estimates for each population predicting $\log_e$ 2-hr plasma glucose concentration, after controlling for age and obesity, and estimates of genetic distance from the baseline population, Asaro, Papua New Guinea. PNG, Papua New Guinea; CAL, New Caledonia; WAL, Wallis Islands; SAM, Western Samoa; FIJ, Fiji; KIR, Kiribati. From King et al (1984b), with permission.

The thrifty genotype hypothesis

Both the very high prevalence of NIDDM in certain unusual populations, and also the gradient observed in the ethnicity/admixture studies, require explanation. What could be the mechanism whereby an apparently disadvantageous genotype (predisposing to disease and premature death) can occur with such high frequency? The most plausible explanation, and one which has withstood much critical appraisal, is Neel's 'thrifty genotype hypothesis'. Long before the distinction between IDDM and NIDDM was clearly appreciated, Neel (1962) proposed that for societies living in a harsh and unstable environment, a highly efficient carbohydrate metabolism, maximizing storage of surplus energy, would enhance the probability of

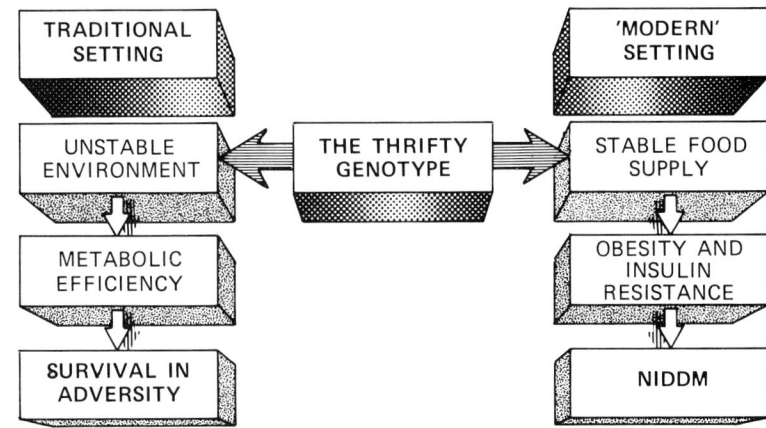

Figure 2. The thrifty genotype hypothesis as proposed by Neel (1962) to explain the high prevalence of diabetes in certain non-Caucasian societies formerly living in harsh and unstable conditions, but now experiencing stable food resources in a modern setting.

survival under adverse circumstances. With the stabilization, and sometimes abundance, of food resources which has often attended industrialization and social change during the 20th century, such a genotype might lead to marked obesity and glucose intolerance in the modern setting (Figure 2).

At the time of its original proposal, Neel found the early onset of formerly fatal IDDM hard to reconcile with his theory. However, the recognition of NIDDM as an aetiologically distinct disease circumvents this problem, since NIDDM has its onset in middle to late adulthood, providing a much less serious barrier to natural selection.

Much modern epidemiological evidence supports Neel's proposal. The communities known to be worst affected by NIDDM today—indigenous North Americans, Micronesian and Polynesian Pacific islanders, Australian Aborigines and migrants from the Indian subcontinent—all lived in harsh environments in the traditional setting, all have undergone marked socio-cultural change recently, and all now seem predisposed to marked obesity.

While it might be argued that the time in which some of these communities have resided in their traditional situation (probably no more than 5000 years, or 200 generations, in the case of most Pacific Islanders) would have been insufficient to result in such marked genetic differentiation, important genetic differences have been demonstrated between the Nauruans and their nearest Micronesian neighbours in Kiribati (formerly Gilbert Islands). For example, ACP*A attains a gene frequency of 25% in Nauru, as compared with 3% in a sample from Kiribati, and there is an almost six-fold excess in the frequency of complement component BF*F in the Nauruans (R. L. Kirk, personal communication). Similar differences, with respect to the gene(s) predisposing to glucose intolerance, would be more than sufficient to explain the present excess prevalence of NIDDM in the Nauruans and other high-risk populations.

Thus, Neel's theory has provided a useful focus for NIDDM research, particularly in the varied populations of the Pacific. Whether or not the same genes which predispose to glucose intolerance in these communities are those which also determine glucose tolerance in the majority of the world's populations, there is more than enough evidence for genetic influence to warrant further study aimed at resolving the genetics of NIDDM.

THE PRECIPITANTS OF NIDDM

Much attention has been focused on the so-called environmental risk factors for NIDDM. This is entirely appropriate, since such knowledge is of value both to the clinician, in directing his advice to the individual patient, and to the public health worker, who is concerned with disease prevention in the community.

Before considering such factors individually, it is convenient to clarify in this context, firstly, what is meant by the environment, and secondly, what is denoted by the term risk factor. Though both terms are widely used, there is often confusion over their precise definition.

For the purpose of epidemiology, *the environment* has been described as 'all that which is external to the individual human host' (Last, 1983). This definition encompasses not only such concepts as physical and biological agents but also less measurable and direct-acting influences such as social and cultural forces and the behavioural tendencies of individuals. It has also been traditional to consider certain characteristics of the host, such as anthropometric indices, and also immutable factors, most particularly subject's age, under the broad heading of environmental influence. The possibility that some of these factors (e.g. the tendency to obesity) may themselves be subject to genetic determination, which may be linked to the genetics of glucose tolerance, considerably complicates the separation of genetic and precipitating influences in the aetiology of NIDDM.

A *risk factor* is generally accepted to be an attribute, the presence of which, in an individual, is associated with an increased probability of a specified outcome, when compared with an otherwise similar individual who lacks the attribute. The important point to note is that, defined in this way, a risk factor may, or may not, bear a causal relationship with the outcome. If it does, it may be termed a *determinant*. Alternatively, however, a risk factor may be a proxy, or marker, for a determinant with which it is independently associated.

The practical importance of this distinction is that, whereas modification of determinants is likely to lead to disease prevention, modification of non-determinant risk factors may or may not do so, depending on whether the determinant is itself concurrently modified. Therefore, until the true relationship between a risk factor and a disease such as NIDDM is established, risk factor intervention must necessarily remain an empirical exercise.

The following factors are those which are currently suspected of being precipitants of NIDDM.

Obesity

For endocrinologists, the association between diabetes and obesity is probably older than any other. Notwithstanding this, it remains one of the most controversial and interesting topics in diabetes epidemiology. The argument is not so much whether obesity is associated with NIDDM but whether it is a true determinant and, if so, to what extent. The mechanism by which obesity might lead to diabetes is generally assumed to be peripheral insulin insensitivity and/or cellular resistance, in the presence of genetically mediated B cell inadequacy (Keen, 1975).

Of the many studies that have demonstrated the NIDDM/obesity association, that of West and Kalbfleisch (1971) which showed an almost linear relationship between average fatness and prevalence of diabetes among populations of ten countries (Figure 3) is a useful starting point. It should be noted at the outset that negative associations between prevalence of diabetes and concurrent obesity may be criticized on the basis of confounding weight loss in diabetic subjects, either due to treatment or to the disease process. Prospective *incidence* studies are required to assess the true impact of obesity, and there have been several.

In the Pima Indians (Knowler et al, 1981) diabetes incidence was shown to be strongly associated with preceding obesity and with a family history of diabetes, suggesting that obesity is not diabetogenic in the absence of genetic predisposition. This plausible conclusion is supported by a wealth of clinical observations of obese subjects with normal glucose tolerance. In the

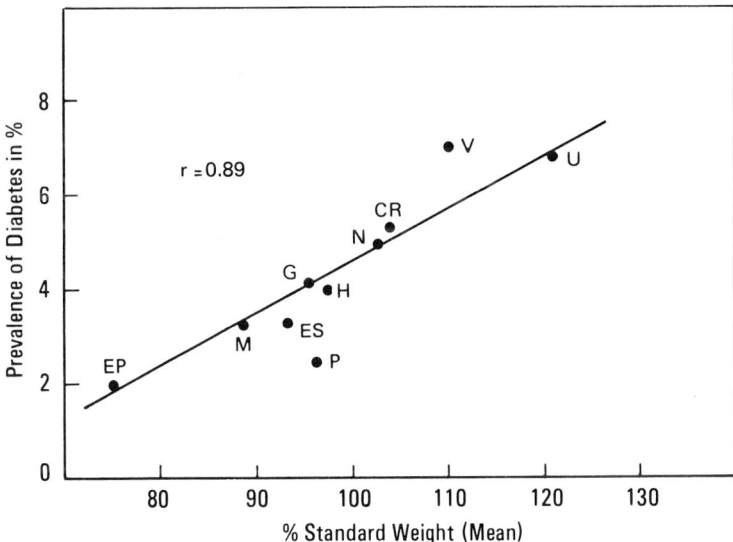

Figure 3. The relationship between average fatness and prevalence of diabetes among populations of ten countries. EP, East Pakistan; M, Malaya; ES, El Salvador; G, Guatemala; P, Panama; H, Honduras; N, Nicaragua; CR, Costa Rica; V, Venezuela; U, Uruguay. From West and Kalbfleisch (1971). (Reproduced with permission from the American Diabetes Association, Inc.)

Nauruans, obesity was shown to be a significant predictor of subsequent diabetes for women, but was of marginal significance in men (Balkau et al, 1985). However, the power of such analyses may be constrained in populations in which obesity is almost universal.

In Caucasian populations, incidence of NIDDM has been associated with preceding obesity in Israeli men (Medalie et al, 1975) and in the Framingham (Wilson et al, 1981) and Tecumseh (Butler et al, 1982) population studies in the USA.

The Tecumseh results (Butler et al, 1982) suggested that diabetes was related to central fat distribution, rather than obesity *per se*, and there is much interest at the present time in the possibility that central, upper body segment (android) obesity, as opposed to more peripheral (gynaecoid) obesity, may be related to a number of chronic disorders including NIDDM, hypertriglyceridaemia and hypertension (Kalkhoff et al, 1983; Krotkiewski et al, 1983; Ohlson et al, 1985).

In the Pima Indians, duration of obesity has emerged as a risk factor for diabetes (Everhart et al, 1986). Modan et al (1986) also came to this conclusion on the basis of Israeli data, and their report sparked off the latest controversy in the saga of NIDDM and obesity. Their study demonstrated a strong association between NIDDM and preceding obesity, and also suggested a dose-response effect, an important criterion of causality. However, Jarrett (1986) interpreted their data as suggesting that only severe obesity was associated with NIDDM, and contended on this basis that obesity could explain only a small proportion of British cases of NIDDM, given anthropometric data from the UK.

Cross-sectional data from Pacific populations (King et al, 1984c) suggest that the association between obesity and diabetes may vary between populations. It is plausible that just as genetic susceptibility to NIDDM may be variable, so may genetic susceptibility to individual risk factors, a concept which is now gaining recognition in other fields of epidemiology (Khoury et al, 1987).

Bennett (1986), commenting on the findings of both the Modan study and those in the Pima Indians, has concluded that insulin resistance may be the principal determinant of both obesity and glucose intolerance. This raises the intriguing possibility that the well-established association between obesity and diabetes is, in fact, non-causal, and that obesity may be a risk factor merely by association. Further support for the primary importance of hyperinsulinaemia has also recently emerged from the Mexican American studies (Haffner et al, 1986).

Thus, recent knowledge has led to further questions and uncertainties, rather than to a clarification of the role of obesity in the aetiology of NIDDM.

Physical inactivity

Exercise is currently a subject of much interest as an adjuvant therapy in the treatment of NIDDM (Wasserman and Vranic, 1987). However, even if exercise can improve glucose tolerance in some NIDDM patients, this is not to say that physical inactivity may be a factor in the aetiology of the disease.

It has been appreciated for some time that in societies which have recently abandoned their traditional life-style, and which have concurrently experienced a major public health problem with respect to NIDDM, sociocultural change has been closely associated with the adoption of sedentary living and markedly reduced habitual physical activity (Zimmet, 1982). Problems which have hampered research in this area include, firstly, the close association between sociocultural change, reduced physical activity, obesity and dietary change and, secondly, the imprecision of methods of assessing habitual physical activity.

Laboratory studies (Krotkiewski et al, 1985) suggest that the effect of exercise training is not a simple one. In subjects with an initially high insulin secretion, improvement in peripheral insulin sensitivity was matched by a reduction of insulin secretion, with no improvement in glucose tolerance. However, in subjects with low insulin secretion initially, training increased insulin secretion and improved glucose tolerance. Another recent report (Lampman et al, 1987) has also cast doubt on the efficacy of physical training alone.

With respect to epidemiological evidence, Taylor et al (1984) showed that diabetes was more prevalent in physically inactive subjects than their active counterparts in Fiji. A wider examination of Pacific data (King et al, 1984c) showed the relationship to be inconsistent. Furthermore, bias due to reduced activity consequent upon the disease state could not be ruled out in either of these cross-sectional analyses.

Perhaps the strongest evidence of the importance of physical activity in NIDDM is a recent report of the Zuni Diabetes Project (Heath et al, 1987). As with a number of other indigenous Amerindian populations, NIDDM is a serious public health problem for the Zuni of New Mexico. Approximately one-quarter of all adults over the age of 45 years suffer from the disease. In 1983 a community-based exercise programme was initiated among the Zuni. Comparing 30 participants with 56 non-participants in the programme, not only was weight loss greater in the former over a two year period, but participants' mean fasting blood glucose concentration fell substantially, compared with little change in the non-participants. Participants were also more likely to have stopped, or decreased, their medication dosage. While an obvious limitation of this study was the self-selection of the participants, the non-participants were matched on a number of characteristics, e.g. age, sex and duration of disease. The study does show that motivated NIDDM patients can benefit from an exercise programme.

Even if this leads us no closer to understanding the aetiology of NIDDM, it should provide a stimulus for a carefully designed prospective trial of exercise and its influence on glucose tolerance in populations at high risk of NIDDM. In such situations, both primary prevention (averting the development of disease) and secondary prevention (reversal of existing disease) may be more effective than in Caucasian and other societies in which NIDDM is less prevalent. It is also possible that physical inactivity may be a more potent precipitant of glucose intolerance in high-risk communities such as the American Indians than in the lower-risk Caucasian subjects who were included in the recent laboratory studies.

Diet

Just as the relationship between sociocultural change and glucose intolerance has led to the consideration of the importance of reduced levels of physical activity in the aetiology of NIDDM, so it has also been taken as possible evidence of the importance of diet. Urbanization of formerly traditional communities almost invariably involves them in a dietary change towards a higher proportion of refined carbohydrate and fats, and reduced dietary fibre.

As in the case of physical exercise, study of this association has been hampered by the relative imprecision of dietary assessment. A recent survey of a Canadian Amerindian population failed to demonstrate an association between dietary change and glucose tolerance (Szathmary et al, 1987) and the area remains as uncertain as it is potentially important.

As has been pointed out in a more detailed review of this particular topic (Mann, 1985) while public opinion has long supported the notion that a high intake of sucrose and other refined carbohydrates is a major aetiological factor in diabetes, there is in fact no evidence of a direct causal role for any specific nutrient in the aetiology of NIDDM.

Both case-control and prospective studies have failed to incriminate sugar consumption, while the debate over dietary fibre and fats continues. However the latter, even if not determinants of the disease, may play a role in its progression by enhancing risk of cardiovascular complications.

More plausible, aetiologically, is that excessive total caloric intake may have an indirect action on glucose tolerance, through obesity, in susceptible individuals. Once again, this emphasises the possibility of a close inter-relationship between diet, obesity and exercise in the aetiology of the disease.

Psychosocial stress

Acute stress is known to precipitate cardiovascular morbidity and, traditionally, there has been a tendency for epidemiological theory concerning NIDDM to adopt conventional cardiovascular risk factors for the purpose of generating provisional aetiological hypotheses. An association between the onset of IDDM and preceding severe life events has been reported (Robinson and Fuller, 1986) and an experiment with a diabetes-prone strain of rats (Carter et al, 1987) recently demonstrated earlier onset of IDDM in a group subjected to a variety of environmental stressors, compared with an otherwise comparable control group.

Both direct and indirect evidence appears entirely lacking for a role of stress in the development of NIDDM, and the apparently low prevalence of diabetes reported during both the two World Wars (West, 1978) provides little encouragement—though no direct refutation—to protagonists of this theory. However, the proposition is likely to continue to receive attention, and could be usefully included in future studies of twin pairs, and in the long-term epidemiological surveillance of communities exposed to natural disaster and the participants in human conflicts.

Age

In almost every population, the prevalence of NIDDM increases with age. Thus, with increasing longevity, NIDDM can be expected to become a growing burden to many of the world's populations, even if age-specific incidence and prevalence were to stay at their present levels.

While age is an immutable function of living, it can be considered usefully as a risk factor for NIDDM in one respect. If the influences of various risk factors interact in their effect, or if the final expression of the disease is dependent upon multiple assaults and a critical threshold, the age effect on pancreatic function might be modified, or even eliminated, by the concurrent modification of other risk factors for which intervention is feasible.

Support for this notion comes from the results of the few studies which have been performed in societies little affected by a modern lifestyle. A total absence of NIDDM at all ages, and an absence of age-effects on glucose tolerance in females, have been demonstrated in two semi-traditional communities in the highlands of Papua New Guinea (King et al, 1984d).

Other possible precipitants, and future directions for aetiological research

Cryptic viruses have been suggested as possible agents in the development of several chronic diseases, and their role in NIDDM cannot be dismissed.

Unlike IDDM, in which viruses are suspected of playing a major aetiological role, there is neither evidence, nor an obvious mechanism for NIDDM, in support of such a notion. However, greater understanding of the latency of some infectious processes is resulting in a growing unification of the traditionally exclusive fields of infectious and chronic disease epidemiology. Kuller (1987) has gone so far as to suggest that multifactorial theories concerning chronic diseases may reflect ignorance, rather than reasoned biological argument. Theoretically, this could be so for NIDDM.

There is much interest at present in the inter-relationship between NIDDM and other chronic disorders such as hypertension, hypercholesterolaemia and hypertriglyceridaemia. The co-existence of these conditions may indicate common genetic influences, common environmental determinants, a causal sequence among the conditions themselves, or a combination of these.

Whilst the nature of these relationships is, as yet, far from clear, this area of study has the potential to create a new level of understanding of chronic disease aetiology. This may, in turn, prove to be in close accord with the current World Health Organization initiative (Epstein and Holland, 1983) for an integrated approach to the control of NIDDM and other chronic diseases. Prevention of these conditions would be of major consequence to public health at the end of the twentieth century and beyond.

SUMMARY

NIDDM appears to be a disease of complex aetiology. Although specific genetic markers for the disease have yet to be defined, there is clear evidence for genetic predisposition, with high concordance in monozygous twins. However, concordance is incomplete, and there are therefore additional, non-genetic, mechanisms which are responsible for increasing the risk of the disease in susceptible subjects.

At the present time, the most plausible environmental precipitants appear to be the inter-related triad of obesity, low levels of habitual physical exercise and diet. The power of environmental determinants, and their interaction one with another, may also be subject to individual genetic determination, and may not act in a similar manner in all populations.

Some non-Caucasian populations, which have undergone marked socio-cultural change, are now extremely susceptible to NIDDM. This is probably the result of evolutionarily heightened genetic predisposition, compounded by strong environmental influence resulting from the recent changes in their human ecology. Since prevalence is strongly related to age, NIDDM also represents a growing problem to the world's industrialized societies, for many of which longevity is now the major demographic trend.

Research into the aetiology of NIDDM must not only continue, it must also explore new directions, and attain greater scientific depth and sophistication, if it is to make a useful contribution to the eventual prevention and control of the disease.

REFERENCES

Baird JD (1973) The role of obesity in the development of clinical diabetes. *Publications of the Royal College of Physicians, Edinburgh* **42:** 83–99.

Balkau B, King H, Zimmet P & Raper LR (1985) Factors associated with the development of diabetes in the Micronesian population of Nauru. *American Journal of Epidemiology* **122:** 594–605.

Barnett AH, Eff C, Leslie RDG & Pyke DA (1981) Diabetes in identical twins: a study of 200 pairs. *Diabetologia* **20:** 87–93.

Bennett PH (1986) More about obesity and diabetes. *Diabetologia* **29:** 753–754 (letter).

Briggs BR, Botha MC, Jackson WPU & Du Toit ED (1980) The histocompatibility (HLA) antigen distribution in South African blacks (Xhosa). *Diabetes* **29:** 68–70.

Brosseau JD, Eelkema RC, Crawford AC & Abe TA (1979) Diabetes among the three affiliated tribes: correlation with degree of Indian inheritance. *American Journal of Public Health* **69:** 1277–1288.

Butler WJ, Ostrander LD, Carman WJ et al (1982) Diabetes mellitus in Tecumseh, Michigan: prevalence, incidence, and associated conditions. *American Journal of Epidemiology* **116:** 971–980.

Carter WR, Herrman J, Stokes K & Cox DJ (1987) Promotion of diabetes onset by stress in the BB rat. *Diabetologia* **30:** 674–675.

Chakraborty R, Ferrell RE, Stern MP, Haffner SM, Hazuda HP & Rosenthal M (1986) Relationship of prevalence of non-insulin-dependent diabetes mellitus to Amerindian admixture in the Mexican Americans of San Antonio, Texas. *Genetic Epidemiology* **3:** 435–454.

Epstein F & Holland WW (1983) Prevention of chronic diseases in the community—one disease versus multiple-disease strategies. *International Journal of Epidemiology* **12:** 135–137.

Everhart JE, Pettitt DJ, Slaine KR & Knowler WC (1986) Duration of obesity as a risk factor for non-insulin-dependent diabetes mellitus. *American Journal of Epidemiology* **124:** 525.

Gardner LI, Stern MP, Haffner SM et al (1984) Prevalence of diabetes in Mexican Americans:

relationship to percent of gene pool derived from native American sources. *Diabetes* **33:** 86–92.

Haffner SM, Stern MP, Hazuda HP, Pugh JA & Patterson JK (1986) Hyperinsulinemia in a population at high risk for non-insulin-dependent diabetes mellitus. *New England Journal of Medicine* **315:** 220–224.

Hammond MG & Asmal AC (1980) HLA and insulin-dependent diabetes in South African Indians. *Tissue Antigens* **15:** 244–248.

Heath GW, Leonard BE, Wilson RH, Kendrick JS & Powell KE (1987) Community-based exercise intervention: Zuni diabetes project. *Diabetes Care* **10:** 579–583.

Jarrett RJ (1986) Obesity and Type 2 (non-insulin-dependent) diabetes. *Diabetologia* **29:** 407–408 (letter).

Kalkhoff RK, Harty AH, Rupley D, Kissebah AH & Kelber S (1983) Relationship of body fat distribution to blood pressure, carbohydrate tolerance and plasma lipids in healthy obese women. *Journal of Laboratory and Clinical Medicine* **102:** 621–627.

Keen H (1975) The incomplete story of obesity and diabetes. In Howard A (ed) *Recent advances in obesity research: Proceedings of the first international congress on obesity*, pp 116–127. London: Newman.

Khoury MJ, Stewart W & Beaty TH (1987) The effect of genetic susceptibility on causal inference in epidemiologic studies. *American Journal of Epidemiology* **126:** 561–567.

King H, Zimmet P, Pargeter K, Raper LR & Collins V (1984a) Ethnic differences in susceptibility to non-insulin-dependent diabetes: a comparative study of two urbanized Micronesian populations. *Diabetes* **33:** 1002–1007.

King H, Zimmet P, Bennett P, Taylor R & Raper LR (1984b) Glucose tolerance and ancestral genetic admixture in six semitraditional Pacific populations. *Genetic Epidemiology* **1:** 315–328.

King H, Zimmet P, Raper LR & Balkau B (1984c) Risk factors for diabetes in three Pacific populations. *American Journal of Epidemiology* **119:** 396–409.

King H, Heywood P, Zimmet P et al (1984d) Glucose tolerance in a highland population in Papua New Guinea. *Diabetes Research* **1:** 45–51.

Knowler WC, Bennett PH, Hamman RF & Miller M (1978) Diabetes incidence in the Pima Indians: a 19-fold greater incidence than in Rochester, Minnesota. *American Journal of Epidemiology* **108:** 497–504.

Knowler WC, Bennett PH, Pettit PJ & Savage PJ (1981) Diabetes incidence in Pima Indians: contributions of obesity and parental diabetes. *American Journal of Epidemiology* **113:** 144–156.

Kobberling J (1971) Studies on the genetic heterogeneity of diabetes mellitus. *Diabetologia* **7:** 46–49.

Krotkiewski M, Bjorntorp P, Sjostrom L & Smith U (1983) Impact of obesity on metabolism in men and women: importance of regional adipose tissue distribution. *Journal of Clinical Investigation* **72:** 1150–1162.

Krotkiewski M, Lonnroth P, Mandroukas K et al (1985) The effects of physical training on insulin secretion and effectiveness and on glucose metabolism in obesity and Type 2 (non-insulin-dependent) diabetes mellitus. *Diabetologia* **28:** 881–890.

Kuller LH (1987) Relationship between acute and chronic disease epidemiology. *Yale Journal of Biology and Medicine* **60:** 363–376.

Lampman RM, Schteingart DE, Santinga JT et al (1987) The influence of physical training on glucose tolerance, insulin sensitivity, and lipid and lipoprotein concentrations in middle-aged hypertriglyceridaemic, carbohydrate intolerant men. *Diabetologia* **30:** 380–385.

Last JM (1983) *A dictionary of epidemiology*. New York, Oxford, Toronto: Oxford University Press.

Leslie RDG & Pyke DA (1978) Chlorpropamide alcohol flushing: a dominantly inherited trait associated with diabetes. *British Medical Journal* **2:** 1519–1521.

Mann JI (1985) Diabetes mellitus: some aspects of aetiology and management. In Trowell HC, Burkitt D & Heaton K (eds) *Refined carbohydrate foods, dietary fibre and disease*, 2nd edn. London: Academic Press.

Medalie JH, Papier CM, Goldbourt U et al (1975) Major factors in the development of diabetes mellitus in 10 000 men. *Archives of Internal Medicine* **135:** 811–817.

Modan M, Karasik A, Halkin H et al (1986) Effect of past and concurrent body mass index on prevalence of glucose intolerance and Type 2 (non-insulin-dependent) diabetes and on insulin response: the Israeli study of glucose intolerance, obesity and hypertension. *Diabetologia* **29**: 82–89.

National Diabetes Data Group (1979) Classification and diagnosis of diabetes mellitus and other categories of glucose intolerance. *Diabetes* **28**: 1039–1057.

Neel JV (1962) Diabetes mellitus: a 'thrifty' genotype rendered detrimental by progress? *American Journal of Human Genetics* **14**: 353–362.

Newman B, Selby JV, King M-C, Slemenda C, Fabsitz R & Friedman GD (1987) Concordance for Type 2 (non-insulin-dependent) diabetes mellitus in male twins. *Diabetologia* **30**: 763–768.

Ohlson L-O, Larsson B, Svardsudd K et al (1985) The influence of body fat distribution on the incidence of diabetes mellitus: 13.5 years of follow-up of the participants in the study of men born in 1913. *Diabetes* **34**: 1055–1058.

Owerbach D & Nerup J (1982) Restriction fragment length polymorphism of the insulin gene in diabetes mellitus. *Diabetes* **31**: 275–277.

Owerbach D, Thomsen B, Johansen K et al (1983) DNA insertion sequences near the insulin gene are not associated with maturity-onset diabetes of young people. *Diabetologia* **25**: 18–20.

Reid DD, Hamilton PJS, Keen H, Brett G, Jarrett RJ & Rose G (1974) Cardiorespiratory disease and diabetes among middle-aged male civil servants. *Lancet* **i**: 469–473.

Robinson N & Fuller JH (1986) Severe life events and their relationship to the aetiology of insulin-dependent (Type 1) diabetes mellitus. *Pediatric and Adolescent Endocrinology* **15**: 129–133.

Rotwein PS, Chirgwin J, Province M et al (1983) Polymorphism in the 5′ flanking region of the human insulin gene: a genetic marker for non-insulin-dependent diabetes. *New England Journal of Medicine* **308**: 65–71.

Serjeantson SW, Ryan DP, Ram P et al (1981) HLA and non-insulin-dependent diabetes in Fiji Indians. *Medical Journal of Australia* **1**: 462–463.

Serjeantson SW, Ryan DP, Zimmet P et al (1982) HLA antigens in four Pacific populations with non-insulin-dependent diabetes mellitus. *Annals of Human Biology* **9**: 69–84.

Serjeantson SW, Owerbach D, Zimmet P, Nerup J & Thoma K (1983) Genetics of diabetes in Nauru: effects of foreign admixture, HLA antigens and the insulin-gene-linked poly-morphism. *Diabetologia* **25**: 13–17.

Serjeantson SW & Zimmet P (1984) Diabetes in the Pacific: evidence for a major gene. In Baba S, Gould M & Zimmet P (eds) *Diabetes mellitus: recent knowledge on aetiology, complications and treatment*, pp 23–30. Sydney: Academic Press.

Simpson NE (1968) Diabetes in the families of diabetics. *Canadian Medical Association Journal* **98**: 427–432.

Stern MP, Gaskill SP, Hazuda HP, Gardner LI & Haffner SM (1983) Does obesity explain excess prevalence of diabetes among Mexican Americans? Results of the San Antonio Heart Study. *Diabetologia* **14**: 272–277.

Szathmary EJE, Ritenbaugh C & Goodby C-SM (1987) Dietary change and plasma glucose levels in an Amerindian population undergoing cultural transition. *Social Science and Medicine* **24**: 791–804.

Taylor R, Ram P, Zimmet P, Raper LR & Ringrose H (1984) Physical activity and prevalence of diabetes in Melanesian and Indian men in Fiji. *Diabetologia* **27**: 578–582.

Wasserman DH & Vranic M (1987) Exercise and diabetes. In Alberti KGMM & Krall LP (eds) *The Diabetes Annual/3*, pp 527–559. Amsterdam, New York, Oxford: Elsevier.

West KM (1978) Epidemiology of diabetes and its vascular lesions, pp 280–281. New York: Elsevier.

West KM & Kalbfleisch JM (1971) Influence of nutritional factors on prevalence of diabetes. *Diabetes* **20**: 99–108.

Williams DRR, Moffitt PS, Fisher JS & Bashir HV (1987) Diabetes and glucose tolerance in New South Wales coastal Aborigines: possible effects on non-Aboriginal genetic admix-ture. *Diabetologia* **30**: 72–77.

Williams RC, Bennett PH, Butler WJ et al (1981) HLA-A2 and Type 2 (insulin-dependent) diabetes mellitus in Pima Indians: an association of allele frequency with age. *Diabetologia* **21**: 460–463.

Wilson PW, McGee DL & Kannel WB (1981) Obesity, very low density lipoproteins, and glucose intolerance over fourteen years: The Framingham Study. *American Journal of Epidemiology* **114:** 697–704.

World Health Organization Expert Committee on Diabetes Mellitus (1980) Second Report. *Technical Report Series* **646.** Geneva: World Health Organization.

World Health Organization (1985) Diabetes mellitus. Report of a study group. *Technical Report Series* **727.** Geneva: World Health Organization.

Yamashita TS, Mackay W, Rushforth NB, Bennett PH & Houser H (1984) Pedigree analyses of non-insulin-dependent diabetes in the Pima Indians suggest a dominant mode of inheritance. *American Journal of Human Genetics* **36:** 183S.

Zimmet P (1982) Type 2 (non-insulin-dependent) diabetes—an epidemiological overview. *Diabetologia* **22:** 399–411.

Zimmet P, King H, Taylor R et al (1984) The high prevalence of diabetes mellitus, impaired glucose tolerance and diabetic retinopathy in Nauru—the 1982 survey. *Diabetes Research* **1:** 13–18.

2

Role of insulin resistance in the pathogenesis of Type 2 (non-insulin-dependent) diabetes mellitus

JOHN E. GERICH

For insulin to exert its actions on carbohydrate metabolism, the hormone must be secreted from the islet B cell, diffuse from the islet extracellular space into the circulation, and reach its target tissues intact. The insulin molecule must then bind to its receptor, and this event at the plasma membrane must trigger an intracellular signal (e.g. generation of a second messenger or receptor-induced protein phosphorylation) that in turn initiates changes in certain biochemical processes (e.g. translocation of glucose transporters, increases or decreases of enzyme activity) which regulate the uptake and flux of glucose through different metabolic pathways (Figure 1). Any abnormality in this sequence can result in decreased

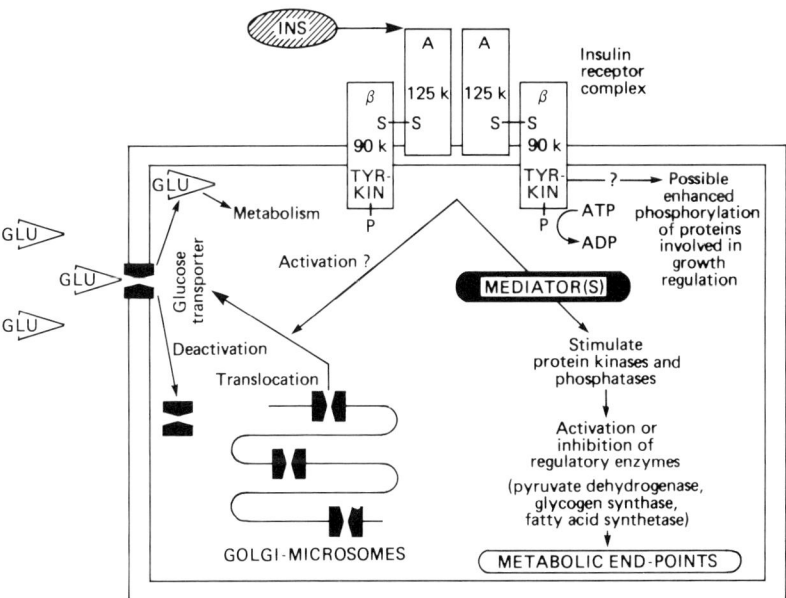

Figure 1. Sequence of cellular events in insulin action adapted from Truglia et al (1985), with permission.

insulin action and hyperglycaemia unless appropriate compensatory mechanisms intervene.

A common cause of diminished insulin action in humans is deficient insulin secretion such as that resulting from the reduced islet B cell mass of patients with Type 1 (insulin-dependent) diabetes. In rare instances, impaired release of insulin may be caused by synthesis of an abnormal insulin molecule (Olefsky et al, 1980) or lack of conversion of proinsulin to insulin (Gabbay et al, 1976).

Tissue resistance to insulin (for example in acromegaly or Cushing's syndrome) and accelerated degradation of insulin (as in hyperthyroidism) can also lead to diminished insulin action when the compensatory capacity of the B cell is limited or when defects in the above sequence of events make it impossible for even increased amounts of insulin to exert a normal biological effect (for example, acanthosis nigricans with antireceptor antibodies) (Flier et al, 1979).

The most commonly encountered clinical situations associated with insulin resistance are obesity and Type 2 (non-insulin-dependent) diabetes (Reaven et al, 1976; DeFronzo et al, 1983). In recent years, there has been considerable controversy concerning the relative roles of impaired B cell function and insulin resistance in the pathogenesis of Type 2 diabetes (Fujita et al, 1975; Olefsky, 1981; Rizza et al, 1981a; Bogardus et al, 1984a; Fajans, 1987). Part of the reason for this controversy lies in the imprecision of methods used to assess B cell function and insulin resistance. Other reasons for the controversy include the failure of many investigators to draw a distinction between impaired B cell function and diminished insulin secretion and the failure to take into consideration the fact that Type 2 diabetes is a heterogenous disorder (Efendic et al, 1984) and that B cell function and tissue insulin sensitivity may vary during the course of Type 2 diabetes.

The major issues regarding B cell function and insulin resistance in Type 2 diabetes are:

1. Which defect initiates the change from normal glucose tolerance to impaired glucose tolerance to overt hyperglycaemia?
2. What are the causes of these abnormalities on a molecular basis?
3. Which defect is the more important determinant of hyperglycaemia?
4. To what extent does one abnormality beget or exacerbate the other?
5. What is the relative importance of hepatic or peripheral tissue insulin resistance for fasting and postprandial hyperglycaemia?

This review will attempt to summarize our current understanding of some of these issues and indicate what kind of future studies are needed to resolve present controversies.

EVIDENCE FOR INSULIN RESISTANCE

If one defines insulin resistance as a condition in which a normal concentration of insulin produces less than a normal response (Khan, 1978), there is now indisputable evidence that nearly all patients with Type 2 diabetes have some degree of insulin resistance. The evidence for this may be briefly summarized as follows: most patients with Type 2 diabetes are obese, obesity itself is associated with insulin resistance (Kolterman et al, 1980; Bogardus et al, 1984b). Even in the absence of obesity, patients with Type 2 diabetes are hyperglycaemic despite normal or increased circulating insulin levels (Bogardus et al, 1984b). Many of these patients have exaggerated increases in plasma glucose levels after oral (Chiles and Tzagournis, 1970) or intravenous glucose (Efendic et al, 1980) despite 'normal' or increased plasma insulin responses. Obviously, those plasma insulin concentrations are not exerting the same effect as they would in a person without diabetes.

More sophisticated studies using the limb balance technique (Rabinowitz and Zierler, 1962; Jackson et al, 1973; DeFronzo et al, 1985), splanchnic balance technique (Felig et al, 1978) and the in vivo and in vitro isotopic techniques (Kolterman et al, 1981; DeFronzo et al, 1982; Ciaraldi et al, Yki-Jarvinen et al, 1987a; Campbell et al, 1988) have demonstrated that people with Type 2 diabetes have decreased muscle and adipose tissue glucose uptake, and decreased suppression of hepatic glucose output compared to non-diabetic individuals when studied at identical insulin levels. Furthermore, patients with hyperglycaemia have increased rates of hepatic glucose output and decreased rates of glucose clearance despite normal or increased circulating insulin levels (Kolterman et al, 1981; DeFronzo et al, 1982, 1985; Ciaraldi et al, 1982; Yki-Jarvinen et al, 1987a; Campbell et al, 1988).

TYPE 2 DIABETES—A HETEROGENOUS DISORDER

When studying a group of patients with diabetes, investigators hope that they have chosen a representative sample of the population of diabetic patients so that the results which they obtain accurately reflect the general situation in Type 2 diabetes. However, it is now recognized that Type 2 diabetes is a heterogenous disorder (Efendic et al, 1984). As shown in Figure 2, among families of patients with comparable degrees of glucose intolerance, different (low, high, normal) plasma insulin patterns can be observed after oral glucose. This presumably reflects different degrees of impaired insulin secretion and/or insulin resistance. This heterogeneity must be taken into consideration when interpreting data of studies on the pathogenesis of Type 2 diabetes. The results of studies can be influenced by selection of patients and their data may not be an accurate reflection of diabetes in general. It is quite likely that abnormalities in insulin secretion and insulin resistance may play considerably different roles in different subsets of patients with Type 2 diabetes.

DISTINCTION BETWEEN IMPAIRED B CELL FUNCTION AND IMPAIRED INSULIN SECRETION

It has been proposed that the finding of normal or increased circulating plasma insulin levels in patients with Type 2 diabetes provides indisputable

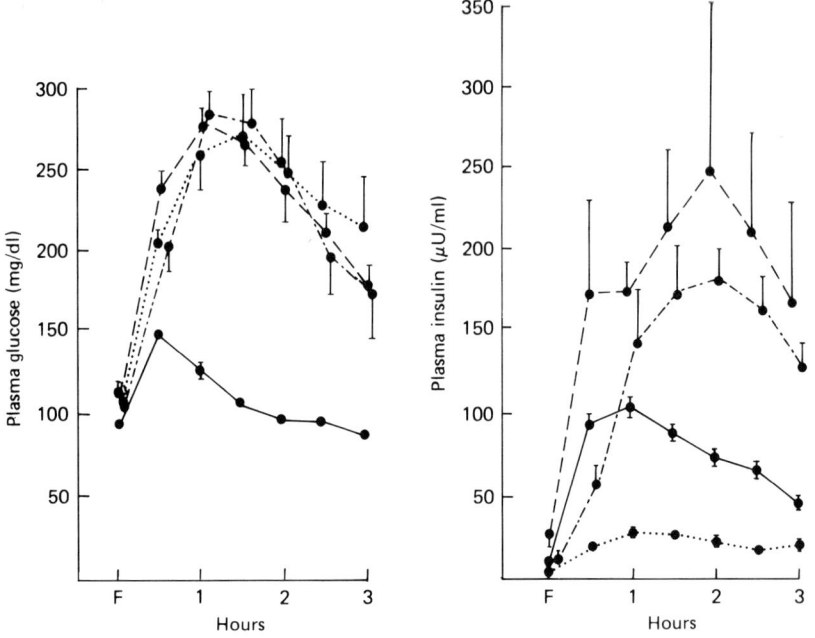

Figure 2. Heterogeneity of plasma insulin responses in families with Type 2 diabetes from Fajans (1987), with permission. (——) 150 control subjects, (. . . .) 9 members MODY Pedigree RW, (––) 5 members MODY Pedigree Te, (–·–·) 5 members MODY Pedigree H.

evidence that insulin resistance rather than impaired insulin secretion is the major factor responsible for the metabolic abnormalities of this condition. Such a conclusion, however, ignores the fact that these circulating insulin levels may be inappropriate for the prevailing hyperglycaemia and thus a defect in islet B cell function may be present. For example, Perley and Kipnis (1967) studied patients with Type 2 diabetes who, apparently, had normal plasma insulin levels during an oral glucose tolerance test. However, when subjects without diabetes were made comparably hyperglycaemic, it was demonstrated that the diabetic subject had subnormal plasma insulin responses (Figure 3). Other studies in which a comparable stimulus for insulin secretion was presented to diabetic and non-diabetic individuals have demonstrated a defect in islet B cell function in patients with Type 2 diabetes (Ward et al, 1984; Dimitriadis et al, 1985). Thus, hyperinsulinaemia in the face of hyperglycaemia does not necessarily exclude the presence of impaired islet B cell function.

This issue is, of course, relevant to the question of which defect (impaired insulin secretion or insulin resistance) precedes the other and which defect contributes more to the metabolic abnormalities of Type 2 diabetes. Insulin resistance has been quantitated in patients with Type 2 diabetes under

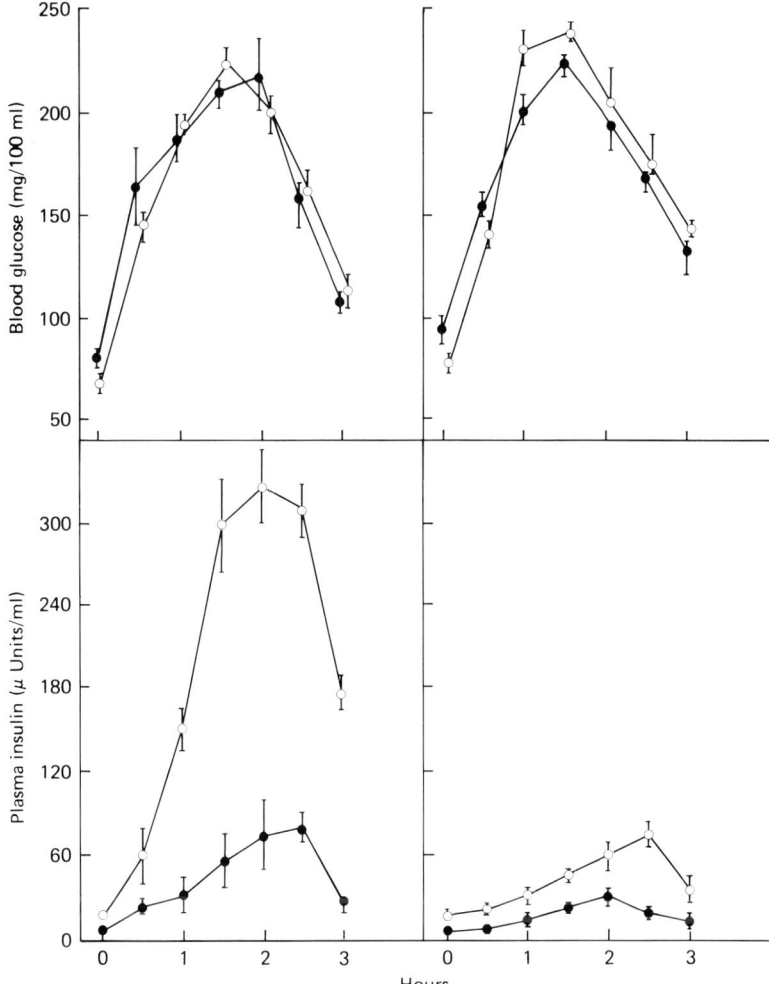

Figure 3. Demonstration of impaired B cell responses in patients with Type 2 diabetes from Perley & Kipnis (1967) by copyright permission of the American Society for Clinical Investigation. Normal (●), obese (○). Left panel—non-diabetic, right panel—diabetic.

carefully controlled conditions in which plasma glucose and plasma insulin levels have been made identical to those of subjects without diabetes using the insulin-glucose clamp technique (Kolterman et al, 1981; DeFronzo et al, 1982; Bogardus et al, 1984a; Donner et al, 1985; Campbell et al, 1988) but few studies have examined islet B cell function in Type 2 diabetes under such controlled conditions (Perley and Kipnis, 1967; Ward et al, 1984; Dimitriadis et al, 1985). When this has been done, impaired B cell function has been demonstrated.

THE INITIAL LESION—IMPAIRED B CELL FUNCTION OR INSULIN RESISTANCE

There are several potential sequences by which the interactions between impaired B cell function and insulin resistance may lead to the development of Type 2 diabetes. Some of these are illustrated in Figure 4. First of all there may be a primary, perhaps genetically determined, B cell functional defect. At some time this defect may progress to the situation in which episodes of mild elevations in plasma glucose levels occur. These glucose levels may still be in what is considered the normal range and the defect in B cell function could be as subtle as mild delay in early postprandial insulin release (Fujita et al, 1975) (e.g. elevated threshold for stimulation of secretion). This hyperglycaemia would require additional insulin secretion, giving rise to episodes of hyperinsulinaemia and perhaps more insulin being secreted than would be necessary if B cell function were normal. Simulated glucose sensor modelling studies have shown such a sequence of events to be plausible (Sorensen et al, 1982). This increased insulin secretion over a period of time could lead to exhaustion of B cell reserve in an islet with already impaired B cell function. The hyperinsulinaemia could also induce insulin resistance (Mandarino et al, 1984a; Marangou et al, 1986). The transient episodes of hyperglycaemia themselves could adversely affect B cell function (Leahy et al, 1986; Rossetti et al, 1987) and could also induce insulin resistance as shown by studies of Yki-Jarvinen et al (1987b). The combination of these factors reinforcing one another (e.g. hyperinsulinaemia causing insulin resistance, insulin resistance requiring greater insulin secretion) could ultimately lead to sustained severe hyperglycaemia associated with either greater than normal, normal or subnormal circulating insulin levels depending on the patient's B cell reserve.

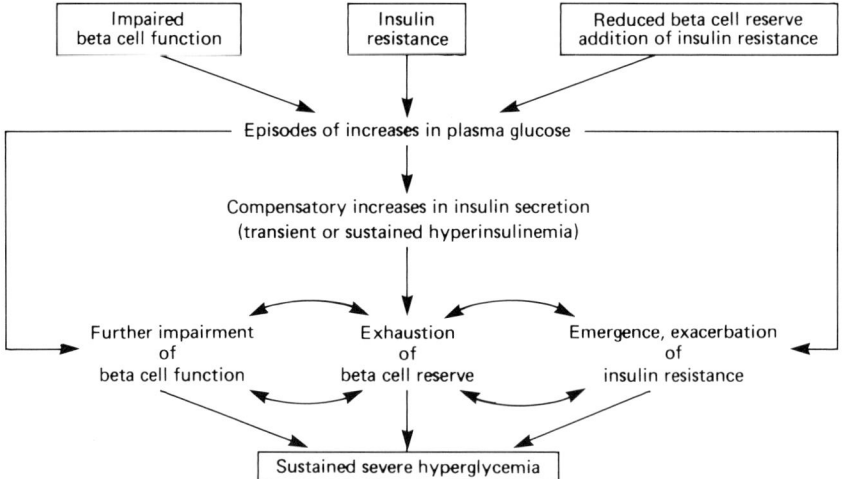

Figure 4. Potential interactions of impaired B cell function and insulin resistance which result in Type 2 diabetes.

A second potential sequence of events might start with the patient having some degree of insulin resistance. This could be genetically preprogrammed or could be secondary to development of obesity. This insulin resistance at some time may cause episodes of increased plasma glucose levels so as to initiate a compensatory increase in insulin secretion and sustained hyper-insulinaemia. Again, the increases in plasma glucose levels may be mild and within the normal range. The prolonged hyperinsulinaemia could further exacerbate the underlying insulin resistance and ultimately lead to exhaustion of B cell reserve to the point where sustained hyperglycaemia emerges.

A third potential sequence of events might start with a patient in whom there is a genetically determined defect in B cell reserve. This defect could be such that without addition of insulin resistance and the need for a compensatory increase in insulin secretion, it could remain clinically silent. Were such a patient, however, to become obese or have some other cause of insulin resistance (e.g. infection, pregnancy), B cell exhaustion might occur. Initially, the patient might compensate by secreting an increased amount of insulin in the post-absorptive state and have fasting hyperinsulinaemia because the B cell was working at near maximal, albeit reduced, capacity but would not be able to secrete additional appropriately increased amounts of insulin after meals. The reinforcing effects of transient or mild hyper-glycaemia and prolonged hyperinsulinaemia on B cell function and insulin resistance could lead to sustained severe hyperglycaemia—the same clinical picture as observed with the other two potential sequences.

Evidence from cross-sectional studies

Several cross-sectional studies (Savage et al, 1975; Bogardus et al, 1984a; Fajans, 1987) have examined insulin secretion or insulin resistance (usually not both) of individuals with varying degrees of glucose tolerance. The assumption of these studies is that these different groups represent different stages in the evolution of diabetes. As illustrated in Figure 5, these studies have generally found that as mean fasting and postprandial plasma glucose levels increase, plasma insulin levels also increase up to a point beyond which as fasting and postprandial glucose levels increase further, plasma insulin levels decrease back to 'normal' absolute levels and ultimately to below normal levels (Savage et al, 1975; Bogardus et al, 1984a; Fajans, 1987). These results have been interpreted to indicate that insulin resistance precedes the development of impaired insulin secretion.

Although it would be reasonable to conclude that some degree of insulin resistance was present preceding the development of diabetes, these obser-vations neither exclude the possibility of coexistent, and perhaps, antedecent defect in the B cell function nor do they indicate that the insulin resistance was necessarily the cause for the subsequent development of diabetes. Many individuals with insulin resistance (e.g. those who are obese) do not develop diabetes. Cross-sectional studies using intravenous injec-tions of glucose to assess islet B cell function have demonstrated that logarithmic decrements in first phase insulin secretion occur with only

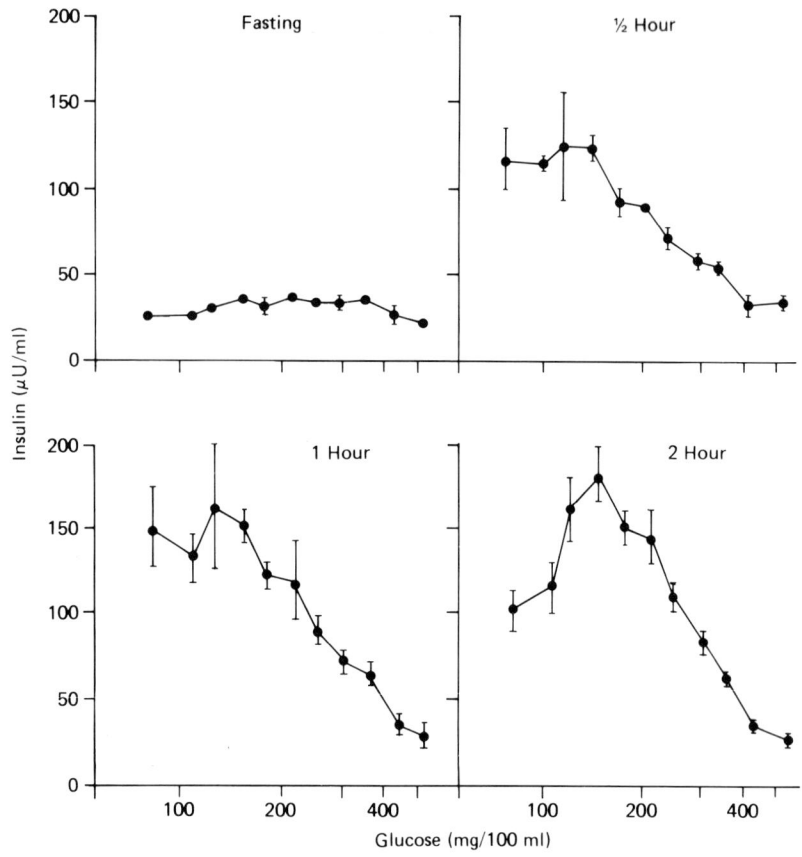

Figure 5. Relationship between glucose tolerance and plasma insulin from Savage et al (1975) reproduced with permission from the American Diabetes Association, Inc.

moderate increases in fasting glucose levels (Brunzell et al, 1976). The results of these cross-sectional studies are compatible with either impaired B cell function or insulin resistance being the initial defect present and B cell exhaustion occurring after some degree of sustained hyperglycaemia.

Studies in patients at risk to develop diabetes

Several studies have examined either fasting plasma insulin levels and/or post-glucose plasma insulin responses in populations with increased risk of developing diabetes. Mexican Americans, a population with an increased risk of developing Type 2 diabetes, were found to have a greater post-glucose plasma insulin response when compared with non-Hispanic Caucasian Americans after correction for such factors as obesity, age, sex and fat distribution (Haffner et al, 1986). In Pima Indians (Savage et al, 1975) and Micronesians (Balku et al, 1985), hyperinsulinaemia has been found to predict conversion from normal to impaired glucose tolerance. In contrast, in the Japanese low plasma insulin responses were found to predict conversion (Kosaka et al, 1977; Kadowaki et al, 1984) and in a Scandinavian population, Cerasi et al (1973) found decreased plasma insulin responses to glucose in relatives of patients with Type 2 diabetes. There are several possible explanations for these conflicting results. For example, they may simply reflect the heterogeneity of diabetes or the subjects may have been studied at different stages in the evolution of their disease. In another study, Cerasi and Luft (1967) examined the plasma insulin responses to an intravenous glucose challenge in non-diabetic identical twins of patients with Type 2 diabetes. Although they suggested that their data indicated that the B cell response was gentically determined and that a low insulin response was a prerequisite for the development of diabetes, there was no significant difference between the responses of the non-diabetic twin and those of a non-diabetic control group. The lack of simultaneous evaluation of insulin resistance limits the value of the above studies in determining whether insulin resistance or impaired B cell function is the initial defect.

Two recent studies (Ward et al, 1985; O'Rahilly et al, 1986) have examined indices of insulin secretion and insulin resistance in subjects at increased risk of developing Type 2 diabetes in an attempt to identify defects which precede the onset of Type 2 diabetes. Ward et al (1985) administered intravenous glucose tolerance tests to eight subjects with a history of gestational diabetes and analysed the results using the minimal model developed by Bergman and his colleages (1981). Although the number of subjects studied was small, it was nevertheless demonstrated that the subjects who had had gestational diabetes had greater fasting plasma insulin levels (despite comparable plasma glucose levels), reduced first-phase insulin responses to the intravenous glucose, and a reduced tissue sensitivity to insulin. These studies thus demonstrated that impaired B cell function can exist in the presence of fasting hyperinsulinaemia and that both insulin resistance and impaired B cell function precede the onset of overt diabetes. The first-phase insulin response was reduced 50% while tissue insulin sensitivity was reduced 66%. Whether or not the impairment in insulin sensitivity was significantly different from that of B cell function was not evaluated. A difficulty in the interpretation of this study is that some of the subjects who had had gestational diabetes still had impaired glucose tolerance.

O'Rahilly et al (1986) studied 154 first-degree relatives of patients with Type 2 diabetes by infusing them with glucose and analysing the changes in plasma insulin and glucose with reference to the normal values for B cell function and tissue insulin sensitivity predicted by a model (Hosker et al, 1985). Some of the first-degree relatives had excessive increases in plasma glucose concentrations and their results were compared with 75 of the other relatives who had plasma glucose responses ± 1 standard deviation of 64 control subjects with no first-degree relative having diabetes. The 28 subjects with excessive plasma glucose responses were found to have both reduced B cell function and reduced tissue insulin sensitivity. Compared with the controls, B cell function was reduced by 59% and tissue sensitivity was reduced 34%. Whether these degrees of impairment were significantly different was not evaluated. However, the subjects with excessive plasma glucose responses were subdivided into tertiles based on their responses and the B cell function and tissue sensitivity of each tertile was compared with those of the other relatives. All three tertiles had significantly impaired B cell function, whereas only the tertile with the greatest plasma glucose responses was considered to have significantly impaired tissue insulin sensitivity. It was concluded that the primary defect was B cell dysfunction.

However, several factors must be considered to determine the validity of this conclusion. First, it is assumed that the model has equal sensitivity for detecting impaired B cell function and impaired tissue insulin sensitivity. This remains to be demonstrated. Second, the relatives with plasma glucose responses ± 1 standard deviation of the controls had B cell sensitivity 109% of normal but tissue insulin sensitivity was only 85% of normal. One could interpret these data to indicate that insulin resistance preceded impaired B cell function and whether or not glucose tolerance deteriorated depended on simultaneous worsening of both. Finally, there was apparently less of a correlation between deterioration in B cell dysfunction among tertiles of plasma glucose responses than worsening of tissue insulin sensitivity.

In summary, few studies have simultaneously examined alterations of B cell function and tissue sensitivity prior to onset of impaired glucose tolerance and those performed to date have demonstrated coexistence of abnormalities of both processes without clear cut evidence of priority in temporal sequence or severity.

Studies in patients with impaired glucose tolerance

There are considerable data on plasma insulin after oral or intravenous glucose in patients with impaired glucose tolerance. As summarized recently by DeFronzo et al (1983), there are at least 25 reports including approximately 1100 subjects. The conclusions of these studies are anything but unanimous. One-third of studies concluded that insulin secretion was reduced, one-third concluded that insulin secretion was not different from that in subjects with normal glucose tolerance and one-third of studies concluded that insulin responses were greater than normal. Several factors could explain these varying conclusions including differences in definition of impaired glucose tolerance, patient selection and matching and true heterogeneity of Type 2 diabetes. Furthermore, it must be remembered that not all patients with impaired glucose tolerance will progress to overt diabetes.

Nevertheless, the overall data of these studies permit several conclusions. First, about two-thirds of patients with impaired glucose tolerance do not have reduced circulating insulin levels. Thus, in these individuals, insulin resistance must be present to account for some of the impaired glucose tolerance. Second, had B cell function been unimpaired, patients with impaired glucose tolerance should have greater than normal plasma insulin levels because they had a greater than normal stimulus for insulin secretion during the oral glucose tolerance test. The fact that only one-third of subjects were reported to have greater than normal responses indicates, therefore, that the majority of patients with impaired glucose tolerance have some degree of impaired B cell function which must contribute to their impaired glucose tolerance.

Insulin resistance has not been directly or quantitatively assessed in a large number of subjects with impaired glucose tolerance. Where insulin resistance has been assessed, virtually all studies have demonstrated that insulin resistance is evident at this stage although not necessarily in all subjects (Harano et al, 1981; Kolterman et al, 1981; Bogardus et al, 1984a; Ward et al, 1985; O'Rahilly et al, 1986). Longitudinal studies examining changes in islet B cell function and insulin sensitivity as individuals progress from normal to abnormal glucose tolerance are needed. It is, of course, important that the tests used to evaluate B cell function and insulin sensitivity have equal sensitivity for detecting changes.

WHICH IS MORE IMPORTANT—IMPAIRED INSULIN SECRETION OR INSULIN RESISTANCE?

This question can be addressed on two levels. First, which is essential for development of diabetes and second, which defect contributes more to a diabetic person's hyperglycaemia? One could argue that no matter how much insulin resistance were present, a person would not become diabetic unless his pancreas failed to compensate. It generally takes more than a 90% pancreatectomy to produce diabetes, thus the normal pancreas has a tremendous reserve. Furthermore, not all individuals with marked obesity and presumably severe insulin resistance develop diabetes. Thus, prolonged insulin resistance by itself may not be a sufficient cause for development of diabetes. On the other hand, reduction in insulin secretion by itself (e.g. Type 1 diabetes) is a sufficient cause for development of diabetes. Viewed in these terms, impaired insulin secretion would appear to be more important. Indeed, in a long-term follow-up of nearly 300 individuals with impaired glucose tolerance, an initially decreased plasma insulin response was found to be predictive of the subsequent development of diabetes (Kadowaki et al, 1984).

On the other hand, although impaired B cell function may be necessary for emergence of overt diabetes, the degree of fasting and postprandial hyperglycaemia found in a given person with this disorder will be a function of the ambient insulin concentration and the degree of insulin resistance present. Both these factors may differ considerably among patients. For example, as a generalization, when equally hyperglycaemic lean and obese individuals are examined, the lean individuals are less insulin resistant and thus in this group impaired B cell function would be more important than it might be in obese individuals who are more insulin resistant and have greater circulating insulin levels (Perley and Kipnis, 1967). Within these groups there can also be considerable heterogeneity. Insulinopoenia, when it occurs, can itself result in insulin resistance as evidenced from studies of patients with Type 1 diabetes (Yki-Jarvinen and Koivisto, 1986) and animals made diabetic by experiment (Bevilacqua et al, 1985). Hyperinsulinaemia also can lead to insulin resistance (Mandarino et al, 1984a; Marangou et al,

1986). At different stages and different periods of the disease, the relative contribution of impaired insulin secretion and insulin resistance may vary. Consider the patient receiving a thiazide diuretic whose potassium depletion further limits his ability to secrete insulin or the borderline patient who becomes overtly diabetic during a pregnancy because of third trimester insulin resistance.

It is currently impossible to say whether impaired B cell function or insulin resistance is the more important determinant of fasting and postprandial hyperglycaemia in patients with Type 2 diabetes. Further studies will need not only to quantify the degree of abnormality of each of these factors but also to determine their impact. It is likely that approaches such as those of Bergman et al (1981) and Turner and his colleagues (as reported in Hosker et al, 1985) will prove of value in this regard.

SITE OF TISSUE INSULIN RESISTANCE

It was initially thought that a decreased number of insulin receptors was the primary cause of insulin resistance of Type 2 diabetes (Olefsky, 1976). Patients with Type 2 diabetes were reported to have reduced numbers of insulin receptors on their adipocytes, presumably reflecting the situation on other insulin sensitive tissues (Kolterman et al, 1981). It had also been reported that sulphonylurea treatment, which improved glycaemic control in patients with Type 2 diabetes, was associated with increased insulin receptor binding (Olefsky and Reaven, 1976) implying a cause–effect relationship. Subsequent studies in which subjects were carefully age-, weight-, and sex-matched, however, have failed to confirm these postulates (Maloof and Lockwood, 1981; Kashiwagi et al, 1983; Lonroth et al, 1983; Mandarino et al, 1984b; Bolinder et al, 1985) and now it is generally believed that the insulin resistance of Type 2 diabetes is located at some step in the sequence of events distal to the binding of insulin with its receptor.

Liver, muscle and adipose tissue are the major insulin sensitive tissues involved in glucose homeostasis in man. Although adipose tissue is a minor factor in the direct disposal of glucose, probably accounting for less than 5%, it can indirectly influence production of glucose by the liver and utilization of glucose by muscle via its release of glycerol and lactate, which can serve as gluconeogenic substrates, and via the release of free fatty acids, whose oxidation in liver may promote gluconeogenesis (Williamson et al, 1966) and whose oxidation in muscle may reduce glucose disposal (Ferrannini et al, 1983).

Individuals with Type 2 diabetes have increased hepatic glucose output (Kolterman et al, 1981; DeFronzo et al, 1982; Campbell et al, 1988) and reduced muscle glucose clearance (Rabinowitz and Zierler, 1962; DeFronzo et al, 1985). The presence of elevated plasma free fatty acids suggests that there may be increased rates of lipolysis as well (Chen et al, 1987). Since all these abnormalities are found despite increased or normal plasma insulin concentrations, their presence constitutes prima facie evidence for liver muscle and adipose tissue insulin resistance in Type 2 diabetes.

Currently there is controversy concerning the major tissue site of insulin resistance in this disorder. Some investigators have proposed that the predominant site is muscle (Kolterman et al, 1981; DeFronzo et al, 1985; Donner et al, 1985), whereas others consider the liver to be the most important tissue involved (Best et al, 1982; Kelley et al, 1988; Campbell et al, 1988). It is most likely that insulin resistance in both tissues contributes to the disordered glucose metabolism found in this condition but that hepatic insulin resistance is the predominant factor responsible for fasting hyperglycaemia.

Relative severity of insulin resistance of liver and muscle

The main assumptions underlying the proposal that muscle is the major site of insulin resistance are that insulin resistance in muscle is greater than that in liver and that muscle is the major organ regulating glucose disposal. Studies of limb glucose balance and glucose disposal during glucose clamp experiments form one of the bases for the contention that muscle is the of insulin resistance. Studies (Kolterman et al, 1981) examining the dose-response characteristics for insulin-stimulated glucose disposal conditions in which more than 90% of glucose uptake occurs in extrahepatic tissues have demonstrated that patients with NIDDM have markedly reduced insulin sensitivity (ED_{50}) and/or responsiveness (V_{max}). These observations and the correlations found between impaired glucose disposal and both fasting and postprandial hyperglycaemia (Kolterman et al, 1981) support the concept that peripheral tissues are the major site of the insulin resistance in NIDDM.

This conclusion implies that peripheral tissues are more resistant to insulin than the liver. However, the relative severity of hepatic insulin resistance in NIDDM has only recently been established. A major reason for this stems from the fact that the experimental conditions used in previous studies have not permitted an assessment of the dose-response characteristics for suppression of glucose production by insulin. In some studies, suppression of hepatic glucose production was examined at only one insulin concentration (Kimmerling et al, 1976; Scarlett et al, 1982; DeFronzo et al, 1985). In other studies, which used more than one insulin concentration, the lowest concentration of insulin resulted in near maximal suppression of glucose production (Kolterman et al, 1981; Bogardus et al, 1984a).

In a study comparing suppressibility of hepatic glucose output and stimulation of leg glucose uptake (DeFronzo et al, 1985), it was found that suppression of hepatic glucose output was decreased by about 10%, whereas stimulation of leg glucose uptake was reduced by 50%. It was concluded that muscle was more resistant than liver. A problem with the interpretation of these studies is that the insulin concentration used (<100 mU/l) is more than sufficient to produce maximal suppression of the hepatic glucose output but only produces about half-maximal muscle glucose uptake (Rizza et al, 1981b). In other words, the experimental conditions were optimized for detecting differences in muscle glucose metabolism but not liver glucose metabolism. Moreover, the concentrations of insulin used were supraphysiological; under usual daily conditions, plasma insulin levels do not normally exceed 60 mU/l and if they do so, it is only transiently.

Recently, Campbell et al (1988) have conducted euglycaemic clamp experiments which circumvented most of the shortcomings of previous studies. These studies examined the dose-response characteristics of suppression of hepatic glucose output and stimulation of glucose uptake (mostly in muscle) in normal volunteers and carefully matched subjects with Type 2 diabetes. As shown in Figure 6, the ED_{50} for the suppression of hepatic glucose output and for the stimulation of glucose uptake were increased to a similar extent in patients with Type 2 diabetes, thus demonstrating that liver and muscle were equally resistant to insulin in this condition.

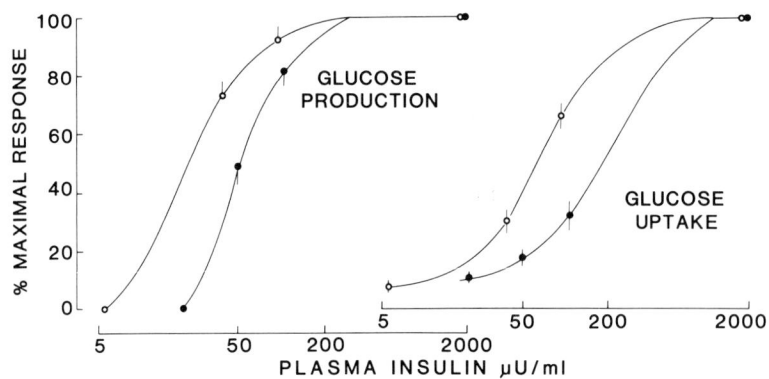

Figure 6. Insulin dose-response characteristics for suppression of hepatic glucose output and stimulation of peripheral glucose uptake in patients with Type 2 diabetes and non-diabetic volunteers. Data from Campbell et al (1988). (○—○) Non-diabetic subjects ($n = 14$), (●—●) NIDDM subjects ($n = 14$).

Relative importance of muscle and liver for glucose homeostasis

Postabsorptive state

In the postabsorptive state (after a 12–14 h fast), plasma insulin averages 5–15 mU/l and most glucose utilization occurs in non-insulin-sensitive tissues with brain alone accounting for about 55% (Della-Porta et al, 1964) and muscle only about 25% (Andres et al, 1956). Therefore, in the postabsorptive state, insulin does not exert a major influence on muscle glucose utilization. In contrast, all glucose delivery into the circulation comes from the liver under these conditions, and insulin is the only hormone restraining hepatic glucose output. Under these circumstances, a small decrease or increase in plasma insulin will result in a marked change in hepatic glucose output without a decrease in peripheral glucose utilization (Miles et al, 1980;

Rizza et al, 1981b). Thus in the postabsorptive state, the effects of insulin on the liver are more important than its effects on muscle for maintaining normal homeostasis. Since muscle and liver are equally insulin resistant in Type 2 diabetes, one would, therefore, expect insulin resistance of the liver to have a greater impact on glucose homeostasis in the postabsorptive state. In support of this concept are a number of studies (Best et al, 1982; Campbell et al, 1988) which have demonstrated a correlation between increased rates of hepatic glucose output and fasting plasma glucose levels in patients with Type 2 diabetes.

Postprandial state

After ingestion of a mixed meal or glucose load, plasma insulin normally increases to a maximum of 60–80 mU/l after one hour and returns to post-absorptive values between 3 and 4 hours (Kelley et al, 1988; Ferrannini et al, 1988). During this interval the average plasma insulin concentration is only about 30 mU/l. Because of the insulin dose-response characteristics for liver and muscle, hepatic glucose output will be near maximally suppressed for a substantial period, whereas glucose utilization will not be even half-maximally stimulated (Rizza et al, 1981b). Thus, potential abnormalities in insulin secretion and insulin sensitivity might affect liver glucose kinetics more than muscle glucose kinetics.

The extent to which such changes may affect postprandial glucose homeostasis depends upon which tissues are primarily responsible for dis-position of the carbohydrate load. Until recently this has been controversial, but several studies (Jackson et al, 1973; Kelley et al, 1988; Ferrannini et al, 1988) summarized in Figure 7 have clarified this issue. Nearly 30% of an oral

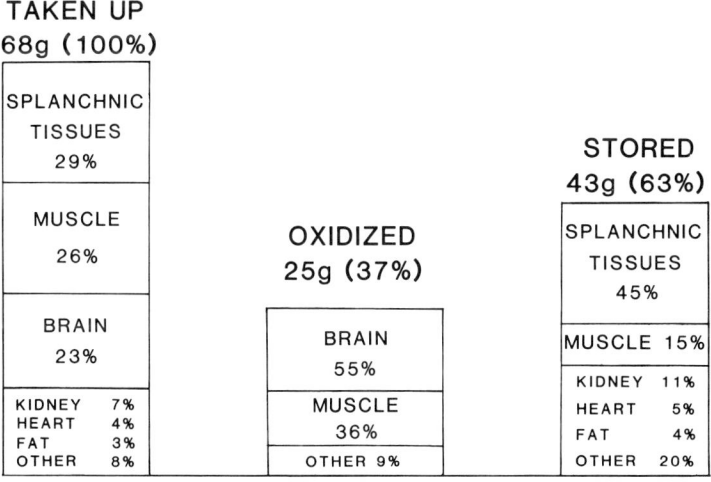

Figure 7. Metabolic fate of an oral glucose load. Data from Kelley et al (1988).

glucose load is taken up by splanchnic tissues. This still leaves 70% of the oral glucose load to be accounted for, and conceivably muscle could be the predominant tissue responsible. As it turns out, however, muscle is approximately as important as the liver. Because release of endogenous glucose from the liver is suppressed nearly 60% postprandially, exogenous glucose from the oral load must be used to satisfy tissue glucose requirements normally satisfied by endogenous glucose from the liver. As a consequence, brain glucose uptake accounts for nearly 25% of the disposition of the oral glucose load with other tissues accounting for about 20% of the load (Kelley et al, 1988). Studies measuring glucose uptake across the forearm after oral carbohydrate administration (Jackson et al, 1973; Kelley et al, 1988) indicate that only about 25% of the oral load is taken up by muscle. Thus, in the postprandial situation, the liver appears to have at least as important a role as muscle in the maintenance of normal homeostasis.

Taking into consideration the fact that the liver is the prime regulator of glucose homeostasis in the postabsorptive state and that liver and muscle are about equally important in the postabsorptive state, it would seem that overall the liver is the more important insulin sensitive tissue. Consequently, the insulin resistance of Type 2 diabetes should have a greater impact on glucose homeostasis via the liver rather than muscle.

CLINICAL IMPLICATIONS

Our current, though incomplete, understanding of the pathogenesis of Type 2 diabetes has implications for our present and future treatment of this disorder. First of all, the demonstration of adverse effects of hyperglycaemia *per se* on islet B cell function and tissue responses to insulin suggest that restoring euglycaemia by temporary insulin treatment may improve insulin secretion and decrease insulin resistance and render patients capable of achieving adequate glycaemia on a diet with or without sulphonylurea treatment (Yki-Jarvinen et al, 1988). Second, regardless of which comes first, impaired B cell function or insulin resistance, improvement of one defect will usually be accompanied by improvement in the other (Best et al, 1982; Scarlett et al, 1982). Third, where it is obvious that one defect predominates, e.g. insulin resistance in the obese Type 2 patient with fasting hyperinsulin-aemia, therapy should primarily be directed toward reversing that defect or at least diminishing its magnitude. Diminution of the insulin resistance of obesity will markedly improve glycaemic control (Savage et al, 1979a, b). Obviously, the development of effective appetite suppressants (or satiety stimulants) would be of great help in the management of most patients with Type 2 diabetes.

Finally, although there are as yet no specific agents available to treat insulin resistance, we can anticipate that in the future there will be. For example, work is being done on the development of analogues of insulin which are hepatic specific. Use of these insulins might reproduce more closely the normal portal-peripheral insulin gradient with relative diminution of peripheral hyperinsulinaemia, a risk factor for atherosclerosis.

Glucagon antagonists are being investigated. These agents, by blocking the effects of glucagon, should decrease the overproduction of glucose by the liver in Type 2 diabetes. The demonstration that accelerated gluconeogenesis accounts for nearly all of the increased hepatic glucose output in Type 2 diabetes (Consoli et al, 1987) suggests that agents which block gluconeogenesis may be useful. The biguanide, metformin, and inhibitors of fatty acid oxidation are currently under investigation for this purpose.

REFERENCES

Andres R, Cader G & Zierler K (1956) The quantitatively minor role of carbohydrate in oxidative metabolism by skeletal muscle in intact man in the basal state. Measurements of oxygen and glucose uptake and carbon dioxide and lactate production in the forearm. *Journal of Clinical Investigation* **35:** 671–682.

Balku B, King H, Zimmet P & Raper L (1985) Factors associated with the development of diabetes in the Micronesian population of Nauru. *American Journal of Epidemiology* **122:** 594–605.

Bergman R, Phillips J & Cobelli C (1981) Physiologic evaluation of factors controlling glucose tolerance in man: measurement of insulin sensitivity and B-cell glucose sensitivity from the response to intravenous glucose. *Journal of Clinical Investigation* **68:** 1456–1467.

Best J, Judzewitsch R, Pfeifer M, Beard J, Halter J & Porte D (1982) The effect of chronic sulfonylurea therapy on hepatic glucose production in noninsulin-dependent diabetes. *Diabetes* **31:** 333–338.

Bevilacqua S, Barrett E, Smith D et al (1985) Hepatic and peripheral insulin resistance following streptozotocin-induced insulin deficiency in the dog. *Metabolism* **34:** 817–825.

Bogardus C, Lillioja S, Howard B, Reaven G & Mott D (1984a) Relationships between insulin secretion, insulin action and fasting plasma glucose concentration in nondiabetic and noninsulin-dependent diabetic subjects. *Journal of Clinical Investigation* **74:** 1238–1246.

Bogardus C, Lillioja S, Mott D, Reaven G, Kashiwagi A & Foley J (1984b) Relationship between obesity and maximal insulin stimulated glucose uptake in vivo and in vitro in Pima Indians. *Journal of Clinical Investigation* **73:** 800–805.

Bolinder J, Ostman J & Arner P (1985) Effects of intravenous and oral glucose administration on insulin action in human fat cells. *Diabetes* **34:** 884–890.

Brunzell J, Robertson R, Lerner R et al (1976) Relationships between fasting plasma glucose levels and insulin secretion during intravenous glucose tolerance tests. *Journal of Clinical Endocrinology and Metabolism* **42:** 222–229.

Campbell P, Mandarino L & Gerich J (1988) Quantification of the relative impairment in actions of insulin on hepatic glucose production and peripheral glucose uptake in noninsulin-dependent diabetes mellitus. *Metabolism* **37:** 15–22.

Cerasi E & Luft R (1967) Insulin response to glucose infusion in diabetic and nondiabetic monozygotic twin pairs: genetic control of insulin response. *Acta Endocrinologica* **55:** 330–345.

Cerasi E, Efendic S & Luft R (1973) Dose-response relation between plasma insulin and blood glucose levels during oral glucose loads in prediabetic and diabetic subjects. *Lancet* **1:** 794–797.

Chen Y, Swislocki A & Reaven G (1987) Resistance to insulin suppression of plasma free fatty acid concentrations and insulin stimulation of glucose uptake in noninsulin-dependent diabetes mellitus. *Journal of Clinical Endocrinology and Metabolism* **64:** 17–21.

Chiles R & Tzagournis M (1970) Excessive serum insulin response to oral glucose in obesity and mild diabetes. *Diabetes* **19:** 458–464.

Ciaraldi T, Kolterman O, Scarlett J, Kao M & Olefsky J (1982) Role of glucose transport in the postreceptor defect of noninsulin-dependent diabetes mellitus. *Diabetes* **31:** 1016–1022.

Consoli A, Nurjhan N, Kennedy F & Gerich J (1987) Accelerated gluconeogenesis accounts for all of the increase in basal hepatic glucose output of noninsulin-dependent diabetes mellitus. *Diabetes* **36 (supplement 1):** 4A.

DeFronzo RA, Simonson D & Ferrannini E (1982) Hepatic and peripheral insulin resistance: a common feature of Type II (noninsulin-dependent) and Type I (insulin-dependent) diabetes mellitus. *Diabetologia* **23:** 313–319.

DeFronzo RA, Ferrannini E & Koivisto V (1983) New concepts in the pathogenesis and treatment of noninsulin-dependent diabetes mellitus. *American Journal of Medicine* **74 (supplement 1A):** 52–81.

DeFronzo RA, Gunnarsson R, Bjorkman O, Olsson M & Wahren J (1985) Effects of insulin on peripheral and splanchnic glucose metabolism in noninsulin-dependent (Type II) diabetes mellitus. *Journal of Clinical Investigation* **76:** 149–155.

Della Porta P, Maiola A, Negri V & Rossella E (1964) Cerebral blood flow and metabolism in therapeutic insulin coma. *Metabolism* **13:** 131–140.

Dimitriadis G, Pehling G & Gerich J (1985) Abnormal glucose modulation of islet A- and B-cell responses to arginine in noninsulin-dependent diabetes mellitus. *Diabetes* **34:** 541–547.

Donner C, Fraze E, Chen Y & Reaven G (1985) Quantitation of insulin-stimulated glucose disposal in patients with noninsulin-dependent diabetes mellitus. *Diabetes* **34:** 831–835.

Efendic S, Wajngot A, Cerasi E & Luft R (1980) Insulin release, insulin sensitivity and glucose tolerance. *Proceedings of National Academy of Science* **77:** 7425–7429.

Efendic S, Luft R & Wajngot A (1984) Aspects of the pathogenesis of Type II diabetes. *Endocrine Review* **5:** 395–410.

Fajans S (1987) MODY—a model for understanding the pathogenesis and natural history of Type II diabetes. *Hormone and Metabolic Research* **19:** 591–599.

Felig P, Wahren J & Hendler R (1978) Influence of maturity-onset diabetes on splanchnic glucose balance after oral glucose ingestion. *Diabetes* **27:** 121–126.

Ferrannini E, Barrett EJ, Bevilacqua S & DeFronzo RA (1983) Effects of fatty acids on glucose production and utilisation in man. *Journal of Clinical Investigation* **72:** 1737–1747.

Ferrannini E, Simonson D, Katz L et al (1988) The disposal of an oral glucose load in patients with noninsulin-dependent diabetes. *Metabolism* **37:** 79–85.

Flier J, Kahn C & Roth J (1979) Receptors, antireceptor antibodies and mechanisms of insulin resistance. *New England Journal of Medicine* **300:** 413–419.

Fujita Y, Herron A & Seltzer H (1975) Confirmation of impaired early insulin response to glycemic stimulus in nonobese mild diabetes. *Diabetes* **24:** 17–28.

Gabbay K, DeLuca D, Fisher J, Mako M & Rubenstein A (1976) Familial hyperproinsulinemia: an autosomal dominant defect. *New England Journal of Medicine* **294:** 911–915.

Haffner S, Stern M, Hazuda H, Pugh J & Patterson J (1986) Hyperinsulinemia in a population at high risk for noninsulin-dependent diabetes mellitus. *New England Journal of Medicine* **315:** 220–224.

Harano Y, Ohgaku S, Kosugi K et al (1981) Clinical significance of altered insulin sensitivity in diabetes mellitus assessed by glucose, insulin and somatostatin infusion. *Journal of Clinical Endocrinology and Metabolism* **52:** 982–987.

Hosker J, Mathews D, Rudenski A et al (1985) Continuous infusion of glucose with model assessment: measurement of insulin resistance and B-cell function in man. *Diabetologia* **28:** 401–411.

Jackson R, Perry G, Rogers J, Advani U & Pilkington T (1973) Relationship between the basal glucose concentration, glucose tolerance and forearm glucose uptake in maturity-onset diabetes. *Diabetes* **22:** 751–761.

Kadowaki T, Miyake Y, Hagura R et al (1984) Risk factors for worsening to diabetes in subjects with impaired glucose tolerance. *Diabetologia* **26:** 44–49.

Kashiwagi A, Verso M, Andrews J, Vasquez B, Reaven G & Foley J (1983) In vitro insulin resistance of human adipocytes isolated from subjects with noninsulin-dependent diabetes mellitus. *Journal of Clinical Investigation* **72:** 1246–1254.

Kelley D, Mitrakou A, Marsh H et al (1988) Skeletal muscle glycolysis, oxidation and storage of an oral glucose load. *Journal of Clinical Investigation* **81:** 1563–1571.

Khan C (1978) Insulin resistance, insulin insensitivity and insulin unresponsiveness: a necessary distinction. *Metabolism* **27 (supplement 2):** 1893–1902.

Kimmerling G, Javorski W, Olefsky J & Reaven G (1976) Locating the site(s) of insulin resistance in patients with nonketotic diabetes mellitus. *Diabetes* **25:** 673–678.

Kolterman O, Insel J, Saekow M & Olefsky J (1980) Mechanisms of insulin resistance in human obesity: evidence for receptor and postreceptor defects. *Journal of Clinical Investigation* **65**: 1272–1284.

Kolterman O, Gray R, Griffin J et al (1981) Receptor and postreceptor defects contribute to the insulin resistance in noninsulin-dependent diabetes mellitus. *Journal of Clinical Investigation* **68**: 957–969.

Kosaka K, Hagura R & Kuzuya T (1977) Insulin responses in equivocal and definite diabetes, with special reference to subjects who had mild glucose intolerance but later developed definite diabetes. *Diabetes* **26**: 944–952.

Leahy J, Cooper H, Deal D & Weir G (1986) Chronic hyperglycemia is associated with impaired glucose influence on insulin secretion: a study of normal rats using chronic in vivo glucose infusions. *Journal of Clinical Investigation* **77**: 908–915.

Lonroth P, DiGirolamo M, Krotiewski M & Smith U (1983) Insulin binding and responsiveness in fat cells from patients with reduced glucose tolerance and Type II diabetes. *Diabetes* **32**: 748–754.

Maloof B & Lockwood D (1981) In vitro effects of a sulfonylurea on insulin action in adipocytes: potentiation of insulin-stimulated hexose transport. *Journal of Clinical Investigation* **68**: 85–90.

Mandarino L, Baker B, Rizza R, Genest J & Gerich J (1984a) Infusion of insulin impairs human adipocyte glucose metabolism in vitro without decreasing adipocyte insulin receptor binding. *Diabetologia* **27**: 358–363.

Mandarino L, Campbell P, Gottesman I, Gerich J (1984b) Abnormal coupling of insulin receptor binding in noninsulin-dependent diabetes. *American Journal of Physiology* **247**: E688–E692.

Marangou A, Weber K, Boston R et al (1986) Metabolic consequences of prolonged hyperinsulinemia in humans: evidence for induction of insulin insensitivity. *Diabetes* **35**: 1383–1389.

Miles J, Rizza R, Haymond M & Gerich J (1980) Effect of acute insulin deficiency of glucose and ketone body turnover in man: evidence for the primacy of overproduction of glucose and ketone bodies in the genesis of diabetic ketoacidosis. *Diabetes* **29**: 926–930.

Olefsky J (1976) The insulin receptor: its role in insulin resistance of obesity and diabetes. *Diabetes* **25**: 1154–1161.

Olefsky J (1981) Insulin resistance and insulin action: an in vitro and in vivo perspective. *Diabetes* **30**: 148–162.

Olefsky J & Reaven G (1976) Effects of sulfonylurea therapy on insulin binding to mononuclear leukocytes of diabetes patients. *American Journal of Medicine* **60**: 89–95.

Olefsky J, Saekow M, Tager H & Rubenstein A (1980) Characterisation of a mutant human insulin species. *Journal of Biological Chemistry* **255**: 6098–6105.

O'Rahilly S, Rudenski A, Burnett M et al (1986) Beta-cell dysfunction, rather than insulin insensitivity, is the primary defect in familial Type II diabetes. *Lancet* **2**: 360–364.

Perley J & Kipnis D (1967) Plasma insulin responses to oral and intravenous glucose: studies in normal and diabetic subjects. *Journal of Clinical Investigation* **46**: 1954–1962.

Rabinowitz D & Zierler K (1962) Forearm metabolism in obesity and its response to intra-arterial insulin. *Journal of Clinical Investigation* **41**: 2173–2181.

Reaven G, Berstein R, Davis B & Olefsky J (1976) Nonketotic diabetes mellitus: insulin deficiency or insulin resistance. *American Journal of Medicine* **60**: 80–88.

Rizza R, Mandarino L & Gerich J (1981a) Mechanism and significance of insulin resistance in noninsulin-dependent diabetes mellitus. *Diabetes* **30**: 990–995.

Rizza R, Mandarino L & Gerich J (1981b) Dose-response characteristics for the effects of insulin on production and utilisation of glucose in man. *American Journal of Physiology* **240**: E630–E639.

Rossetti L, Shulman G, Zawalich W & DeFronzo RA (1987) Effect of chronic hyperglycemia on in vivo insulin secretion in partially pancreatectomized rats. *Journal of Clinical Investigation* **80**: 1037–1044.

Savage P, Dippe S, Bennett P et al (1975) Hyperinsulinemia and hypoinsulinemia: insulin responses to oral carbohydrate over a wide spectrum of glucose tolerance. *Diabetes* **24**: 362–368.

Savage P, Bennion L, Flock E et al (1979a) Diet-induced improvement of abnormalities in insulin and glucagon secretion and in insulin receptor binding in diabetes mellitus. *Journal of Clinical Endocrinology and Metabolism* **48**: 999–1007.

Savage P, Bennion L & Bennett P (1979b) Normalisation of insulin and glucagon secretion in ketosis-resistant diabetes mellitus with prolonged diet therapy. *Journal of Clinical Endocrinology and Metabolism* **49**: 830–833.

Scarlett J, Gray R, Griffin J, Olefsky J & Kolterman O (1982) Insulin treatment reverses the insulin resistance of Type II diabetes mellitus. *Diabetes Care* **5**: 353–363.

Sorensen J, Colton C, Hillman R & Soeldner J (1982) Use of a physiologic pharmokinetic model of glucose homeostasis for assessment of performance requirements for improved insulin therapies. *Diabetes Care* **5**: 148–157.

Truglia JA, Livingston JN & Lockwood DH (1985) Insulin resistance: receptor and post-binding defects in human obesity and non-insulin-dependent diabetes mellitus. *American Journal of Medicine* **79**: 13–22.

Ward W, Bolgiano D, McKnight B, Halter J & Porte D (1984) Diminished B-cell secretory capacity in patients with noninsulin-dependent diabetes mellitus. *Journal of Clinical Investigation* **74**: 1318–1328.

● Ward W, Johnston C, Beard J, Benedettgi T, Halter J & Porte D (1985) Insulin resistance and impaired insulin secretion in subjects with histories of gestational diabetes mellitus. *Diabetes* **34**: 861–869.

Williamson J, Kreisberg R & Felts P (1966) Mechanism for the stimulation of gluconeogenesis by fatty acids in perfused rat liver. *Proceedings of National Academy of Science (USA)* **56**: 247–254.

Yki-Jarvinen H & Koivisto V (1986) National course of insulin resistance in Type I diabetes. *New England Journal of Medicine* **315**: 224–230.

Yki-Jarvinen H, Kubo K, Zawadski J et al (1987a) Dissociation of in vitro sensitivities of glucose transport and antilipolysis to insulin in NIDDM. *American Journal of Physiology* **253**: E300–E304.

Yki-Jarvinen H, Helve E & Koivisto V (1987b) Hyperglycemia decreases glucose uptake in Type I diabetes. *Diabetes* **38**: 892–896.

● Yki-Jarvinen H, Nikkila E, Helve E & Taskinen M (1988) Clinical benefits and mechanisms of a sustained response to intermittent insulin therapy in Type II diabetic patients with secondary drug failure. *American Journal of Medicine* **84**: 185–192.

3

Pathogenesis of NIDDM—a disease of deficient insulin secretion

R. C. TURNER
D. R. MATTHEWS
A. CLARK
S. O'RAHILLY
A. S. RUDENSKI
J. LEVY

Type 2 diabetes is probably caused by the interaction of several different genetic and environmental factors. It has a strong hereditary basis and a key pathophysiological question is whether the majority of patients with Type 2 diabetes have a unique major genetic defect causing this predisposition, and whether this primarily affects beta cell function or insulin resistance. This question is of clinical importance, since identification of a major gene would allow an assessment of the risk of diabetes in relatives of affected patients and in the general population. If the disease is polygenic without a major pre-disposing gene, identification of those at risk will be more difficult.

Diabetes mellitus is characterized both by increased excursions of postprandial glucose concentrations and by a raised fasting plasma glucose level. Both features could be the result of deficient beta cell function, impaired insulin sensitivity or a combination of the two processes. Factors controlling the secretion of insulin and its action are complex, so that inherited abnormalities could affect several aspects of either system, in different combinations, and thus precipitate diabetes (Fajans et al, 1986). In populations who remain thin and fit diabetes is uncommon. A sedentary life style, with over-eating and development of obesity, are important precipitating factors acting through impaired insulin sensitivity. Although these factors are extremely important in the genesis of the disease, is it likely that they can only lead to diabetes in genetically predisposed individuals.

IS THERE A MAJOR SUSCEPTIBILITY GENE?

Since insulin resistant states do not invariably precipitate diabetes (e.g. only a proportion of those with acromegaly or Cushing's disease become diabetic) it is likely that the genetic predisposition exists only in a sub-section of the general population.

The studies of Pyke and colleagues on twins have shown nearly 100% concordance of Type 2 diabetes in monozygotic twins. In the few instances in which an identical twin of a Type 2 diabetic has appeared to be normal, a glucose tolerance test has revealed glucose intolerance (Barnett et al, 1981). These studies indicate that inheritance has a major role, but have given no indication whether this is monogenic or polygenic.

Two populations with a particularly high prevalence of diabetes associated with obesity, the Nauruans (Raper et al, 1984) and the Pima Indians (Rushforth et al, 1971), show a bimodality of glucose tolerance. This indicates a major predisposing gene to the disease.

The study by Kobberling and colleagues of the prevalence of known diabetes in families suggests that nearly 50% of the first degree relatives of Type 2 diabetics would develop the disease if they lived to the age of 80 (Kobberling et al, 1985). Similar data have been obtained in Japan (Matsuda and Kuzuya, 1984). This prevalence raises the possibility of dominant inheritance of a susceptibility gene, although it cannot necessarily distinguish between polygenic and monogenic inheritance.

A recent study of families of Caucasian Type 2 diabetic patients, investigating first degree relatives with a glucose tolerance test, suggested that 'early-onset Type 2 diabetes' presenting before the age of 40 might represent patients who had 'double-gene dose' (O'Rahilly et al, 1987). In most cases both parents of these subjects had glucose intolerance or diabetes, and a high proportion of their siblings (67%) were similarly affected. As many parents of the affected subjects were glucose intolerant rather than diabetic, it suggests that Type 2 diabetes may be a disorder in which a single gene on its own (in a non-obese patient) could be expressed only as life-long glucose intolerance. With additional impaired insulin sensitivity from any cause, genetic or environmental, the gene defect may result in clinical diabetes in middle or old age. The data raise the possibility that if a patient has a double-gene dose, diabetes might present in the 3rd or 4th decades in obese subjects and in later decades in normal weight subjects. In the UK, Type 2 diabetics who present at an early age are particularly obese in relation to their peers (UKPDS, 1988). Further studies are needed to assess whether this pattern of inheritance can be confirmed and whether it is widely applicable. Against this hypothesis is the lack of reports of a very high prevalence of diabetes in offspring of conjugal diabetic parents (Kahn et al, 1969; Tattersall et al, 1975), but this might reflect the fact that most studies have included parents with both Type 1 and Type 2 diabetes, and heterogeneity between parents would mean that homozygosity for a particular gene in offspring would be uncommon. In India, a high prevalence of Type 2 diabetes is found in offspring of conjugal Type 2 diabetic patients (Viswanathan et al, 1985). In Kuwait, which has a high incidence of Type 2 diabetes, early-onset Type 2 diabetes is common (Richens et al, 1988) and one can postulate that a high population prevalence of a gene would increase the chance of the appearance of a 'double gene dose', leading to early-onset presentation, particularly if environmental factors, such as sedentary life or marked obesity are present.

DOES IMPAIRED BETA CELL FUNCTION HAVE A PRIME ROLE?

Table 1 details the three main possibilities, (1) the predisposition to diabetes is from a single 'beta cell failure gene', (2) a single 'insulin resistant gene' or (3) is a heterogeneous disorder with many genetic and environmental predispositions. We suggest that the available evidence indicates a major susceptibility gene affects beta cell function, although other factors are needed to produce overt diabetes. Not all patients will have the same genetic predisposition. It is recogized that some will have occult Type 1 diabetes (Groop et al, 1988). Nevertheless, the majority may have a homogeneous hereditary basis. To determine whether beta cell dysfunction or impaired insulin sensitivity has a primary role, it is necessary to study patients at an early stage before hyperglycaemia has induced secondary effects. It then appears that beta cell dysfunction is a prominent defect.

Table 1. Three major theories of aetiology/pathophysiology of Type 2 diabetes.

(I) Major predisposing B-cell susceptibility gene
accounts for familial inheritance of diabetes
a gene frequency of perhaps 10–15% in Caucasian populations
made clinically overt by interaction with impaired insulin sensitivity from any cause e.g. genetic disorders, sedentary life, obesity, steriod or other hormonal disorders

(II) Major pre-disposing insulin resistance susceptibility gene
accounts for familial inheritance of diabetes
a gene frequency of perhaps 10–15% in Caucasian populations
made clinically overt by interplay with other factors such as obesity
if sufficiently severe will lead to impaired beta-cell function in either all or possibly only susceptible subjects

(III) Heterogeneous polygenic/environmental disorder
in which there are
(a) *many B-cell defects, including, for example*
    defects of neural control
    glucose metabolism
    ATP regulated K^+ channel
    cyclic AMP and other signal transducers
    calcium handling
    Betagranule/microtubule/membrane transport
    extracellular amyloid accumulation
    failure of regeneration of beta-cells
    occult Type 1 immunological disturbance
    occult haemachromatosis
    occult chronic pancreatitis
(b) *many insulin sensitivity defects including, for example*
    defects of insulin receptor binding
    insulin receptor tyrosine kinase
    signal transduction mechanisms
    glucose transporter defects
    enzyme regulation defects e.g. glycogen synthase pyruvate dehydrogenase
    steroid metabolism
    counter-regulatory hormones
(c) obesity/sedentary lifestyle
    which can amplify any specific beta-cell or insulin sensitivity defects

Quantitative defect of insulin secretion

Twenty years ago Cerasi and Luft reported that patients with Type 2 diabetes, who had near normal fasting plasma glucose concentrations, had an impaired insulin response to a high plasma glucose concentration maintained by an intraveneous glucose infusion (Cerasi and Luft, 1967). They suggested (a) that 20% of the normal population might be affected in this manner and (b) that it was an inherited characteristic. However, the prevalence of diabetes is considerably less than 20%, so other factors must operate before diabetes becomes overt.

The observation of decreased insulin production would seem to differ from the findings of Yalow and Berson (1960), who, in the first paper reporting immunoreactive insulin measurements, found maturity-onset diabetic patients had raised insulin concentrations both in the basal state and after oral-glucose ingestion. However, it was shown subsequently that the major association of hyperinsulinaemia was with obesity rather than diabetes. In a classical study, Perley and Kipnis (1967) compared normal and overweight

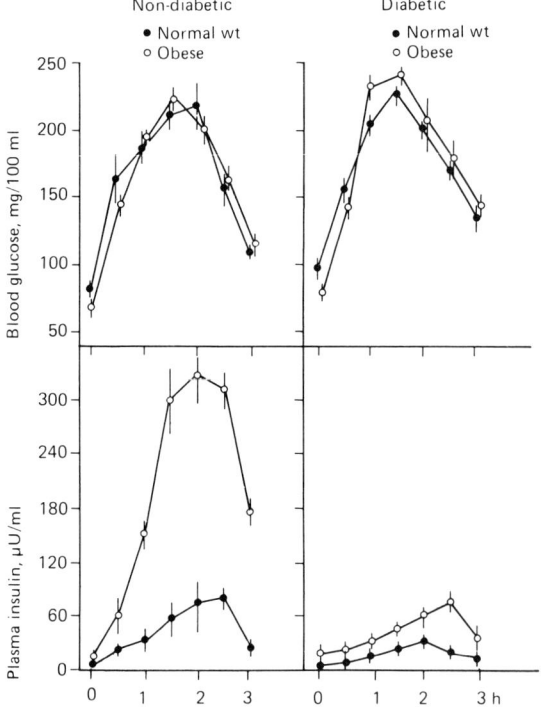

Figure 1. Plasma insulin responses of 12 normal and 12 obese non-diabetic subjects, and 12 normal weight and 11 obese subjects with glucose intolerance. All were given an infusion of glucose to maintain in each person the 'diabetic' glucose profile obtained by an oral glucose tolerance test in subjects with glucose intolerance. Both normal weight and obese 'diabetic' subjects had an impaired insulin response compared with their similarly obese controls. From Perley & Kipnis (1967), with permission.

non-diabetic and diabetic patients (who had near-normal fasting plasma glucose concentrations) at identical glucose concentrations produced by a glucose infusion. When a normal glucose tolerance test was mimicked by the infusion, normal-weight diabetic patients had a marked impairment of insulin response. Although obese diabetics appeared to have high levels compared with normal weight, non-diabetic patients, they were lower than the plasma insulin levels of their appropriate control group of obese non-diabetic subjects. When Perley and Kipnis infused more glucose, to induce the raised plasma levels found in diabetic patients, non-diabetic subjects markedly increased their insulin secretion whereas the normal-weight or obese diabetics, had an overtly impaired response (Figure 1). The diabetic

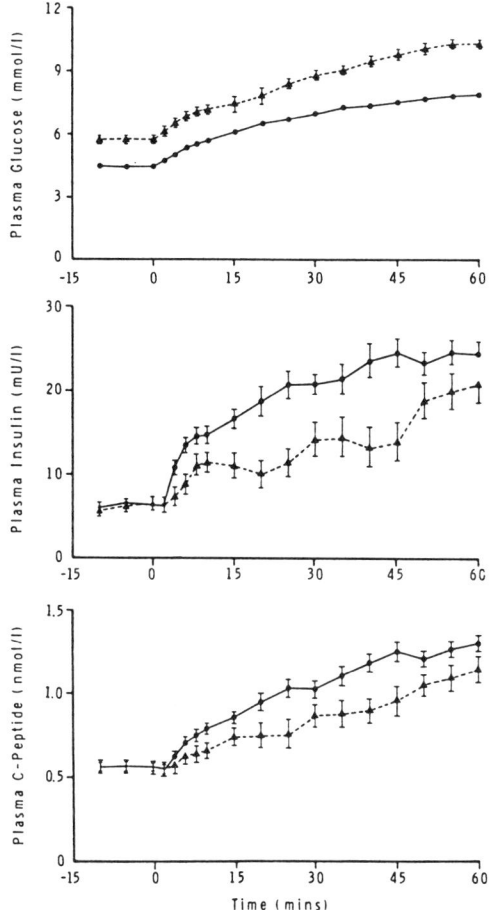

Figure 2. Impaired insulin and C-peptide responses in 28 glucose intolerant first degree relatives of Type 2 diabetic patients (▲ . . . ▲) to a continuous glucose infusion (5 mg kg ideal body weight min^{-1}) compared with 75 age and weight matched relatives with normal glucose tolerance (●——●) (mean ± SEM). From O'Rahilly et al (1986), with permission.

patients particularly had an impaired initial response, and this was also apparent in the initial 30 min following oral glucose in Yalow and Berson's obese diabetic patients. The lack of an initial response in diabetic patients is also seen as a diminished 'first phase' response to intravenous glucose, which is markedly reduced if the fasting plasma glucose is raised, particularly when it is 6 mmol/l or higher (Lerner and Porte, 1972).

Recently, studies of first degree relatives of Type 2 diabetics have shown that subjects with minimal glucose intolerance had a reduced insulin response compared with normoglycaemic relatives or with normal, age and weight matched, non-diabetic subjects (O'Rahilly et al, 1986). Quantitation using a mathematical model of glucose–insulin relationships (continuous infusion of glucose with model assessment, CIGMA) showed that these patients had a marked reduction of beta cell function and similar insulin insensitivity to age and weight matched non-diabetic relatives (Figure 2). This suggested that beta cell dysfunction, rather than impaired insensitivity, may be the first detectable abnormality in the evolution of Type 2 diabetes and therefore may be the site of the inherited defect.

Lack of insulin pulsatility

Type 2 diabetic patients not only have a quantitative defect in insulin production, but also lack the regular, 14-min cycles of basal insulin secretion which occur in non-diabetic subjects. Brief, irregular pulses of insulin secretion are found in diabetic patients including those who after diet therapy have normal basal glucose concentrations (Lang et al, 1981). This abnormality may represent a primary disorder of islet function, since minimally hyperglycaemic first degree relatives of Type 2 diabetic patients, who have presumably never been hyperglycaemic, have also been shown to lack pulsatility of insulin release (O'Rahilly et al, 1988a).

Impaired insulin response as a predictor of diabetes

Kadowaki and colleagues (1984) have studied patients with impaired glucose tolerance, in order to determine which patients later progressed to develop diabetes. It was found those who had an impaired insulin response to intravenous glucose were prone to diabetes, whereas those who had a normal insulin response tended to remain with impaired glucose tolerance.

Progressive beta cell dysfunction

A longitudinal study of beta cell function in Type 2 diabetic patients treated by diet alone, has been made over a six year period using a mathematical model of fasting glucose–insulin relationships. During the six year period, the patients had a slight reduction in body weight, an increase in fasting plasma glucose concentration and a decrease in beta cell function by 15% normal function per decade (Rudenski et al, 1988). While this decrease in beta cell function could theoretically be secondary to hyperglycaemia, a primary, progressive defect of beta cell function is a candidate for the worsening diabetes.

DOES INSULIN RESISTANCE HAVE A PRIMARY ROLE?

Insulin resistance has a primary role in particular insulin resistant states, such as in gross defects of the insulin receptor (Kadowaki et al, 1988). However, many patients with severe insulin resistance do not develop diabetes and insulin resistance *per se* is unlikely to be the sole cause of diabetes in most patients. Nevertheless, most diabetic patients have some degree of insulin resistance contributing to hyperglycaemia and without this insulin resistance, many patients would probably have had subclinical rather than clinical diabetes.

Reaven and colleagues investigated apparently normal subjects who were found to have glucose intolerance when the normal population was screened. They were found to have unequivocal insulin resistance with high basal and postprandial insulin concentrations. In patients with greater fasting hyperglycaemia, the insulin responses were impaired, and a 'horse-shoe' response (with first a greater and then a lesser insulin response with increasing hyperglycaemia) was taken to indicate a secondary beta cell defect, with the cells decompensating when over-loaded, analogous to Starling's law for the heart (Reaven, 1984). While this explanation seems correct for their patients, it is possible glucose intolerant patients obtained by screening the normal population have a different insulin sensitivity defect from glucose intolerant patients who are first degree relatives of Type 2 diabetic patients. One population may be characterized by insulin resistance and glucose intolerance which usually does not progress, whereas a diabetes prone population may become 'hypo-insulinaemic' and progress to diabetes. The prospective study of Kadowaki et al (1984), described above, has shown that patients who are thought to be characterized by insulin resistance do not usually progress to develop diabetes.

There is a high prevalence of diabetes in some ethnic populations and both Mexican (Haffner et al, 1986) and Asian (Mohan et al, 1986) populations have also been shown to have a high prevalence of impaired insulin sensitivity. Insulin resistance has been shown to have a major role in the development of diabetes in Pima Indians (Nagulesparan et al, 1982) with a suggestion of a trimodal distribution (Bogardus et al, 1988). While insulin resistance in these populations is likely to be an important contributor to their diabetes, it does not necessarily indicate that their insulin resistance is the only or the major inherited disorder leading to diabetes.

Insulin resistance in many diabetic patients is in part related to their obesity, although there is not a close correlation between obesity and insulin resistance in normal or diabetic patients (Olefsky et al, 1985). Many inherited and lifestyle factors affect insulin action, and it is possible that it will be more heterogeneous in nature than the beta cell defect, although some populations, such as Pima Indians, might have a particularly high prevalence of one or two genetic influences. Candidate genes include mutants of the insulin receptor (Kadowaki et al, 1988) or of a glucose-transporter gene (Li et al, 1988). Both abnormalities may be factors leading to the clinical presentation of diabetes. This does not necessarily mean either is the major autosomal susceptibility gene for Type 2 diabetes, although it would imply that it is at least one factor potentiating the development of insulin resistance and diabetes in some patients.

INTERACTION BETWEEN BETA CELL DYSFUNCTION AND IMPAIRED INSULIN SENSITIVITY

The relative importance of these two factors can be estimated with the aid of a theoretical model of metabolism. Each patient with Type 2 diabetes has, for a given state of nutrition, a 'set' basal plasma glucose concentration which is maintained over-night and is reproducible from night-to-night (Holman and Turner, 1980). The steady-state glucose concentration is determined by a negative-feedback loop between the hepatocytes and the pancreatic beta cells, the 'hepa-beta feedback loop'. Factors controlling glucose uptake by the periphery have an additional influence on the 'set' of this feedback loop which is determined by (i) the efficiency of the beta cell response to glucose and (ii) the efficiency of the hepatic and peripheral response to insulin.

The degree to which impaired beta cell function and insulin resistance can contribute to the fasting plasma glucose concentrations can be illustrated, in a semi-quantitative manner, by a mathematical model of the interactions of glucose and insulin (Turner et al, 1982). Figure 3 shows the predictions of such a model. It appears that marked beta cell dysfunction on its own is needed to induce a raised fasting plasma glucose in the order of 6 mmol/l, since the normal pancreas has excess capacity. A beta cell capacity reduced to 25 or 50% of normal gives only slight basal hyperglycaemia, which is sufficient to stimulate the reduced capacity to maintain the basal plasma insulin concentration within the normal range. In any feedback loop, compensation is not complete and the model predicts that in a normal-weight diabetic, who does not have marked insulin resistance, mild hyperglycaemia would be maintained by a slightly subnormal insulin production. There is some corroborative evidence from basal plasma C-peptide concentrations to support this (Holman and Turner, 1980). It is evident that a normal basal plasma insulin concentration does not signify an unaffected beta cell. In a patient with basal hyperglycaemia a normal basal plasma insulin levels signifies an *impaired* beta cell response compared with the response to the same glucose level of a normal person. The 'hepa-beta feedback loop' is analogous to other negative feedback loops in endocrinology, such as the perturbations of ACTH and TSH in Addison's disease and hypothyroidism respectively (Turner et al, 1987).

The model suggests that insulin resistance on its own, proportional to that found in pronounced obesity (i.e. 100% overweight is associated with a 3–5 fold increased insulin resistance), produces a large increase in fasting insulin concentration, stimulated by only a small rise in basal plasma glucose

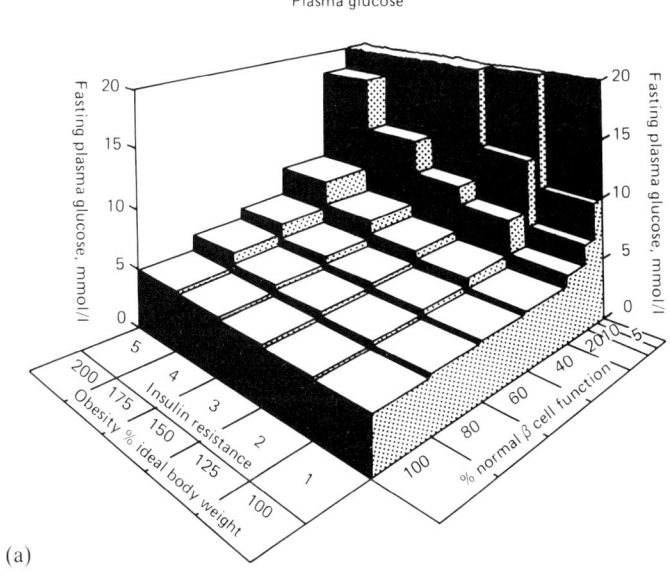

(a)

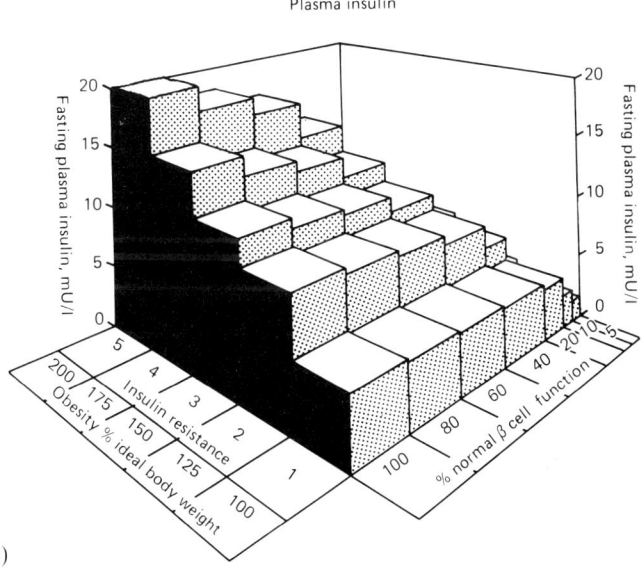

(b)

Figure 3. A mathematical model of the interaction of insulin and glucose metabolism predicts the basal, fasting plasma glucose and insulin levels which arise from different degrees of beta cell dysfunction and insulin resistance. Insulin resistance on its own produces little glycaemia because of the markedly increased insulin response. However, if there is moderate beta cell dysfunction, insulin resistance can markedly increase glycaemia. From Turner et al (1987), with permission.

concentration. In this model a raised basal plasma insulin is a secondary rather than a primary phenomenon. Some animal models suggest that a hypothalamic defect can directly increase the basal plasma insulin concentration and that this can induce insulin resistance (Jeanrenaud et al, 1985), but there is no evidence that this occurs in man.

Studies of many diabetic populations have suggested that both normal and over-weight diabetics have raised fasting plasma insulin concentrations, with increased insulin resistance contributing to the hyperglycaemia (Reaven, 1984; Olefsky et al, 1985). According to the model, although insulin resistance on its own induces only slight hyperglycaemia, it produces a dramatic increase in glucose concentration when cell function is sufficiently impaired to induce a basal plasma glucose concentration just above the normal range. For example, if a patient with a fasting plasma glucose of 6 mmol/l were to become obese, resulting in a halving of the insulin sensitivity, the fasting plasma glucose would rise to 10 mmol/l. In such a patient, dieting to halve the insulin resistance will reverse the effect. There would be a similar improvement in the plasma glucose response if treatment with sulphonylurea were to double the efficiency of beta cell function (Hosker et al, 1985). This model underlines the degree to which diabetes could be due to defects of both insulin secretion and insulin action.

SECONDARY EFFECTS OF HYPERGLYCAEMIA ON BETA CELL FUNCTION AND INSULIN ACTION

Insulin resistance is in part secondary to hyperglycaemia, and it improves when the fasting plasma glucose is reduced by insulin therapy (Garvey et al, 1985). Hyperglycaemia also leads to impaired beta cell function, and reduction in the plasma glucose in Type 2 diabetic patients enhances their beta cell response (Turner et al, 1976). Whilst this might arise in part because the beta cells no longer function over their most sensitive range, it seems likely that the hyperglycaemia itself can affect the beta cells. Thus glycaemia can 'feed forward' to impair both beta cell function and insulin sensitivity (Figure 4). In a model of Type 2 diabetes in rats induced by partial pancreatectomy, streptozotocin or by a glucose infusion, a marked decrease in the insulin response was produced by mild hyperglycaemia (Weir et al, 1986). This secondary defect can be clinically important, as patients presenting with ketoacidosis have functioning beta cells which are 'exhausted' by the high plasma glucose concentration. When the plasma glucose concentration is reduced to near-normal, the beta cells respond over a three week period, and this contributes to the 'honeymoon period' in Type 1 diabetes.

Hyperglycaemia can also affect islet structure, as shown by fibrosis of the remaining islets when diabetes is produced in rats by 95% partial pancreatectomy (Clark et al, 1982). The degree to which this is important in the genesis of beta cell dysfunction is uncertain, but is it possible that prolonged hyperglycaemia could in some individuals produce irreversible beta cell damage (Figure 4).

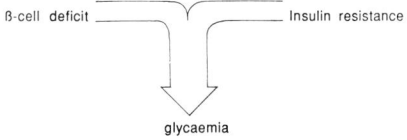

(I) "SIMPLE INTERACTION", SYNERGISTICALLY INCREASING GLYCAEMIA

β-cell deficit ——— Insulin resistance

glycaemia

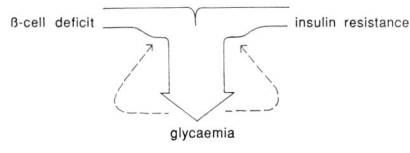

(II) GLYCAEMIA "FEED-FORWARD" ENHANCING BOTH DEFECTS

(including reversible β-cell "exhaustion" and glucose-transporter defects).

β-cell deficit ——— insulin resistance

glycaemia

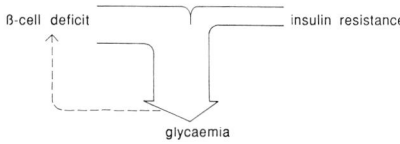

(III) GLYCAEMIA "β-CELL WEAR OUT"

(with irreversible β-cell damage from prolonged glycaemia)

β-cell deficit ——— insulin resistance

glycaemia

Figure 4. Three modes of interaction of deficient beta-cell function and impaired insulin sensitivity.

ISLET PATHOLOGY

Quantitative studies of islets in Type 2 diabetes have shown only a moderate decrease in the total number of beta cells. This suggests that the defect in beta cell function is a qualitative and not a quantitative defect.

Is there a glucose-specific beta cell defect?

Many studies have shown that diabetic patients with raised fasting plasma glucose levels have a marked impairment of the insulin response to intravenous glucose, but an apparently normal insulin response to either a mixed meal (Turner et al, 1977), intravenous isoprenaline (Halter et al, 1979), arginine (Palmer et al, 1976) or tolbutamide (Vague and Moulin, 1982). This raised the possibility that Type 2 diabetic patients have a functional defect of their beta cells, possibly a specific loss of a 'glucose receptor' mechanism. However, beta cell responses to stimuli are dependent on the prevailing glucose concentration; in normal islets, the higher the plasma glucose the greater the insulin response to non-glucose stimuli and the lesser response to glucose (Halter et al, 1979). The loss of the insulin response to glucose is probably a secondary feature, since an identical pattern can be demonstrated in animal models with either a reduced number of beta cells, induced by partial pancreatectomy or streptozotocin, or with a normal number of beta cells with hyperglycaemia induced by a glucose infusion (Weir et al, 1986).

Might islet amyloid be pathogenic?

Islet amyloid was first noted by Opie in 1901, and indeed his observation of 'hyaline material' in the pancreas of two diabetic patients first indicated that islet pathology was connected with diabetes. The 'hyaline material' was subsequently shown to be a localized amyloid, not associated with systemic amyloidisis. Although amyloid is found in 50–90% of diabetic patients over the age of 40, it is occasionally found in normal subjects, suggesting that it might be a feature of ageing rather than of diabetes. However, in spontaneously diabetic *Macaca nigra* monkeys islet amyloid precedes the onset of hyperglycaemia (Howard, 1986). It is possible that the islet amyloid in apparently normal subjects may represent a sub-clinical stage of diabetes.

The amyloid is situated between the beta cells and the capillaries with the fibrils occurring in deep clefts in the beta cells (Clark et al, 1987) (Figure 5).

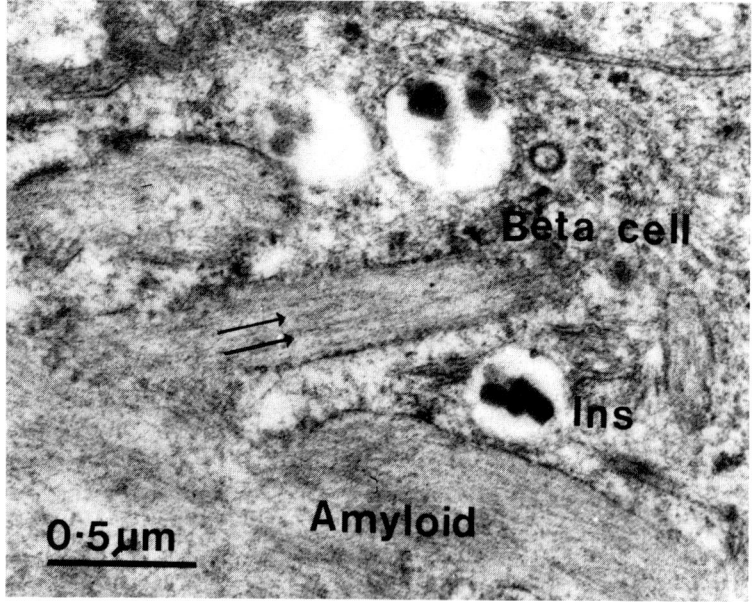

Figure 5. Electron micrograph of intra islet amyloid showing invaginations (arrows) into the beta cell containing granules (Ins).

An inherited disease which is expressed late in life is curious, and it is possible that progressive deposition of amyloid disrupts islet architecture and leads to impaired beta cell function. This would be analogous to the inherited defect of the low-density lipoprotein (LDL) receptor, which only presents as angina or a myocardial infarct after the development of cholesterol deposits in the arterial wall over several decades.

Recently two independent groups have isolated the formative 37 amino-acid peptide of islet amyloid. It was extracted only from pancreases of diabetic patients and therefore was termed 'diabetes-associated peptide' (DAP) (Cooper et al, 1987). A probably identical peptide has been characterized by Westermark et al (1987) from the amyloid of an insulinoma, 'insulinoma amyloid polypeptide' (IAPP), a term later changed to a 'islet amyloid polypeptide'. It has 46% homology with calcitonin gene-related peptide (Westermark et al, 1987), and it also has a distant homology with the insulin A-chain (Cooper et al, 1987).

The amyloid peptide probably originates from islet beta cells since immunoreactivity for the peptide has been shown in beta cells of both non-diabetic and Type 2 diabetic subjects (Clark et al, 1987; Westermark et al, 1987). The factors inducing the formation of amyloid are unknown. Two hypotheses can be considered. The first is that there is a single base–pair substitution, leading to replacement of an amino acid in the normal occurring peptide. This might result in beta-pleating of the substituted peptide, DAP, leading to progressive amyloid deposition. However, the occurrence of amyloid within many, but not all, insulinomas suggests that the peptide is a normal beta cell constituent, which accumulates when abnormal beta cell function induces abnormal release of DAP. Thus amyloid may accumulate, either because of a primary defect of beta cell function or because of abnormal beta cell function secondary to prolonged hyperglycaemia. Increased insulin secretion secondary to insulin resistance, such as found in obesity, might increase beta cell production of DAP and increase islet amyloid formation.

Is there abnormal neural or paracrine control of islet function?

The islets have extensive neural connections, and it is known that the 'cephalic' phase of insulin secretion, as food is received, is neural in origin. The lack of normal insulin pulsatility in Type 2 diabetes (Lang et al, 1981) might indicate either a neural defect or a paracrine disturbance, but no direct or indirect evidence is available.

WHERE WILL PROGRESS BE MADE?

Detailed studies of family members of Type 2 diabetic patients, before the onset of hyperglycaemia, will help to determine whether beta cell dysfunction or insulin resistance is a major inherited abnormality. However, the identification of a major susceptibility gene will probably be obtained by a molecular biological approach (O'Rahilly et al 1988b). Identification of families in which there is apparently dominant inheritance will be crucial, so that it will be possible to determine whether restriction fragment length polymorphisms (RFLPs) for a particular gene will segregate with the disease. It should then be possible to determine whether a particular gene has a predominant role and whether this mainly affects beta cell function or insulin sensitivity.

SUMMARY

Type 2 diabetes is a familial disease and studies of both Caucasian and Japanese families have raised the possibility that a major susceptibility gene is involved. The majority of patients have both beta cell dysfunction and impaired insulin sensitivity but studies of relatives of Type 2 diabetic patients suggest that beta cell dysfunction is an early feature of the disease. Impaired insulin sensitivity, from acromegaly, Cushing's disease or steroid therapy, induces diabetes only in a small proportion of the population, and they may be those who have an inherited cell defect. We postulate that a single beta cell defect gene, on its own, may be insufficient to cause overt diabetes and would lead to life-long glucose intolerance unless associated with other defects such as impaired insulin sensitivity. The nature of such a postulated beta cell defect is uncertain. Whilst it has been reported to be specific to glucose, and not to non-glucose stimuli, this feature may be secondary to hyperglycaemia. The occurrence of islet amyloid in 70–90% of Type 2 diabetic patients, and rarely in the normal population, raises the possibility that amyloid deposition causing disruption of the islet is a factor which might affect beta cell function. Amyloid formation may be a primary abnormality or could be secondary to beta cell dysfunction induced by hyperglycaemia. A major susceptibility gene might predispose a proportion, perhaps 10–15%, of a Caucasian population towards diabetes. The subsequent development of diabetes in a particular patient is likely to depend on many factors including other genetic factors, a sedentary life style and obesity. In different populations different genetic influences may operate, including abnormalities of insulin receptor genes and glucose transporter genes, which may allow a beta cell abnormality to become expressed clinically.

REFERENCES

Barnett AH, Spiliopoulos AJ, Pyke DA et al (1981) Metabolic studies in unaffected co-twins of non-insulin dependent diabetics. *British Medical Journal* **282:** 1656–1658.

Bogardus C, Lillioja S, Nyomba BL et al (1988) Evidence for a single gene, co-dominant mode of inheritance of insulin resistance in Pima Indians. *Diabetes* **37 (supplement 1):** 91A.

Cerasi E & Luft R (1967) The plasma insulin response to glucose infusion in healthy subjects and in diabetes mellitus. *Acta Endocrinology* **55:** 278–304.

Clark A, Bown E, King T, Vanhegan RI & Turner RC (1982) Islet changes induced by hyperglycaemia in rats: effect of insulin or chlorpropamide therapy. *Diabetes* **31:** 319–325.

Clark A, Cooper GJS, Lewis CE et al (1987) Islet amyloid formed from diabetes-associated peptide may be pathogenic in type 2 diabetes. *Lancet* **ii:** 231–234.

Cooper GJS, Willis AC, Clark A et al (1987) Purification and characterisation of a peptide from amyloid-rich pancreases of type 2 diabetic patients. *Proceedings of the National Academy of Sciences USA* **84**: 8628–8632.

Fajans SS (1986) Heterogeneity of insulin secretion in Type II diabetes. *Diabetes and Metabolism Reviews* **2**: 347–361.

Garvey WT, Olefsky JM, Griffin J, Hamman RF & Kolterman OG (1985) The effect of insulin treatment on insulin secretion and insulin action in type II diabetes mellitus. *Diabetes* **34**: 222–234.

Groop L, Miettinen A, Groop P-H et al (1988) Organ-specific autoimmunity and HLA–DR antigens as markers for B-cell destruction in patients with type II diabetes. *Diabetes* **37**: 99–103.

Haffner SM, Stern MP, Hazuda HP, Pugh JA & Patterson JK (1986) Hyperinsulinaemia in a population at high risk for non-insulin-dependent diabetes mellitus. *New England Journal of Medicine* **315**: 220–224.

Halter JB, Graf RJ & Porte D Jr (1979) Potentiation of insulin secretory responses by plasma glucose levels in man: evidence that hyperglycemia in diabetes compensates for impaired glucose potentiation. *Journal of Clinical Endocrinology and Metabolism* **48**: 946–954.

Holman RR & Turner RC (1979) The maintenance of basal plasma glucose and insulin concentrations in maturity-onset diabetes. *Diabetes* **28**: 227–230.

Holman RR & Turner RC (1980) The basal plasma glucose: a simple, relevant index of maturity-onset diabetes. *Clinical Endocrinology* **14**: 279–286.

Hosker JP, Burnett MA, Davies EG & Turner RC (1985) Sulphonylurea therapy doubles beta-cell response to glucose in type 2 diabetic patients. *Diabetologia* **28**: 809–814.

Howard CF (1986) Longitudinal studies on the development of diabetes in individual *Macaca nigra. Diabetologia* **29**: 301–306.

Jeanrenaud B, Halimi S & van de Werve G (1985) Neuro-endocrine disorders seen as triggers of the triad: obesity—insulin resistance—abnormal glucose tolerance. *Diabetes/Metabolism Reviews* **1** (3): 261–291.

Kadowaki T, Miyake Y, Hagura R et al (1984) Risk factors for worsening to diabetes in subjects with impaired glucose tolerance. *Diabetologia* **26**: 44–49.

Kadowaki T, Bevins CL, Cama A et al (1988) Two mutant alleles of the insulin receptor gene in a patient with extreme insulin resistance. *Science* **240**: 787–789.

Kahn CR, Soeldner JS, Gleason RE et al (1969) Clinical and chemical diabetes in the offspring of diabetic couples. *New England Journal of Medicine* **281**: 343–346.

Kobberling J, Tillil H & Lorenz H-J (1985) Genetics of type 2A- and type 2B- diabetes mellitus. *Diabetes Research and Clinical Practice* **1(supplement 1)**: s311.

Lang DA, Matthews DR & Turner RC (1981) Brief, irregular oscillations of basal plasma insulin and glucose concentrations in diabetic man. *Diabetes* **30**: 435–439.

Lerner RL & Porte D Jr (1972) Acute and steady-state insulin responses to glucose in non-obese diabetic subjects. *Journal of Clinical Investigation* **51**: 624–631.

Li SR, Baroni MG, Oelbaum RS, Stock J & Galton DJ (1988) Association of genetic variant of the glucose transporter with non-insulin-dependent diabetes mellitus. *Lancet* **ii**: 368–370.

Matsuda A & Kuzuya T (1984) Family history of Japanese patients with non-insulin-dependent diabetes. Differential implications of diabetes in parents and in siblings. *Endocrinology Japon* **31**: 335–341.

Mohan V, Sharp PS, Cloke HR et al (1986) Serum immunoreactive insulin responses to glucose load in Asian Indian and European Type 2 (non-insulin-dependent) diabetic patients and control subjects. *Diabetologia* **29**: 235–237.

Nagulesparan M, Savage PJ, Knowler WC, Johnson GC & Bennett PH (1982) Increased in vivo insulin resistance in nondiabetic Pima Indians compared with Caucasians. *Diabetes* **31**: 952–956.

Olefsky JM, Ciaraldi TP & Kolterman OG (1985) Mechanisms of insulin resistance in non-insulin-dependent (type II) diabetes. *American Journal of Medicine* **79(supplement 3B)**: 12–22.

Opie E (1901) The relation of diabetes mellitus to lesions of the pancreas. Hyaline degeneration of the islets of Langerhans. *Journal of Experimental Medicine* **5**: 527–540.

O'Rahilly SP, Nugent Z, Rudenski AS et al (1986) Beta-cell dysfunction, rather than insulin insensitivity, is the primary defect in familial type 2 diabetes. *Lancet* **ii**: 360–363.

O'Rahilly SP, Spivey RS, Holman RR et al (1987) Type II diabetes of early onset: a distinct clinical and genetic syndrome? *British Medical Journal* **294**: 923–928.

O'Rahilly SP, Turner RC & Matthews DR (1988a) Impaired pulsatile secretion of insulin in relatives of patients with non-insulin-dependent diabetes. *New England Journal of Medicine* **318**: 1225–1230.

O'Rahilly SP, Wainscoat JS & Turner RC (1988b) Review: Type 2 (non-insulin-dependent) diabetes mellitus. New genetics for old nightmares. *Diabetologia* **31**: 407–414.

Palmer JP, Benson JW, Walter RM & Ensinck JW (1976) Arginine-stimulated acute phase of insulin and glucagon secretion in diabetic subjects. *Journal of Clinical Investigation* **58**: 565–570.

Perley MJ & Kipnis DM (1967) Plasma insulin responses to oral and intravenous glucose: studies in normal and diabetic subjects. *Journal of Clinical Investigation* **46**: 1954–1962.

Raper LR, Taylor R, Zimmet P, Milne B & Balkau B (1984) Bimodality in glucose tolerance distributions in the urban Polynesian population of Western Samoa. *Diabetes Research* **1**: 19–26.

Reaven GM (1984) Insulin secretion and insulin action in non-insulin-dependent diabetes mellitus: Which defect is primary? *Diabetes Care* **7(supplement 1)**: 17–24.

Richens ER, Abdella N, Jayyab AK, Al-Saffar M & Behbehani K (1988) Type 2 diabetes in Arab patients in Kuwait. *Diabetic Medicine* **5**: 231–234.

Rudenski AS, Hadden DR, Atkinson AB et al (1988) Natural history of pancreatic islet B-cell function in type 2 diabetes mellitus studied over six years by homeostasis model assessment. *Diabetic Medicine* **5(1)**: 36–41.

Rushforth NB, Bennett PH, Sternberg AG, Burch TA & Miller M (1971) Diabetes in the Pima Indians; evidence of bimodality in glucose tolerance distributions. *Diabetes* **20**: 756–765.

Tattersall R & Fajans SS (1975) Diabetes and carbohydrate tolerance in 199 offspring of 37 conjugal diabetic parents. *Diabetes* **24**: 452–462.

Turner RC, McCarthy ST, Holman RR & Harris E (1976) Beta cell function improved by supplementing basal insulin secretion in mild diabetes. *British Medical Journal* **1**: 1252–1254.

Turner RC, Mann JI, Simpson RD, Harris E & Maxwell R (1977) Fasting hyperglycaemia and relatively unimpaired meal responses in mild diabetes. *Clinical Endocrinology* **6**: 253–264.

Turner RC, Holman RR, Matthews DR & Peto J (1982) Relative contributions of insulin deficiency and insulin resistance in maturity-onset diabetes. *Lancet* **i**: 596–598.

Turner RC, Rudenski AS, Holman RR, Matthews DR & O'Rahilly SP (1987) Quantitative modelling of the endocrine diseases as exemplified by diabetes. *Clinical Endocrinology* **26**: 107–116.

UK Prospective Diabetes Study. Multi-centre Study (1988) IV Characteristics of newly presenting type 2 diabetic patients: Male preponderance and obesity at different ages. *Diabetic Medicine* **5**: 154–159.

Vague P & Moulin JP (1982) The defective glucose sensitivity of the B-cell in non-insulin-dependent diabetes: improvement after 24 hours of normoglycemia. *Metabolism* **31**: 139–142.

Viswanathan M, Mohan V, Snehalatha C & Ramachandran A (1985) High prevalence of type 2 (non-insulin-dependent) diabetes among the offspring of conjugal type 2 diabetic parents in India. *Diabetologia* **28**: 907–910.

Weir GC, Leahy JL & Bonner-Weir S (1986) Experimental reduction of B-cell mass implications for the pathogenesis of diabetes. *Diabetes and Metabolism Reviews* **2**: 125–161.

Westermark P, Wernstedt C, Wilander E et al (1987) Amyloid fibrils in human insulinoma and islets of Langerhans of the diabetic cat are derived from a neuropeptide-like protein also present in normal islet cells. *Proceedings of the National Academy of Sciences USA* **84**: 3881–3885.

Yalow RS & Berson SA (1960) Immunoassay of endogenous plasma insulin in man. *Journal of Clinical Investigation* **39**: 1157–1175.

4

The natural history of non-insulin-dependent diabetes mellitus

B. M. SINGH
J. D. RUTTER
M. G. FITZGERALD

To the purist the natural history of a disease such as non-insulin-dependent diabetes mellitus (NIDDM) would be the course which the untreated disease follows. To study this would, of course, be unethical and of necessity consideration of the natural history of NIDDM must be of the treated disease. This in turn must reflect a dynamic rather than a static situation as treatments come and go with considerations of their efficacy and as accent upon particular forms of treatment alters with the fashions of clinical practice.

In order to delineate the natural history of NIDDM a fundamental prerequisite is the need to classify patients accurately into the two major types of diabetes proposed by the WHO (WHO, 1980). The difficulties of this in practice will be well known to any physician faced with deciding treatment in the diabetic clinic and it is a problem inherent in a number of studies dealing with aspects of the natural history of NIDDM. Many groups have used age at onset and form of treatment as guidelines for classification although this is recognised to be arbitrary (Keen, 1986). The expedient of considering those over the age of 40 years to be predominantly of the NIDDM group seems acceptable and has been employed of necessity in this review.

PITFALLS IN DETERMINING THE NATURAL HISTORY

In addition to difficulties of classification there are several other major confounding factors in elucidating the natural history of NIDDM. First, the criteria for the diagnosis of diabetes have changed (WHO, 1980) so that results of early studies, however meticulously undertaken, are not entirely transposable to today's NIDDM population. Second, there is the problem of selection of data derived from patients attending hospital diabetic clinics because of inevitable referral bias (Melton et al, 1984). Third, for longitudinal population studies the number of patients with diabetes or developing diabetes is often relatively small. The temptation is to study populations with a high prevalence of diabetes but these are often genetically distinct. Finally, and perhaps most importantly, most studies rely on mortality statistics from certification of death. Here we are faced with the major problem of reliability of death certificate information and with the well recognized non-coding of diabetes especially in older patients with multiple pathology. Thus of 2134 deaths observed in the British Diabetic Association cohort, diabetes was not mentioned on 33% of death certificates (Fuller et al, 1983a). Where the primary underlying cause of death was macrovascular disease diabetes was mentioned on 62% of certificates but only on 51% for neoplasms and 18% for accidents so introducing another source of bias (Fuller et al, 1983a).

Nevertheless a clearer picture of the natural history of NIDDM is emerging. It will become evident that we must pursue this where possible not from the time of diagnosis nor the phase of asymptomatic hyperglycaemia but from the pre-diabetic phase. It can also be considered at several levels and while a mechanistic approach blurs the impact of NIDDM upon the individual it allows consideration of public health implications and preventative and therapeutic strategies for the population as a whole. The natural history of NIDDM cannot be divorced from its aetiological and pathogenic mechanisms and these are considered in detail in other chapters.

MACROVASCULAR DISEASE, MORTALITY AND MORBIDITY

Mortality

It seems perverse to start a review of the natural history of any disease at its end but by considering mortality in patients with diabetes mellitus first we have a definitive end point about which to assemble the pieces of a complex and as yet incomplete puzzle.

Kessler (1971) reported the mortality rate of a cohort of 21 447 patients with diabetes recruited as new attenders at the Joslin Clinic in Boston, Massachusetts between 1930 and 1956 and followed to 1960. The observed number of deaths remained significantly in excess of expected for the general population in each five year period from 1930. Standardized mortality ratios ranged from 1.6 to 2.1 and tended to worsen despite the introduction of insulin during this period. Within this overall framework the pattern of mortality altered dramatically as death attributable directly to diabetes fell rapidly from 1936 while that from coronary heart disease rose briskly from 1940. These two causes accounted almost entirely for the excess of mortality.

Results from our own clinic support these findings. Data were collected on all patients attending for the first time at the Diabetic Clinic of the General Hospital, Birmingham between 1960 and 1968 and traced to 1975. Of 1943 males and 2290 females who were entered, 95.3% of males and 94.6% of females were followed up in 1975. Their mortality was compared to the general population by age and sex using English Life Tables adjusted to reflect local West Midlands regional mortality (Table 1). An analysis by cause of death demonstrated 70% of deaths were related to circulatory diseases, predominantly ischaemic heart disease and cerebrovascular disease (Table 2). Of note in our data is that female mortality as a percentage exceeded that of males with striking differences for ischaemic heart disease. In relation to other diseases, males were observed to have a lower risk of death from cancer (observed/expected): male—96/129.3 (74%), female—99/102.3 (97%), mainly because of reduced death from lung cancer (male—27/55.9 (48%)). Both sexes showed diminished mortality from bronchitis (male—8/50.4 (16%), female—4/17.8 (22%)). These observations have also been made in other published data but remain unexplained (Kessler, 1971; Kannel and McGee, 1979; Fuller et al, 1983a) though a decreased mortality from certain diseases must be expected when that from others is in excess. A number of studies broadly agree the excess mortality of NIDDM to be approximately twofold and that ischaemic heart disease and cerebro-

Table 1. Actual and expected deaths, analysed by age and sex, amongst 1943 male and 2290 female diabetic patients followed from first attendance between 1960–68 at the Diabetic Clinic of the General Hospital, Birmingham to 1975.

Attained Age	Actual Deaths	Expected Deaths	Actual/Expected %
Males			
Under 40	10	2.8	357
40–49	16	10.0	160
50–59	81	59.4	136
60–69	232	183.5	126
70–79	237	191.9	124
80+	77	68.7	112
Total	653	516.3	126
Females			
Under 40	2	1.2	167
40–49	9	4.5	200
50–59	74	24.7	300
60–69	204	102.1	200
70–79	349	228.5	153
80+	227	171.3	133
Total	865	532.3	163

Table 2. Ischaemic heart disease and cerebrovascular disease actual/expected deaths (%) by age group and sex in the General Hospital cohort.

Age Group	<59	60–69	70–79	80+
		Ischaemic Heart Disease		
Males	54/23.6 (229)	87/57.1 (152)	86/53.6 (160)	20/16.2 (130)
Females	33/ 3.7 (892)	83/22.2 (374)	128/54.1 (237)	75/38.2 (196)
		Cerebrovascular Disease		
Males	11/ 4.5 (244)	32/18.1 (177)	41/27.1 (151)	14/12.5 (112)
Females	10/ 2.9 (345)	32/14.2 (225)	76/45.6 (167)	61/39.5 (154)

vascular disease are the pre-eminent causes of death in NIDDM (see Panzram, 1987 for a recent review). Another well documented finding is the narrowing of excess mortality with increasing age. Thus in general NIDDM reduces life expectancy by 5–10 years but NIDDM diagnosed in the elderly (>70 years) has little significant impact (Marks and Krall, 1971; Panzram and Zabel-Langhennig, 1981).

Morbidity

Morbidity data for macrovascular disease are more difficult to ascertain. In the prospective Framingham study (Garcia et al, 1974) morbidity ratios in diabetic patients for age adjusted incidence for coronary heart disease, cerebrovascular disease and intermittent claudication were 1.9, 2.4 and 4.5 respectively. In a retrospective study (Knuiman et al, 1986), in which NIDDM was more accurately characterized than in the previously described studies, 53% of patients had evidence of macrovascular disease. The major factor that influenced the prevalence of macrovascular disease in the study of Knuiman et al (1986) was age rather than age at diagnosis or duration of diabetes. Other significant risk factors selected by a stepwise logistic regression analysis were glycosylated haemoglobin, plasma cholesterol, HDL cholesterol (negative association) and plasma creatinine but not hypertension or obesity. Garcia et al (1974) were unable to explain the higher incidence of macrovascular disease solely by the influence of significant excess of several risk factors alone and conferred a risk factor for coronary heart disease of 1.7 in men and 4.2 in women attributable to diabetes *per se*. The impact of diabetes was worsened when associated with high cholesterol, low HDL cholesterol, systolic hypertension, cigarette consumption and ECG abnormalities (Garcia et al, 1974; Kannel and McGee, 1979). Similarly for macrovascular disease mortality, in the ten year follow up of diabetic patients in the Whitehall study (Fuller et al, 1983b) 63% of relative risk of coronary heart disease mortality and 52% of stroke mortality was unexplained purely by age, systolic blood pressure and a number of other significant risk factors established for the non-diabetic population even though they are found in excess in the diabetic population.

Effect of age at diagnosis and duration of diagnosed disease

Hirohata et al (1967) considered mortality by age at diagnosis and duration of diabetes in 3853 patients of the Joslin Clinic cohort. They found patients under the age of 20 years at diagnosis experienced little excess mortality relative to the general population after 15 years of diabetes although a 17% excess occurred at 25 years. This differed markedly from those patients aged 40 to 59 years at diagnosis whose excess mortality was 20% and 35% at 15 and 25 years respectively. Entmacher et al (1964) examined the cause of death in 5721 diabetic patients by age at onset and duration of disease and observed not only that large vessel disease accounted for approximately 70% of the mortality in patients aged over 40 years of age at diagnosis but that this proportion was little affected by duration of diabetes. Vigorita et al

(1980) examined the relationship between the severity and duration of 'adult onset' diabetes to severity of ischaemic heart disease at autopsy and found no significant association between the two, although the prevalence of disease was greater among diabetics than in age and sex matched non-diabetic controls. Herman et al (1977) found 209 newly diagnosed and 270 previously diagnosed diabetic men following screening of 10 000 Israeli males aged over 40 years. After five years follow up a similar incidence of fatal and non-fatal myocardial infarction and similar morbidity ratios for intermittent claudication were found.

Identifying risk

The consistent lack of effect of duration of metabolic abnormality described above raises the question as to whether diabetes and macrovascular disease are causally related. The large prospective Whitehall Study (Fuller et al, 1983b) defined glucose intolerance following a 50 g oral glucose load as a 2 h blood glucose response above the 95th centile—a level of 5.4 mmol/l. A marked increase in macrovascular mortality was demonstrated in their glucose intolerant group and the study suggested a threshold effect for post-load glucose at the 95th centile for increased stroke and coronary heart disease mortality at ten years. There was an excess of various cardiovascular risk factors in this group but, after adjusting for these, glucose intolerance remained a significant risk. Furthermore, age adjusted coronary heart disease and stroke mortality rates were not significantly different between known diabetics and those with glucose intolerance. The findings of the Honolulu Heart programme, taking the 90th centile cut off for a 1 h post-load glucose level, were similar (Yano et al, 1982) but the Bedford study (Jarrett et al, 1982), while confirming excess ten year coronary heart disease mortality in 'borderline diabetics', also suggested an additional adverse effect of being diabetic.

Thus it is apparent that diabetics and non-diabetics above the 90th to 95th centile for post-load glucose share an increased risk of macrovascular disease or, in other words, diabetes *per se* may not confer this additional risk. Medalie (1979) studied men over 40 years of age who went on to develop diabetes over five years of follow up and found significant factors associated with risk of developing diabetes were age, body mass index, systolic blood pressure, peripheral vascular disease and serum cholesterol. Similar observations were made in the Framingham study (Garcia et al, 1974). Is it the case that macrovascular disease and NIDDM share common antecedent risk factors? Interestingly, a relationship between blood glucose, blood pressure and plasma lipids has been observed even in school children (Florey et al, 1976). Hyperinsulinaemia in the non-diabetic population may also be a common risk factor for the development of both macrovascular disease (Stout, 1985) and NIDDM (Sicree et al, 1987). It is also possible that a common genetic background exists for the development of macrovascular disease in the diabetic and non-diabetic populations particularly in the relationship of the U allele of the 5'-region of the insulin gene flanking DNA sequences (Mandrup-Poulsen et al, 1985).

THE NATURAL HISTORY OF MICROVASCULAR DISEASE

Unlike macrovascular disease, the microvascular complications of diabetes mellitus appear to be specifically related to this condition (Dorf et al, 1976). With the advent of effective therapies and screening programmes much effort is directed to the prevention and detection of these major causes of diabetic morbidity. An understanding of their natural history is central to such pursuits.

Retinopathy

In a series of 10000 diabetic patients studied at diagnosis (Mincu, 1970) 4.8% of 20–40 year olds had retinopathy compared to 15.8% of those diagnosed over 40 years. Reanalysing these observations according to length of preceding symptomatology revealed a prevalence of 2.1% when less than six months but 14.6% when exceeding 12 months. Similarly, of 5157 newly diagnosed diabetics seen at the General Hospital, Birmingham, there was an overall 7.5% prevalence of background retinopathy but this was present in only 1.5% of those aged less than 40 years rising to 10% when 60 years and over (Soler et al, 1969). These findings have been ascribed to the insidious onset of NIDDM and protracted asymptomatic hyperglycaemia. Even at diagnosis, NIDDM patients with retinopathy have a higher percentage of glycosylated haemoglobin and fasting blood glucose levels. Elevated systolic blood pressure is also a recognized association (Owens et al, 1987).

There is an almost linear relationship between duration of diabetes and the prevalence of non-proliferative retinopathy. After 20 years approximately 75% of patients with either NIDDM or IDDM have this complication (Herman et al, 1983; Knuiman et al, 1986) (Figure 1). Once background retinopathy has developed, the prognosis for visual deterioration can be serious. In the era before the use of photocoagulation, Caird and Garrett (1963) found that in NIDDM patients with retinopathy and a visual acuity of 6/18 or better, 40% deteriorated to 6/24–6/60 and 20% were blind after only five years. Of those without retinopathy, 15% showed deterioration and 3% were blind. These data did not distinguish between the two vision-threatening forms of retinopathy—proliferative retinopathy and maculopathy.

The natural history of these forms of retinopathy differs between NIDDM and IDDM. Proliferative retinopathy is more common in patients with IDDM than NIDDM (Figure 1). IDDM patients rarely develop this complication within ten years of diagnosis but have a prevalence of 40–60% after 20 years whereas in NIDDM patients the overall prevalence is about 10%, and 40% of these have a duration of diabetes of less than ten years (Herman et al, 1983). There is a greater tendency for the development of maculopathy in NIDDM. In patients with maculopathy 90% have onset of diabetes over 30 years of age and a third are over 60 years at diagnosis (Kohner and Barry, 1984). 65% of maculopathy develops within 10 years of diagnosis. Since photocoagulation is now well recognized to be an effective form of therapy for both forms of vision threatening retinopathy (British Multicentre Study,

1983; 1984) some change in the natural history of the disease is to be expected. It is less clear whether concentration upon screening and early detection will allow effective treatment at an earlier stage.

As well as duration of diabetes there can be little doubt that there is a relationship between the magnitude of hyperglycaemia and the presence of retinopathy. Several studies support this conclusion in patients with NIDDM (Dorf et al, 1976; Howard-Williams et al, 1984; Nathan et al, 1986; Owens et al, 1987). In a prospective study of 149 NIDDM patients followed over seven years, patients developing retinopathy had higher mean fasting blood glucose concentrations at diagnosis and at one, three and five years. Only 18% of patients with an average fasting blood glucose of less than 6 mmol/l developed retinopathy over the period of follow up compared to 88% of those with fasting blood glucose greater than 14 mmol/l (Howard-Williams et al, 1984). Average random clinic blood glucose levels greater

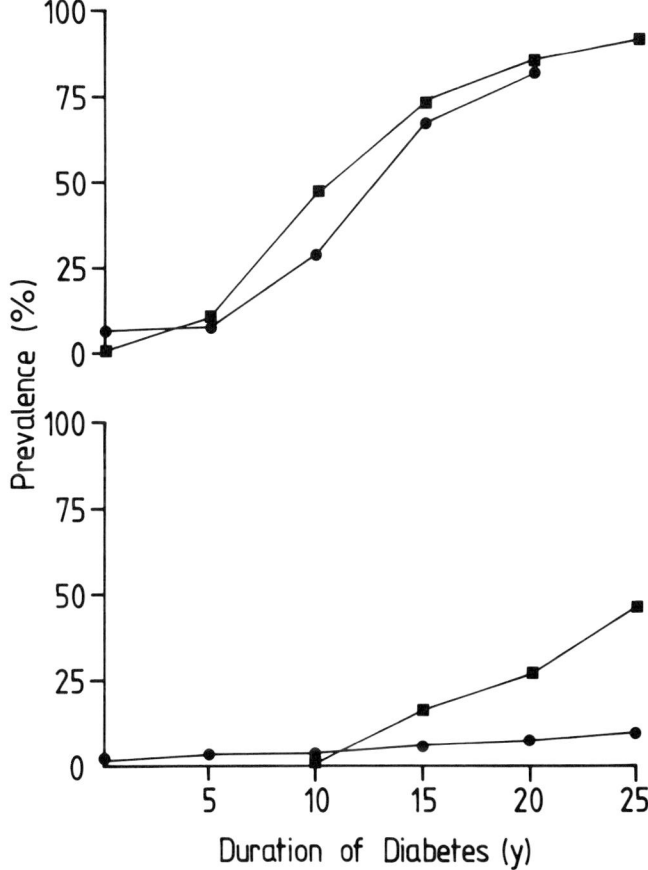

Figure 1. The relationship of duration of diabetes and prevalence of non-proliferative (top panel) and proliferative retinopathy in non-insulin-dependent (●) and insulin-dependent (■) patients. From Herman et al (1983), reproduced with permission from the American Diabetes Association Inc.

than 10 mmol/l were also associated with a marked increased risk of developing retinopathy.

Hypertension may be related to increased risk of retinopathy. In diabetic patients diagnosed over the age of 30 years a relationship of systolic and diastolic blood pressure with retinopathy in patients of 5–14 years duration was demonstrated (Klein et al, 1984). Knowler et al (1980) showed a relationship between systolic hypertension and the development of hard exudates but not haemorrhages in Pima Indians. However, Chahal et al (1985) were unable to demonstrate that those with raised blood pressure showed greater deterioration of retinopathy. Several other risk factors for developing retinopathy have been suggested including low density lipoprotein cholesterol (Dornan et al, 1982), excessive alcohol (Young et al, 1984) and cigarette consumption (Paetkau et al, 1977).

Nephropathy

Proteinuria is the clinical hallmark of diabetic nephropathy and the histological changes of glomerulosclerosis are similar in IDDM and NIDDM. As seen in retinopathy, however, there are a number of striking differences in the natural history of this complication. In contrast to IDDM patients clinical proteinuria (Albustix positive) is often found at diagnosis of NIDDM and the duration of diabetes before the appearance of clinical proteinuria is much shorter (Malins, 1968) (Figure 2). In males with fasting hyper-

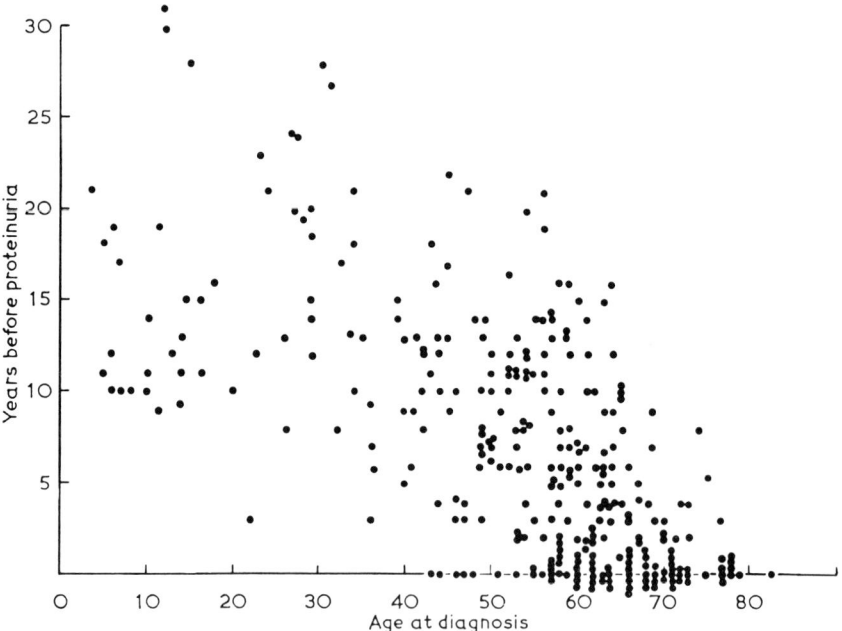

Figure 2. The relationship between age at diagnosis and interval from diagnosis to the appearance of proteinuria. A study of 320 cases. From Malins (1968), with permission.

glycaemia discovered at screening, the presence of subclinical proteinuria (microalbuminuria) is in excess compared to the non-diabetic population (Damsgaard and Mogensen, 1986). As in IDDM the degree of micro-albuminuria in NIDDM is indicative of worsening proteinuria (Schmitz and Vaeth, 1988) and, once present, persistent clinical proteinuria heralds a progressive impairment in renal function (Viberti et al, 1982). Compara-tively little is known about the natural history of this decline in NIDDM patients although it has been suggested it is slower than in IDDM patients with similar proteinuria (Fabre et al, 1982). The prevalence of biochemically impaired renal function increases continuously with duration of diabetes in NIDDM whereas in IDDM it is unusual to find this within ten years of diagnosis (Knuiman et al, 1986).

Though, numerically, NIDDM patients form a substantial proportion of diabetic patients entering renal dialysis programmes in the UK (Retting and Teutsch, 1984; Grenfell et al, 1988), death directly attributable to renal failure, about 3%, is much less common than in IDDM where 40% of patients diagnosed before the age of 20 years die from this complication (Balodimos, 1971). This may be due to excess mortality from macrovascular disease before end stage renal failure is apparent. Once renal failure is established NIDDM and IDDM patients share a similar propensity to macrovascular and other microvascular complications, particularly pro-liferative retinopathy (Grenfell et al, 1988).

Fabre et al (1982) studied 510 patients diagnosed after the age of 40 years over eight years of follow up. 122 patients died but only one of renal disease and, while clinical proteinuria was common, only 8.7% of patients had a glomerular filtration rate (GFR) of less than 60 ml/min. Nevertheless, Jarrett et al (1983) were able to describe a relationship between renal function and subsequent mortality. They studied a small number of NIDDM patients over 13 years and found that initial albumin excretion rates were strong predictors of subsequent mortality even though these were in the microalbuminuria range. Mogensen (1984) followed 232 NIDDM patients over nine years, grouped according to their initial albumin excretion. Those initially in the range less than 15 µg/ml had an excess mortality of 37% compared to non-diabetics, but those in the bands 16–29 µg/ml and 30–140 µg/ml had excess mortality of 76% and 148% respectively. More recently Schmitz and Vaeth (1988) have confirmed this relationship. In all of these studies the excess mortality was due predominantly to macrovascular disease. Increasing age was also a significant risk factor but Jarrett et al (1983) found no independent effect of duration of diabetes while Mogensen (1984) and Schmitz and Vaeth (1988) found only a weak effect.

These observations do not imply a direct relationship. Microalbuminuria is a precursor of overt renal damage and subsequent hypertension which may worsen the cardiovascular risk but equally microalbuminuria may be a sensitive early index of macrovascular disease in NIDDM much as trace proteinuria has been shown to be associated with cardiovascular disease and mortality in the general population (Mogensen, 1984). These considerations make it difficult to interpret the relationship between hypertension and diabetic nephropathy. A weak association has been described between systolic blood pressure and urinary albumin excretion rates in NIDDM (Fabre et al, 1982; Damsgaard and Mogensen, 1986; Schmitz and Vaeth, 1988) but it is not clear that treating hypertension reduces albumin excretion (Corcoran et al, 1987) nor whether it alters the decline in GFR once renal impairment is established as has been suggested in patients with IDDM (Mogensen, 1982). Stronger evidence exists for a relationship between increasing urinary protein loss and poorer glycaemia control (Fabre et al, 1982; Schmitz and Vaeth, 1988). It is recognized that the earliest stages of renal dysfunction in NIDDM may be reversible by improved glycaemic control (Vasquez et al, 1984) but it is not clear what impact this might have on outcome. It is unlikely that even the strictest metabolic control alters outcome once renal impairment is established (Viberti et al, 1983).

Neuropathy

Symmetrical peripheral neuropathy is considered the commonest of the chronic complications of diabetes although estimates of its prevalence vary considerably, largely due to a lack of standardized diagnostic criteria. Thus, in some studies, symptoms without neurological signs or minor neurological signs without symptoms have been accepted as indicating peripheral neuropathy. Often in surveys of diabetic patients with peripheral neuropathy the possible contributions of peripheral vascular disease, alcohol consumption, renal impairment and other metabolic or endocrine disease are not considered. The observation that peripheral neuropathy is more common with increasing age in diabetes (Knuiman et al, 1986) must be considered alongside declining nerve function in the ageing non-diabetic population. Mayne (1965) accepted the presence of peripheral neuropathy when two definite abnormal signs (absent deep reflexes, impaired vibration or position sense) were found or one sign with a definite history of sensory abnormality was present. His data showed a significant trend with age in control ($p < 0.05$) and diabetic patients ($p < 0.01$) and a highly significant difference between the two groups. The overall prevalence of peripheral neuropathy was 69% among diabetic patients and 31% in controls (Table 3).

The effect of duration of diabetes upon the prevalence of peripheral neuropathy is also masked by the lack of controlled studies for age-related variables. Peripheral neuropathy was found in 5–15% of patients at diagnosis over the age of 40 years rising to 40–60% after 25 years of known duration of disease (Pirart, 1977; Knuiman et al, 1986). Knuiman et al

Table 3. Prevalence (%) of peripheral neuropathy by age amongst normal controls and patients with diabetes. Figures in parentheses indicate the number of subjects studied (from Mayne, 1965).

Age Group	Controls		Diabetics	
30–49	0	(8)	6	(16)
50–69	10	(20)	43	(44)
70+	52	(25)	86	(51)

(1986), studying IDDM and NIDDM patients together, found both age at diagnosis and duration of disease were strongly related to the presence of neuropathy. Their data indicated a stronger effect for duration of diabetes suggesting that a five year increase in duration produced an increase in prevalence equivalent to the effect of a 10 year increase in age at diagnosis.

The prevalence of peripheral neuropathy is greater in those with poor glycaemic control (Pirart, 1977). However, Hillson et al (1984), studying deterioration of vibration sensation over five years from diagnosis in 71 NIDDM patients, could only attribute a small but significant effect to the degree of hyperglycaemia, and identified the initial vibration perception threshold as the most significant indicator of deterioration. The known effect of short term improvements in glycaemia with intensive insulin therapy to improve vibration perception thresholds, motor conduction velocity and neuropathic symptoms (Boulton et al, 1982) serve not only to emphasize the importance of good metabolic control but also the need to recognize the presence of acute and chronic effects.

THE NATURAL HISTORY OF THE METABOLIC ABNORMALITIES IN NIDDM

The biochemical criteria for the diagnosis of diabetes mellitus based upon the fasting blood glucose (FBG) and glucose response to an oral glucose load are well defined and delineate the diabetic population from the rest. Indeed the 2 h post glucose challenge plasma glucose level of 11.1 mmol/l is documented as the nadir dividing the bimodal distribution of plasma glucose in a number of human populations (Rushforth et al, 1971; Zimmet and Whitehouse, 1978; Rosenthal et al, 1985). This glucose level remains constant as the population ages. Hence, the distribution does not gradually shift to the right but instead an increasing proportion of the population becomes diabetic. Three studies have examined the prevalence of diabetes by age alone among Caucasians in the UK with remarkably uniform conclusions (Gatling et al, 1985; Mather and Keen, 1985; Neil et al, 1987) (Table 4).

The progression of the NIDDM patient from treatment with diet alone to

Table 4. Age specific prevalence of known diabetes amongst white Caucasians per 1000 population (compiled from Gatling et al, 1985; Mather and Keen, 1985; Neil et al, 1987).

Age Group	Population	Diabetics	Prevalence
0–9	17 754	8	0.5
10–19	23 561	43	1.8
20–29	21 847	88	4.0
30–39	22 361	104	4.6
40–49	18 229	137	7.5
50–59	18 160	249	13.8
60–69	17 255	366	21.3
70–79	13 262	494	37.1
80+	5198	185	35.6

oral hypoglycaemic agents and then insulin to maintain glucose control is well recognized in clinical practice suggesting the mechanisms determining the abnormality of glucose metabolism are changing. Recent evidence allows us not only to consider the natural history of these processes in the NIDDM population but also in those with normal or impaired glucose tolerance (IGT) who may be destined to become diabetic.

A number of studies have shown that the relationship between the 2 h plasma glucose and insulin response to an oral glucose load is non-linear. In subjects with normal glucose tolerance the insulin response increases with the glucose level while in patients with NIDDM there is a progressive decline in the insulin response. The watershed between the two populations falls among those who are categorized as having IGT (Reaven and Miller, 1968; Savage et al, 1975; Zimmet et al, 1978). The importance of the plasma insulin response in predicting deterioration of oral glucose tolerance is increasingly recognized. Among Pima Indians, Knowler and Bennett (1983) suggested hyperinsulinaemia predicted deterioration in glucose tolerance in subjects with initial normal glucose tolerance. Sicree et al (1987) have also studied the plasma insulin response prospectively amongst Nauruans and demonstrated that an initial elevated insulin response was a better predictor of deterioration from normal glucose tolerance than fasting glucose and insulin or the 2 h plasma glucose. Interestingly both studies showed progression from IGT to NIDDM was related to an initial diminished insulin response.

Among those with normal glucose tolerance who go on to develop NIDDM, high insulin responses to oral glucose challenge suggest insulin resistance. Indeed Bogardus et al (1987) have recently documented in Pima Indians with normal glucose tolerance that insulin resistance assessed by the glucose clamp technique was predictive of deterioration to diabetes after 49 months of follow up. Their initial insulin response to meal tolerance was also exaggerated. It has been suggested that insulin resistance but not impaired insulin secretion precedes deterioration of glucose tolerance and that subsequent insulin deficiency is the factor determining conversion to diabetes (Stern, 1988).

Once diabetes has developed the abnormalities of insulin secretion and insulin action are impaired hand in hand in direct relationship to the degree of fasting hyperglycaemia which is relatively constant from day to day in NIDDM patients (Holman and Turner, 1979). Thus in established NIDDM the post-receptor defect of insulin action upon glucose uptake increases with the fasting blood glucose (Kolterman et al, 1981) as does the degree of insulin deficiency (Zimmet et al, 1978). Skyler (1984) has suggested these relationships may determine therapeutic strategy in NIDDM patients. Patients with a FBG less than 7.7 mmol/l with the least impairment of insulin secretion and insulin action can usually be managed on diet alone. Those with a FBG of 7.7–11.1 mmol/l usually require the addition of an oral hypoglycaemic agent. Those with FBG greater than 11.1 mmol/l and certainly those greater than 13.8 mmol/l have a marked abnormality of insulin secretion and will require insulin therapy to maintain acceptable fasting blood glucose concentrations. This stratagem may seem impractical particularly with regard to insulin therapy since it ignores many aspects of an individual patient relevant to a therapeutic decision including age, weight, weight loss and particularly dietary compliance.

In a prospective study in Belfast (Lyons et al, 1984; Hadden et al, 1986) of 223 newly diagnosed diabetic patients aged 40–69 years, particular emphasis was placed upon diet with metabolic goals broadly similar to those outlined by Skyler (1984). After two years 83% of patients were treated with diet alone, 5% with oral hypoglycaemic agents and 12% required insulin therapy. After four years the percentages were 78%, 8% and 14% respectively and after six years 71%, 12% and 17%. Baseline fasting plasma insulin concentrations differentiated those in the various treatment groups six years later with the highest levels in those that remained controlled on diet alone and the lowest in those eventually requiring insulin. Peak insulin responses to oral glucose challenge were also lower in those eventually needing insulin. While this suggested the severity of diabetes is predictable at diagnosis of NIDDM, the period of follow up was relatively short. The natural history of insulin resistance and insulin deficiency in established NIDDM is not known but Rudenski et al (1988) have used a mathematical model of the Belfast data to determine the duration effect of diabetes on insulin secretion and insulin action. In patients remaining controlled with diet therapy they suggested gradually declining B cell function but no alteration in insulin sensitivity over the six year period of follow up.

CONCLUSION

Clinicians close to the day to day management of patients with NIDDM strive to correct hyperglycaemia, hypertension, obesity and hyper-lipidaemia in an effort to prevent diabetic complications and screen for such complications in the knowledge that effective therapies are available when they arise. This approach unquestionably reduces morbidity and mortality. The detached view, however, must teach us that a greater understanding of the pre-diabetic phase and the appropriate direction of health resources and health education to the general population may be equally effective in modifying the natural history of what is an increasingly prevalent disease.

REFERENCES

Balodimos MC (1971) Diabetic nephropathy. In Marble A, White P, Bradley RF & Krall LP (eds) *Joslin's Diabetes Mellitus*, Philadelphia: Lea & Febinger.

Bogardus C, Lillioja S, Foley J et al (1987) Insulin resistance predicts the development of non-insulin-dependent diabetes mellitus in Pima Indians. *Diabetes* **36 (supplement 1):** 47A.

Boulton AJM, Drury J, Clarke B & Ward JD (1982) Continuous subcutaneous insulin infusion in the management of painful diabetic neuropathy. *Diabetes Care* **5:** 386–390.

British Multicentre Study Group (1983) Photocoagulation for diabetic maculopathy. A randomised controlled clinical trial using the xenon arc. *Diabetes* **32:** 1010–1016.

British Multicentre Study Group (1984) Photocoagulation for proliferative diabetic retinopathy: a randomised controlled clinical trial using the xenon arc. *Diabetologia* **26:** 109–115.

Caird FI & Garrett CJ (1963) Prognosis for vision in diabetic retinopathy. *Diabetes* 12: 389–397.

Chahal P, Inglesby D, Sleightholm M & Kohner EM (1985) The effect of blood pressure on the progression of diabetic retinopathy. *Hypertension* 7: 79–83.

Corcoran JS, Perkins JE, Hoffbrand BI & Judkin JS (1987) Treating hypertension in non-insulin-dependent diabetes: a comparison of atenolol, nifedipine, and captopril combined with bendrofluazide. *Diabetic Medicine* 4: 164–168.

Damsgaard EM & Mogensen CE (1986) Microalbuminuria in elderly hyperglycaemic patients and controls. *Diabetic Medicine* 3: 430–435.

Dorf A, Ballintine EJ, Bennett PH & Miller M (1976) Retinopathy in Pima Indians. Relationship to glucose level, duration of diabetes, age at diagnosis of diabetes and age at examination in a population with a high prevalence of diabetes mellitus. *Diabetes* 25: 554–560.

Dornan TL, Carter RD, Bron A, Turner RC & Mann JI (1982) Low density lipoprotein cholesterol: an association with the severity of diabetic retinopathy. *Diabetologia* 22: 167–170.

Entmacher PS, Root HF & Marks HH (1964) Longevity of diabetic patients in recent years. *Diabetes* 13: 373–377.

Fabre J, Balant LP, Dayer PG, Fox HM & Vernet AT (1982) The kidney in maturity onset diabetes mellitus: A clinical study of 510 patients. *Kidney International* 21: 730–738.

Florey C du V, Uppal S & Lowey C (1976) Relationship between blood pressure, weight and plasma sugar and serum insulin levels in school children aged 9–12 years in Westland, Holland. *British Medical Journal* i: 1368–1371.

Fuller JH, Elford J, Goldblatt P & Adelstein AM (1983a). Diabetes mortality: New light on an underestimated public health problem. *Diabetologia* 24: 336–341.

Fuller JH, Shipley MJ, Rose G, Jarrett RJ & Keen H (1983b) Mortality from coronary heart disease and stroke in relation to degree of glycaemia; the Whitehall Study. *British Medical Journal* 287: 867–870.

Garcia MJ, McNamara PM, Gordon T & Kannell WB (1974) Morbidity and mortality in diabetics in the Framingham population. Sixteen year follow up study. *Diabetes* 23: 105–111.

Gatling W, Houston AC & Hill RD (1985). An epidemiological survey: the prevalence of diabetes mellitus in a typical English community. *Journal of the Royal College of Physicians of London* 4: 248–250.

Grenfell A, Bewick M, Parsons V, Snowden S, Taube D & Watkins PJ (1988) Non-insulin-dependent diabetes and renal replacement therapy. *Diabetic Medicine* 5: 172–176.

Hadden DR, Blair ALT, Wilson EA et al (1986) Natural history of diabetes: A prospective study of the influence of intensive dietary therapy. *Quarterly Journal of Medicine* 59: 579–598.

Herman JB, Medalie JH & Goldbourt U (1977) Differences in cardiovascular morbidity and mortality between previously known and newly diagnosed adult diabetics. *Diabetologia* 13: 229–234.

Herman WH, Teutsch SM, Sepe SJ, Sinnock P & Klein R (1983) An approach to the prevention of blindness in diabetes. *Diabetes Care* 6: 608–613.

Hillson RM, Hockaday TDR & Newton DJ (1984) Hyperglycaemia is one correlate of deterioration in vibration sense during the 5 years after diagnosis of Type 2 (non-insulin-dependent) diabetes. *Diabetologia* 26: 122–126.

Hirohata T, MacMahon B & Root HF (1967) The natural history of diabetes. I. Mortality. *Diabetes* 16: 875–881.

Holman RR & Turner RC (1979) Maintenance of basal plasma glucose and insulin concentrations in maturity-onset diabetes. *Diabetes* 28: 227–230.

Howard-Williams J, Hillson RM, Bron A, Awdry P, Mann JI & Hockaday TDR (1984) Retinopathy is associated with higher glycaemia in maturity-onset type diabetes. *Diabetologia* 27: 198–202.

Jarrett RJ, McCartney P & Keen H (1982) The Bedford Survey: Ten year mortality rates in newly diagnosed diabetics, borderline diabetics and normoglycaemic controls and risk factors for coronary heart disease in borderline diabetics. *Diabetologia* 22: 79–84.

Jarrett RJ, Viberti GC, Argyropoulos A, Hill RD, Mahmud U & Murrells TJ (1983) Microalbuminuria predicts mortality in non-insulin-dependent diabetes. *Diabetic Medicine* 1: 17–19.

Kannel WB & McGee DL (1979) Diabetes and glucose tolerance as risk factors for cardio-vascular disease: the Framingham Study. *Diabetes Care* **2:** 120–126.

Keen H (1986) What's in a name? IDDM/NIDDM, Type 1/Type 2. *Diabetic Medicine* **3:** 11–12.

Kessler II (1971) Mortality experience of diabetic patients. *American Journal of Medicine* **51:** 715–724.

Klein R, Klein BE, Moss SE, Davis MD & DeMets DL (1984) The Wisconsin epidemiological study of diabetic retinopathy. III. Prevalence and risk of diabetic retinopathy when age at diagnosis is over 30 years. *Archives of Ophthalmology* **102:** 527–532.

Knowler WC & Bennett PH (1983) Serum insulin concentrations predict changes in oral glucose tolerance. *Diabetes* **32 (supplement 1):** 46A.

Knowler WC, Bennett PH & Ballintine EJ (1980) Increased incidence of retinopathy in diabetics with elevated blood pressure. A six-year follow-up study in Pima Indians. *New England Journal of Medicine* **302:** 645–650.

Knuiman MW, Welborn TA, McCann VJ, Stanton KG & Constable IJ (1986) Prevalence of diabetic complications in relationship to risk factors. *Diabetes* **35:** 1332–1339.

Kohner EM & Barry PJ (1984) Prevention of blindness in diabetic retinopathy. *Diabetologia* **26:** 173–179.

Kolterman OG, Gray RS, Griffin J et al (1981) Receptor and post-receptor defects contribute to insulin resistance in non-insulin-dependent diabetes mellitus. *Diabetes* **30:** 990–995.

Lyons TJ, Kennedy L, Atkinson AB, Buchanan KD, Hadden DR & Weaver JA (1984) Predicting the need for insulin therapy in late onset (40–69) diabetes mellitus. *Diabetic Medicine* **1:** 105–108.

Malins J (1968) *Clinical Diabetes Mellitus*, London: Eyre & Spottiswoode.

Mandrup-Poulsen T, Owerbach D, Nerup J, Johansen K, Ingerslev J & Tybjaerg Hansen A (1985) Insulin-gene flanking sequences, diabetes mellitus and atherosclerosis: a review. *Diabetologia* **28:** 556–564.

Marks HH & Krall LP (1971) Onset, course, prognosis, and mortality in diabetes mellitus. In Marble A, White P, Bradley RF & Krall LP (eds). *Joslin's Diabetes Mellitus*, Philadelphia: Lea & Febiger.

Mather HM & Keen H (1985) The Southall Diabetes Survey: prevalence of known diabetes in Asians and Europeans. *British Medical Journal* **291:** 1081–1084.

Mayne NM (1965) *Diabetic neuropathy: a clinical study*. MD Thesis. University of Birmingham.

Medalie JH (1979) Risk factors other than hyperglycaemia in diabetic macrovascular disease. *Diabetes Care* **2:** 77–84.

Melton LJ, Ochi JW, Palumbo PJ & Chu CP (1984) Referral bias in diabetes research. *Diabetes Care* **7:** 13–18.

Mincu I (1970) Micro- and macroangiopathies and other chronic degenerative complications in newly detected diabetes mellitus. *Reviews of Roumanian Medicine—Medicine Interne* **18:** 155–64.

Mogensen CE (1982) Long term antihypertensive treatment inhibits progression of diabetic nephropathy. *British Medical Journal* **285:** 685–688.

Mogensen CE (1984) Microalbuminuria predicts clinical proteinuria and early mortality in maturity onset diabetes. *New England Journal of Medicine* **310:** 356–360.

Nathan DM, Singer DE, Godine JE, Hodgson Harrington C & Perlmuter LC (1986) Retinopathy in older Type II diabetics. Association with glucose control. *Diabetes* **35:** 797–801.

Neil HAW, Gatling W, Mather HM et al (1987) The Oxford Community Diabetes Study: Evidence for an increase in the prevalence of known diabetes in Great Britain. *Diabetic Medicine* **4:** 539–543.

Owens DR, Jones D, Shannon AG et al (1987) Retinopathy in newly presenting Type 2 (non-insulin-dependent) diabetic patients. *Diabetologia* **29:** 565A.

Paetkau ME, Boyd TAS, Winship B & Grace M (1977) Cigarette smoking and diabetic retinopathy. *Diabetes* **26:** 46–49.

Panzram G (1987) Mortality and survival in Type 2 (non-insulin-dependent) diabetes mellitus. *Diabetologia* **30:** 123–131.

Panzram G & Zabel-Langhennig R (1981) Prognosis of diabetes mellitus in a geographically defined population. *Diabetologia* **20:** 587–591.

Pirart J (1977) Diabetes mellitus and its degenerative complications: A prospective study of 4,400 patients observed between 1947 and 1973. *Diabete et Metabolisme* **3:** 173–182.

Reaven G & Miller R (1968) Study of the relationship between glucose and insulin responses to an oral glucose load in man. *Diabetes* **17:** 560–569.

Retting B & Teutsch SM (1984) The incidence of end-stage renal disease in Type I and Type II diabetes mellitus. *Diabetic Nephropathy* **3:** 26–32.

Rosenthal M, McMahan CA, Stern MP et al (1985) Evidence of bimodality of two-hour plasma glucose concentrations in Mexican Americans: results from the San Antonio Heart Study. *Journal of Chronic Disease* **38:** 5–16.

Rudenski AS, Hadden DR, Atkinson AB et al (1988) Natural history of pancreatic islet B cell function in Type 2 diabetes mellitus studied over six years by homeostasis model assessment. *Diabetic Medicine* **5:** 36–41.

Rushforth NB, Bennett PH, Steinberg AG, Burch TA & Miller M (1971) Diabetes in the Pima Indian. Evidence of bimodality in glucose tolerance distributions. *Diabetes* **20:** 756–765.

Savage PJ, Dippe SE, Bennett PH et al (1975) Hyperinsulinaemia and hypoinsulinaemia: Responses to oral carbohydrate over a wide spectrum of glucose tolerance. *Diabetes* **24:** 362–368.

Schmitz A & Vaeth M (1988) Microalbuminuria: A major risk factor in non-insulin-dependent diabetes. A 10-year follow up study of 503 patients. *Diabetic Medicine* **5:** 126–134.

Sicree RA, Zimmet PZ, King HOM & Coventry JS (1987) Plasma insulin response among Nauruans. Prediction of deterioration in glucose tolerance over 6 years. *Diabetes* **36:** 179–186.

Skyler JS (1984) Non-insulin-dependent diabetes mellitus: A clinical strategy. *Diabetes Care* **7 (supplement 1):** 118–129.

Soler NG, Fitzgerald MG, Malins JM & Summers ROC (1969) Retinopathy at diagnosis of diabetes with special reference to patients under 40 years of age. *British Medical Journal* **3:** 567–569.

Stern MP (1988) Type II diabetes mellitus. Interface between clinical and epidemiological investigation. *Diabetes Care* **11:** 19–26.

Stout RW (1985) Overview of the association between insulin and atherosclerosis. *Metabolism* **34:** 7–12.

Vasquez B, Flock EV, Savage PJ et al (1984) Sustained reduction of proteinuria in Type 2 (non-insulin-dependent) diabetes following diet-induced reduction of hyperglycaemia. *Diabetologia* **26:** 127–133.

Viberti GC, Mackintosh D, Bilous RW & Keen H (1982) Proteinuria in diabetes mellitus: role of spontaneous and experimental variation of glycaemia. *Kidney International* **21:** 714–720.

Viberti GC, Bilous RW, Mackintosh D, Bending JJ & Keen H (1983) Long term correction of hyperglycaemia and progression of renal failure in insulin dependent diabetes. *British Medical Journal* **286:** 598–602.

Vigorita VJ, Moore GW & Hutchins GM (1980) Absence of correlation between coronary arterial atherosclerosis and severity or duration of diabetes mellitus of adult onset. *American Journal of Cardiology* **46:** 535–542.

WHO Expert Committee on Diabetes Mellitus (1980) *Technical Report Series* 646. Geneva: World Health Organisation.

Yano K, Kagan A, McGee D & Rhoads GG (1982) Glucose intolerance and nine-year mortality in Japanese men in Hawaii. *American Journal of Medicine* **72:** 71–80.

Young RJ, McCulloch DK, Prescott RJ & Clarke BF (1984) Alcohol: another risk factor for diabetic retinopathy? *British Medical Journal* **288:** 1035–1037.

Zimmet P & Whitehouse S (1978) Bimodality of fasting and two hour glucose tolerance distributions in a Micronesian population. *Diabetes* **27:** 793–800.

Zimmett P, Whitehouse S, Alford F & Chisholm D (1978) The relationship of insulin response to a glucose stimulus over a wide range of glucose tolerance. *Diabetologia* **15:** 23–27.

5

Enteroinsular axis

JOHN C. BROWN

Release of insulin from the pancreatic B cell is under the control of many regulatory mechanisms including nervous reflexes, circulating peptides and absorbed nutrients. Mechanisms of gastrointestinal origin have become collectively referred to as the 'enteroinsular axis'. This term originally proposed by Unger and Eisentraut (1969) described a regulatory system for the pancreatic B cell in which the hormones of the gastrointestinal tract acted as a 'fine tuning system' for insulin release stimulated by absorbed nutrients. Glucose, amino acids and free fatty acids will all stimulate, to varying degrees, the secretion of insulin, and glucose and free fatty acids will inhibit secretion of glucagon, while amino acids stimulate glucagon release. All of these nutrient groups are also, to a greater or lesser extent, involved in the release of gastrointestinal hormones.

HISTORICAL ASPECTS

Forty years before the term 'enteroinsular axis' appeared in the literature Zunz and Labarre (1929) described the separation from secretin of a gut factor with humoral activity which enhanced the endocrine secretion of the pancreas. Labarre and Still (1930) presented further evidence that the hypoglycaemic factor was other than secretin and Labarre (1932) is credited with introducing the name 'incretin' to describe this gastrointestinal factor. Even earlier studies by Moore, Edie and Abram (1906) had suggested that the duodenum 'supplies a chemical excitant for the internal secretion of the pancreas' and hypothesized that diabetes may be caused by 'the absence of an intestinal excitant of the internal secretion of the pancreas'. However, despite these early references in the literature to the possible existence of a gastrointestinal humoral factor involved in insulin release from the pancreas, it was not until the 1960s that significant advances were made towards the recognition of this particular peptide. The promising studies of Dixon and Wadia (1926) and Laughton and Macallum (1932) in investigating hypoglycaemic properties of duodenal extracts were discredited when Loew, Gray and Ivy (1940) published a series of observations in which they described the failure to isolate a hypoglycaemic substance from the duodenum. They also described that the presence of HCl in the duodenum had no effect on blood sugar levels in either fasting or hyperglycaemic animals.

Adhering strictly to methods previously described by others they prepared several extracts of the mucosa of the small intestine in which hypoglycaemic activity was observed. They concluded the following:

1. Carefully prepared pancreatic tissue-free extracts of intestinal mucosa obtained by a number of methods which have been reported to yield a hypoglycaemic substance have consistently been found to be without effect on the blood sugar level of fasted, unanaesthetized dogs.
2. This, and previous studies, have failed to provide evidence in favour of the theory that the duodenum exerts a hormonal control over carbohydrate metabolism.

Interest in gastrointestinal factors involved in the release of insulin received renewed attention following the development of a radioimmunoassay for insulin. Elrick et al (1964) compared two routes for glucose administration in the same individual, using equal glucose loads, and demonstrated that a significantly greater insulin release was achieved with oral glucose than with intravenous glucose. They suggested that a gastrointestinal factor might be released by the presence of glucose in the stomach or upper small intestine. In the same year, McIntyre et al (1964) compared administration of glucose by the intravenous route with direct jejunal infusion. Even though lower blood glucose levels were achieved following jejunal infusion, a higher plasma insulin response was observed. Again the conclusion from these observations was that a humoral substance was released from the jejunum during glucose absorption and that this agent acted in conjunction with circulating glucose to stimulate insulin release. Perley and Kipnis (1967) estimated that perhaps half of the insulin secreted following an oral glucose load was as the result of gastrointestinal factors.

PHYSIOLOGY

Since the observation that a gastrointestinal factor(s) could be involved in regulation of insulin release, all of the gastrointestinal hormones, at one time or another, have been considered to have insulinotropic effects. Studies with gastrointestinal hormone containing preparations on insulin release have been inconclusive for a variety of reasons. In particular the purity of the preparation used was ill defined, the prevailing degree of glycaemia not controlled or discussed and bolus as opposed to infusion types of experiment were performed, so that non-physiological blood levels were achieved.

Secretin

Earlier observations by Dupré (1964), Pfeiffer et al (1965) and Dupré et al (1969), that secretin had an insulinotropic action in man and that a greater effect was observed during hyperglycaemia than in the fasting state have been subsequently disproved. Lerner and Porte (1970) suggested however, that secretin may have an effect on the readily releasable insulin pool with little or no effect on the second stage of insulin release. Buchanan et al (1968) demonstrated in anaesthetized dogs that doses of secretin which gave excellent exocrine pancreatic responses had no effect on insulin release. These studies, however, were performed in fasting animals in which circulating glucose levels were basal. The inability of glucose administered into the duodenum to stimulate exocrine secretion of the pancreas (Wang and Grossman, 1951) and the inability of glucose (Bloom, 1974; Boden et al, 1975) or a mixed meal (Bloom et al, 1975; Chey et al, 1975) to elevate serum immunoreactive secretin release suggested that secretin was not involved in the enteroinsular axis.

Gastrin

The necessary criteria establishing gastrin as an insulinotropic hormone have also not been satisfied. The insulin response from the pancreas to injections of gastrin is very similar to that seen for secretin. It is monophasic, transitory and unaffected by the prevailing state of glycaemia (Unger et al, 1967; Dupré et al, 1969, Creutzfeldt et al, 1970).

Cholecystokinin-pancreozymin (CCK)

A role for CCK as an insulinotropic agent was first suggested by Dupré and Beck (1966). In these studies a partially purified preparation of CCK was used and it was from this material that gastric inhibitory polypeptide (GIP) was eventually isolated (Brown et al, 1969; 1970). A role for CCK in the enteroinsular axis is still controversial. Studies on the release of CCK from the small intestine using bioassays, have demonstrated that protein hydrolysates and fats are stimulatory (Wang and Grossman, 1951), and the amino acids L-phenylalanine, L-tryptophan (Meyer, 1975) and intraduodenal arginine have a weak stimulatory effect (Konturek et al, 1972). Bioassays have not indicated a secretagogue effect of glucose with respect to CCK release.

Marks and Turner (1977) have suggested that CCK is insulinotropic in the presence of hyperaminoacidaemia, but that it is unlikely to be responsible for the insulinotropic effect of oral glucose, a view held by most researchers in this field.

Glucose-dependent insulinotropic polypeptide/gastric inhibitory polypeptide (GIP)

Since Dupré et al (1973) first demonstrated that the intravenous infusion in man of a highly purified preparation of porcine GIP, in the presence of hyperglycaemia, stimulated insulin release and produced an improvement in glucose tolerance, this hormone has received wide attention as an insulinotropic agent.

The hormone was isolated from an impure preparation of CCK following the observation that it might contain an inhibitor of gastric acid secretion (Brown and Pederson, 1970). Brown et al (1970) described a technique for separation of the gastric inhibitory activity from cholecystokinin activity following partial purification on Sephadex G50. Final purification was achieved using a bioassay for measuring the inhibition of gastric acid secretion (Brown, 1982; Brown et al, 1969, 1970). An amino acid sequence for GIP was reported by Brown and Dryburgh (1971) and later corrected, following studies by Jörnvall et al (1981). Amino acid sequence data is now available for porcine, human and bovine GIP (Figure 1). Confirmation of the sequence of natural porcine GIP has been achieved by synthesis of an analogue which has demonstrated full biological activity.

HOG

Tyr-Ala-Glu-Gly-Thr-Phe-Ile-Ser-Asp-Tyr-Ser-Ile-Ala-Met-

Asp-Lys-Ile-Arg-Gln-Gln-Asp-Phe-Val-Asn-Trp-Leu-Leu-Ala-

Gln-Lys-Gly-Lys-Lys-Ser-Asp-Trp-Lys-His-Asn-Ile-Thr-Gln

HUMAN

Tyr-Ala-Glu-Gly-Thr-Phe-Ile-Ser-Asp-Tyr-Ser-Ile-Ala-Met-

Asp-Lys-Ile-**His**-Gln-Gln-Asp-Phe-Val-Asn-Trp-Leu-Leu-Ala-

Gln-Lys-Gly-Lys-Lys-**Asn**-Asp-Trp-Lys-His-Asn-Ile-Thr-Gln

BOVINE

Tyr-Ala-Glu-Gly-Thr-Phe-Ile-Ser-Asp-Tyr-Ser-Ile-Ala-Met-

Asp-Lys-Ile-Arg-Gln-Gln-Asp-Phe-Val-Asn-Trp-Leu-Leu-Ala-

Gln-Lys-Gly-Lys-Lys-Ser-Asp-Trp-**Ile**-His-Asn-Ile-Thr-Gln

Figure 1. Complete amino acid sequences of porcine (hog), human and bovine GIP. Amino acids in bold face indicate the differences of human and bovine GIP from porcine GIP.

RADIO-IMMUNOASSAY FOR GASTROINTESTINAL PEPTIDES

Radio-immunoassays have been established for most of the gastrointestinal hormones. To satisfy one of the criteria for involvement in the enteroinsular axis, a peptide must be shown to be released by either glucose or amino acids. When glucose is introduced into the duodenum the only gastrointestinal hormone which has been shown to be significantly elevated in plasma is GIP. Some controversy exists as to the absolute values which are measured in plasma, both basal and following stimulation, however, most laboratories agree upon the pattern of release and the overall changes. Mixtures of amino acids, on the other hand, are extremely potent stimulators for the release of gastrin, cholecystokinin, and to a lesser extent secretin and GIP. However, interaction of amino acids and the gastrointestinal hormones at the B cell level has received limited attention.

Recently, some of the problems associated with the radio-immunoassay for GIP have been carefully examined. Jorde et al (1983) measured fasting and postprandial plasma immunoreactive-GIP (IR-GIP) levels in man using seven different antisera. They showed that mean fasting IR-GIP levels varied from 12 to 92 pmol per litre and postprandially from 35 to 235 pmol per litre. Serum fractions were subjected to separation on Sephadex G50 and all antisera used identified three circulating forms of IR-GIP, with the bulk of the IR-GIP diluting at a volume indicating a molecular size of 5 kDa. The studies of Krarup and Holst (1984) involved the use of five different antisera and they compared measurements on porcine and human gastrointestinal mucosal tissue. All of the antisera gave reasonably similar results with the porcine extract, however, the levels for the human extract varied considerably. Most of the antisera used recognized an epitope within the GIP sequence 15 to 42. Moody et al (1984) have reported that there are two substitutions within the human GIP sequence, histidine for arginine at position 18 and asparagine for serine at position 34. It is possible that certain of these antisera raised to porcine GIP which are directed to this part of the molecule would then not accurately measure IR-GIP in human plasma or serum. This could contribute to the equivocal results which exist concerning the measurement of IR-GIP in man.

Circulating IR-GIP levels have been shown to be increased following the ingestion of a mixed meal (Kuzio et al, 1974; Burhol et al, 1980), glucose and other carbohydrates (Cataland et al, 1974), some amino acids (Thomas et al, 1978) and fatty acids (Brown, 1974; Falko et al, 1975).

Response to carbohydrates

Many studies have been performed, demonstrating that when glucose passes into the small intestine there is an immediate increase in circulating levels of IR-GIP (Crockett et al, 1975; Pederson et al, 1975; Morgan et al, 1979). The studies of Morgan et al (1979) also demonstrated that IR-GIP levels were elevated when galactose and sucrose were ingested. Fructose, however, was without effect. The delayed secretion of IR-GIP in response to sucrose was considered to be due to the necessity for hydrolysis of sucrose prior to absorption. Morgan (1979) suggested that release of GIP from the small intestine was dependent on active transport of monosaccharides. Creutzfeldt et al (1983) concluded that sugars which are not transported, such as mannose, or transported and not metabolized, such as 2-deoxyglucose, will not stimulate GIP secretion. Sykes et al (1980) investigated the release of IR-GIP in response to monosaccharides, analogues of monosaccharides and disaccharides, using a rat intestinal perfusion technique. They confirmed the earlier observation of Creutzfeldt and Ebert (1977) when they demonstrated that phloridzin, which inhibited glucose absorption, also abolished the release of IR-GIP. Both sucrose and maltose stimulated IR-GIP release and the failure of lactose to do so, was considered to be due to the fact that the rat has difficulty in metabolizing it.

Response to fats

Triglyceride preparations have been shown to stimulate IR-GIP release. Brown (1974) used the triglyceride suspension (Lipomul) which contains between 34–62% linoleic acid, 19–49% oleic acid, 8–12% palmitic acid, 2.5–4.5% stearic acid, 0.1–1.7% myristic acid and 0.2–1.6% hexadeconic acid without any glucose or carbohydrates (Falko et al, 1975). A suspension of medium chain triglycerides when introduced intraduodenally in dogs via a Mann-Bollman fistula (O'Dorisio et al, 1976) produced only a modest increase in circulating levels of IR-GIP. It is now considered that the long chain fatty acids are the most potent stimulators of GIP release. In none of the studies, in which triglyceride was ingested and a significant release of IR-GIP observed, was there an increase in plasma immunoreactive insulin (IRI) levels. In the experiments in which glucose and other carbohydrates were shown to increase significantly GIP release, there was always a concurrent increase in circulating levels of IRI. Increases seen following galactose ingestion were usually quite small and transient, and Morgan et al (1979) considered that this was because a small rise in blood glucose was usually associated with galactose ingestion.

Response to amino acids

Ingestion of protein as either a meat extract (Brown, 1974) or as fillet steak (Cleator and Gourlay, 1975) did not result in an increase in serum IR-GIP levels. However, mixtures of specific amino acids when introduced directly into the small intestine have been shown to stimulate IR-GIP release. Thomas et al (1978) demonstrated that a mixture of amino acids containing arginine, histidine, isoleucine, lysine and tyrosine produced a marked increase in serum in both IR-GIP and IRI when the mixture was introduced directly into the duodenum. A much weaker response was observed when a mixture of amino acids containing methionine, phenylalanine, tryptophan and valine was used.

EFFECT OF GIP ON INSULIN SECRETION IN MAN

Dupré et al (1973) infused intravenously a highly purified preparation of GIP in normal human volunteers. These experiments were a natural extension of the observations made earlier in which it was shown that highly purified CCK preparations did not stimulate insulin release in both man and rat (Rabinovitch and Dupré, 1972). The dose of GIP which Dupré et al (1973) used in these studies was 1 μg/min for 60 min. The infusion was given together with an intravenous infusion of glucose (0.5 g/min for 60 min) and compared with the same dose of glucose administered alone. A significant improvement in glucose tolerance, coincidental with a marked elevation in plasma levels of IRI were observed (Figure 2). The insulinotropic action of GIP was later shown to be glucose concentration dependent in both rat (Pederson and Brown, 1976) and human (Elahi et al, 1979). It was also observed that there was a glucose concentration threshold below which GIP was not insulinotropic. In the isolated perfused rat pancreas this was shown

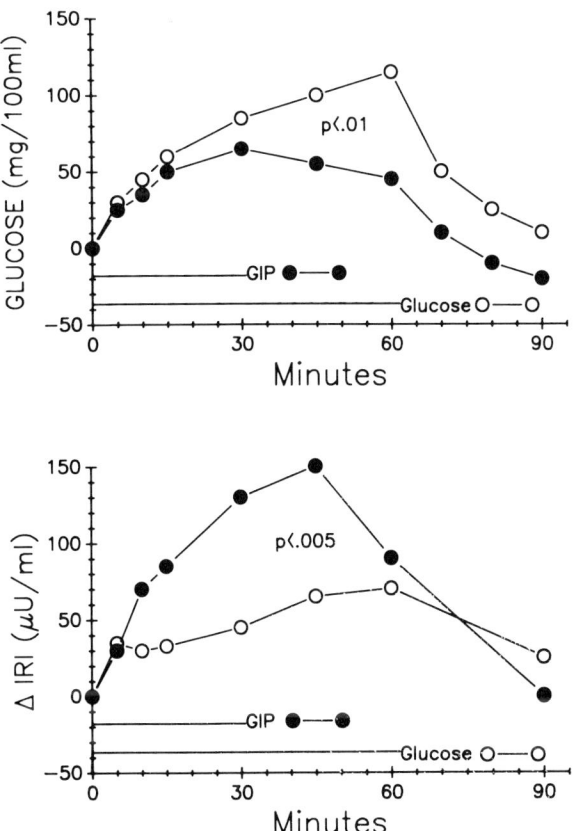

Figure 2. Effect of the intravenous infusion of 1.0 µg per min GIP (filled circle) on IRI release to an intravenous infusion of 0.5 g per minute glucose (unfilled circle) for 60 min in normal human volunteers. From Dupré et al (1973), with permission of the publishers.

to be 4.4 mM (Figure 3), and an equivalent concentration in man has been demonstrated (Elahi et al, 1979). The potentiating effect of GIP was shown to be maximum at a glucose concentration of 16 mM and this was similar to what was observed when glucose alone was the stimulus (Figure 4). However, in the presence of GIP, the maximum insulin release by glucose was several fold higher than that seen with glucose alone (Figure 4). In general,

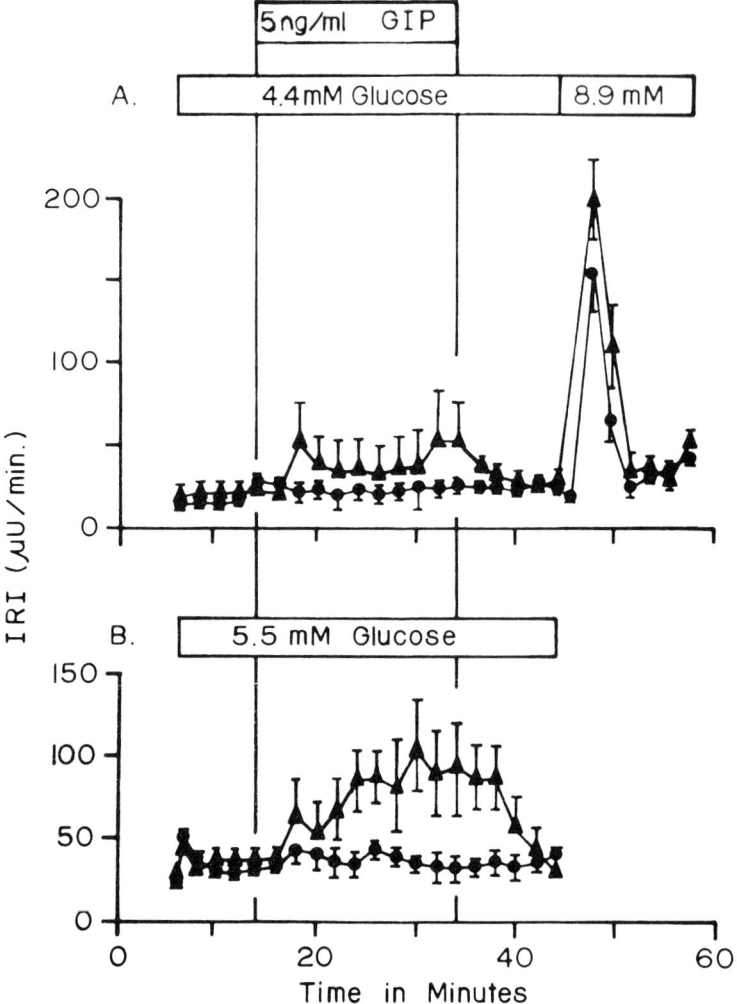

Figure 3. The effect of 5 ng per ml GIP on IRI release from the isolated perfused rat pancreas **A** in the presence of 4.4 mM and **B** 5.5 mM glucose demonstrating the glucose concentration threshold for the insulinotropic action of GIP. ● Control ▲ GIP. From Pederson and Brown (1976), with permission of the publishers.

studies with porcine GIP on insulin release in man have produced similar results to those obtained from the isolated perfused rat pancreas. Elahi et al (1979) clamped the circulating glucose levels in normal human volunteers at 54 and 143 mg/dl above basal glycaemia. The degree of hyperinsulinaemia observed, was dependent upon the glucose concentration used (Figure 5). In similar experiments in which blood glucose levels were kept at basal, GIP was without an insulinotropic effect.

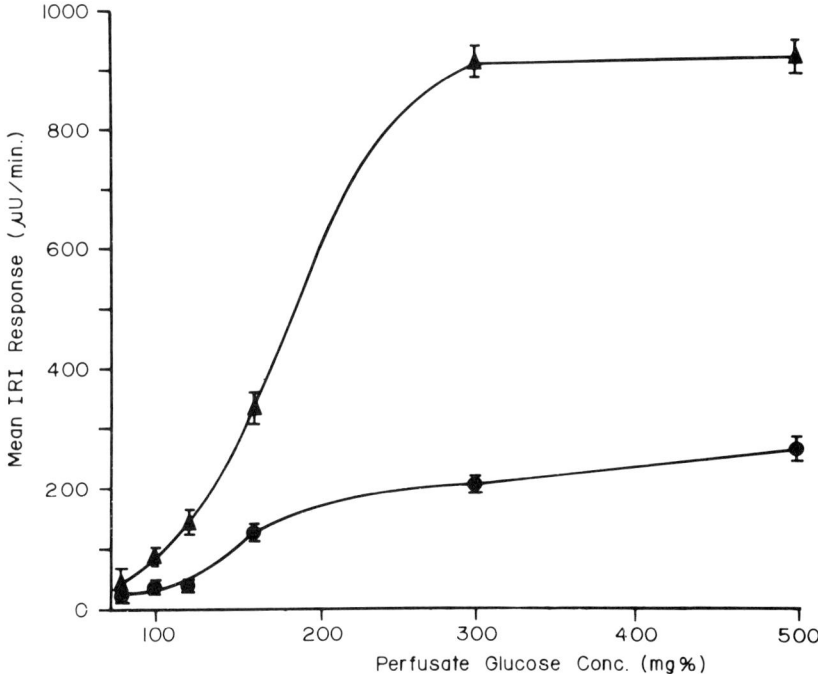

Figure 4. Effect of varying the glucose concentration from 100–500 mg per cent on the IRI release from the isolated perfused rat pancreas to a constant infusion of 5 ng per ml porcine GIP. ▲ Glucose + 5 ng/ml GIP, ● Glucose. From Brown (1982), with permission of the publishers.

PATHOLOGY OF THE ENTEROINSULAR AXIS

The development of a radio-immunoassay appropriate for determination of IR-GIP levels in serum has led to multiple investigations into a possible role for GIP in a variety of pathophysiological situations in which the enteroinsular axis could be involved including non-insulin-dependent diabetes mellitus (NIDDM). Perley and Kipnis (1967) and Cerasi et al (1973) had indicated earlier that the enteroinsular axis was probably hyperactive in maturity onset diabetes. Most of the recent studies which have attempted to correlate a disturbed enteroinsular axis with a pathophysiological situation have concentrated on measurement of IR-GIP levels.

Creutzfeldt et al (1983) reviewed the literature with respect to the enteroinsular axis and pathophysiological situations. The review dealt exclusively with an evaluation of a role for GIP and GIP abnormalities in diseases which could indicate an involvement of the enteroinsular axis. They suggested that because GIP could be considered the main incretin and GIP release to be dependent on nutrient absorption, then a large number of gastrointestinal and metabolic diseases may result in abnormal secretion of GIP. They concluded that in situations where a large number of gastrointestinal and

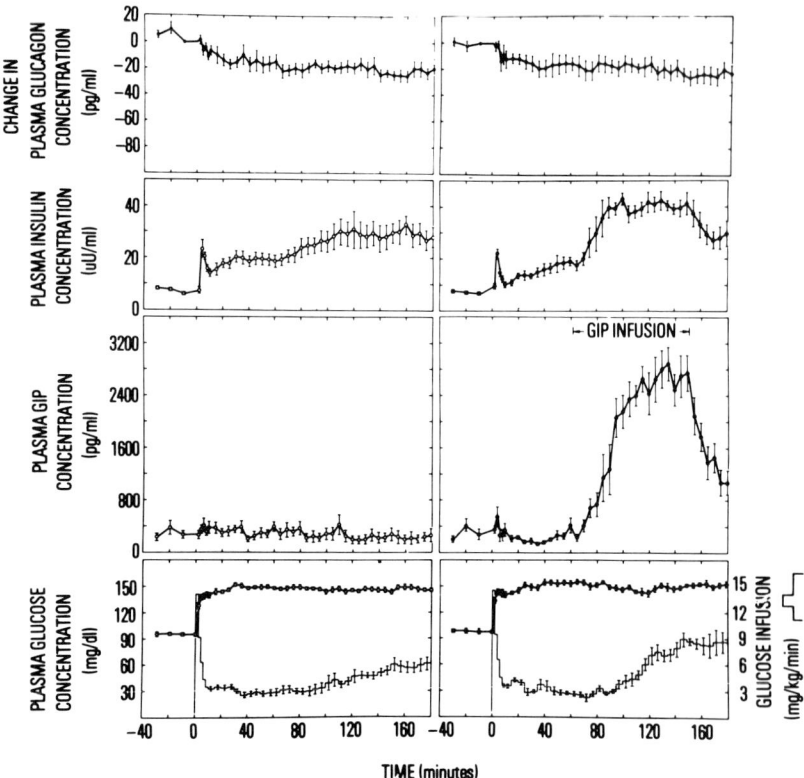

Figure 5. Effect of the infusion of 6.67 ng.kg^{-1}. min^{-1} GIP on IRI, IR-glucagon and glucose infusion required to maintain a stable glycaemia of 54 mg/dl above basal. The results of the GIP infusion are indicated in the right panels. From Elahi et al (1979), with permission of the publishers.

metabolic diseases demonstrated an abnormality in IR-GIP secretion, these changes were rarely of clinical significance and usually secondary to a primary defect. In NIDDM an exaggerated secretion of GIP (Bloom, 1975; Crockett et al, 1976; Ebert et al, 1976; Ross et al, 1977; Salera et al, 1982) have been reported but little correlation between GIP and insulin response has been observed. It was also stated that GIP abnormalities were not identical with disturbances of the enteroinsular axis and that estimation of a defect in the enteroinsular axis can only be achieved by comparing the insulin response to oral glucose with the insulin response produced by an intravenous glucose infusion. A disturbance of the enteroinsular axis has been reported in patients following both jejunoileal bypass and in NIDDM. However, in neither situation can a correlation between incretin, the enteroinsular axis and an IR-GIP response be found. It was concluded that disturbances of the enteroinsular axis are rarely explained by abnormalities in secretion of IR-GIP. From a review of this work, Creutzfeldt et al (1983) concluded that there must be other humoral gut factors or a neural component to the enteroinsular axis which could be involved in these abnormal situations. In all of the studies, no attempt was made to investigate an abnormal response of GIP at the receptor level.

GIP on receptors

The action of GIP at the level of the receptor has received little attention. It is only recently that the existence of GIP binding sites on membranes has been demonstrated. Indeed, success has only been achieved using the hamster transplantable insulinoma (Couvineau et al, 1984; Maletti et al, 1983, 1984) and an insulin secreting β-cell line In [111] (Amiranoff et al, 1984, 1985). Two types of binding sites have been identified, a small population with high affinity and a larger population of low affinity (Amiranoff et al, 1984, 1985). The binding to both these receptor sites was specific in that glucagon, secretin and vasoactive intestinal peptide did not cause displacement of ^{125}I-GIP. It has been suggested that GIP may interact with glucagon receptors in some tissues, in that the peptide was shown to inhibit the binding of ^{125}I-glucagon to adipocytes (Dupré et al, 1976). It has been shown to exert a strong antagonism to the actions of glucagon (Dupré et al, 1976; Ebert and Brown, 1976).

A recent study by Chan et al (1984) using the Zucker 'fatty' (fa/fa rat) investigating the involvement of GIP in the hyperinsulinaemia observed in this animal, has indicated that there could be a disturbance in receptor function. This animal is characterized by hyperphagia, hyperinsulinaemia

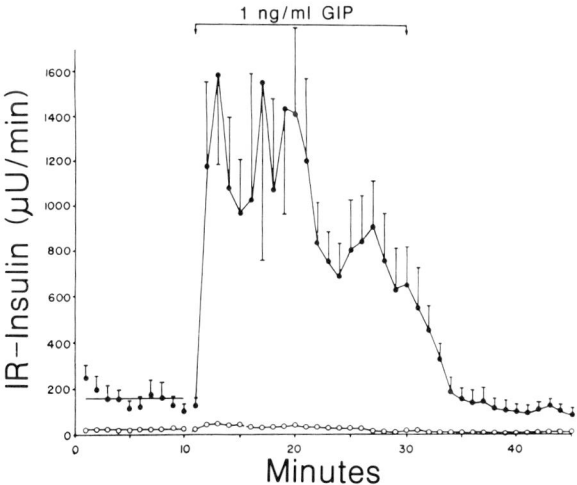

Figure 6. IRI release from the isolated perfused rat pancreas from lean (○) and obese (●) Zucker rats to a square wave stimulus of 1.0 ng per ml GIP in the presence of 4.4 mM glucose. The insulinotropic action of GIP is not glucose concentration dependent in the obese animal. From Chan et al (1984), with permission of the publishers.

and hyperlipidaemia. A comparison of lean and obese Zucker rats has demonstrated that the obese animal has an elevated insulin response to both glucose and GIP. In particular, this study demonstrated that there is a lack of a glucose threshold for the insulinotropic action of GIP in the obese animal. When the pancreas was perfused with glucose at 4.4 mM, GIP acted as a very potent stimulus for insulin release from the obese animals as compared to the lean fitter mates in which GIP was not insulinotropic at this glucose concentration (Figure 6).

SUMMARY

A physiological role for GIP as an insulinotropic hormone involved in the enteroinsular axis has been established and ingestion of glucose, fatty acids and certain amino acids will produce an increase in circulating IR-GIP levels. The insulinotropic action of GIP is glucose concentration dependent in normal animals. A role for GIP in NIDDM is equivocal although several studies have demonstrated elevated serum levels. Animal models have indicated a disturbance of GIP receptor function associated with hyper-insulinaemia, i.e. lowering of the minimum glucose concentration at which GIP is insulinotropic.

REFERENCES

Amiranoff B, Vauclin-Jacques N & Laburthe M (1984) Functional GIP receptors in a hamster pancreatic beta cell line In 111: specific binding and biological effects. *Biochemistry and Biophysics Research Communications* **123:** 671–676.

Amiranoff B, Vauclin-Jacques N & Laburthe M (1985) Interaction of gastric inhibitory polypeptide (GIP) with the insulin-secreting pancreatic beta cell line In 111: characteristics of GIP binding sites. *Life Sciences* **36:** 807–813.

Bloom SR (1974) Hormones of the gastrointestinal tract. *British Medical Bulletin* **30:** 62–67.

Bloom SR (1975) GIP in diabetes. *Diabetologia* **11:** 334.

Bloom SR, Bryant MG & Cochrane JPS (1975) Normal distribution and post prandial release of gut hormones. *Clinical Science and Molecular Medicine* **49:** 3P.

Boden G, Essa M & Owen OE (1975) Effects of intraduodenal amino acids, fatty acids and sugars on secretin concentrations. *Gastroenterology* **68:** 722–727.

Brown JC (1974) Gastric inhibitory polypeptide (GIP). In Taylor S (ed) *Endocrinology 1973*, pp 276–284. London: Heinemann.

Brown JC (1982) Gastric inhibitory polypeptide. In Gross, Grumbach, Labhart, et al (eds) *Monographs on endocrinology*, Berlin: Springer.

Brown JC & Dryburgh JR (1971) A gastric inhibitory polypeptide. II The complete amino acid sequence. *Canadian Journal of Biochemistry* **49:** 867–872.

Brown JC & Pederson RA (1970) A multiparameter study on the action of preparations containing cholecystokinin-pancreozymin. *Scandinavian Journal of Gastroenterology* **5:** 537–541.

Brown JC, Mutt V & Pederson RA (1970) Further purification of a polypeptide demonstrating enterogastrone activity. *Journal of Physiology* **209:** 57–64.

Brown JC, Pederson RA, Jorpes JE & Mutt V (1969) Preparation of a highly active entero-gastrone. *Canadian Journal of Physiology and Pharmacology* **47:** 113–114.

Buchanan KD, Vance JE, Morgan A & Williams RH (1968) Effect of pancreozymin on insulin and glucagon levels in blood and bile. *American Journal of Physiology* **215:** 1293–1298.

Burhol PG, Jorde R & Waldun HL (1980) Radio-immunoassay of plasma gastric inhibitory polypeptide (GIP), release of GIP after a test meal and duodenal infusion of bile and immunoreactive plasma GIP components in man. *Digestion* **20**: 336–345.

Cataland S, Crockett SE, Brown JC & Mazzaferri EL (1974) Gastric inhibitory polypeptide (GIP) stimulation by oral glucose in man. *Journal of Clinical Endocrinology and Metabolism* **39**: 223–228.

Cerasi E, Efendic S & Luft R (1973) Dose-response relation between plasma-insulin and blood-glucose levels during oral glucose loads in prediabetic and diabetic subjects. *Lancet* **i:** 794–797.

Chan CB, Pederson RA, Buchan AMJ, Tubesing KB & Brown JC (1984) Gastric inhibitory polypeptide (GIP) and insulin release in the obese Zucker rat. *Diabetes* **33**: 536–542.

Chey WY, Rhodes RA, Lee KY & Hendricks J (1975) Radio-immunoassay of secretin: Further studies. In Thompson JC (ed) *Gastrointestinal hormones*, pp 269–281. Austin: University of Texas Press.

Cleator JGM & Gourlay RH (1975) Release of immunoreactive gastric inhibitory polypeptide (IR-GIP) by oral ingestion of food substances. *American Journal of Surgeons* **130**: 128–135.

Couvineau A, Amiranoff B, Vauclin-Jacques N & Laburthe M (1984) The GIP receptor on pancreatic beta cell tumor: molecular identification by covalent cross-linking. *Biochemistry and Biophysics Research Communications* **122**: 283–288.

Creutzfeldt W & Ebert R (1977) Release of gastric inhibitory polypeptide (GIP) to a test meal under normal and pathological conditions in man. In Bajaj JS (ed) *Diabetes*, pp 63–75. Amsterdam: Excerpta Medica.

Creutzfeldt W, Feurle G & Ketterer H (1970) Effect of gastrointestinal hormones on insulin and glucagon secretion. *New England Journal of Medicine* **282**: 1139–1141.

Creutzfeldt W, Ebert R, Nauck M & Stöckmann F (1983) Disturbances of the enteroinsular axis. *Scandanavian Journal of Gastroenterology* **18: (supplement 83)** 111–119.

Crockett SE, Cataland S, Falko J & Mazzaferri EL (1975) Gastric inhibitory polypeptide: Responses to variable doses of glucose in normal subjects and abnormal responses to oral glucose in patients with adult onset diabetes mellitus. *Diabetes* **24**: 413.

Crockett SE, Mazzaferri EL & Cataland S (1976) Gastric inhibitory polypeptide (GIP) in maturity-onset diabetes mellitus. *Diabetes* **25**: 931–935.

Dixon W & Wadia JH (1926) The action of intestinal extracts. *British Medical Journal* **i:** 820.

Dupré J (1964) An intestinal hormone affecting glucose disposal in man. *Lancet* **ii:** 672–673.

Dupré J & Beck JC (1966) Stimulation of release of insulin by an extract of intestinal mucosa. *Diabetes* **15**: 555–559.

Dupré J, Rojas L, White JJ, Unger RH & Beck JC (1966) Effects of secretin on insulin and glucagon in portal and peripheral blood in man. *Lancet* **ii:** 26–27.

Dupré J, Curtis JD, Unger RH, Waddell RW & Beck JC (1969) Effects of secretin, pancreozymin or gastrin on the response of the endocrine pancreas to administration of glucose or arginine in man. *Journal of Clinical Investigations* **48**: 748–757.

Dupré J, Ross SA, Watson D & Brown JC (1973) Stimulation of insulin secretion by gastric inhibitory polypeptide in man. *Journal of Clinical Endocrinology and Metabolism* **37**: 826–828.

Dupré J, Greenidge N, McDonald TJ, Ross SA & Rubenstein D (1976). Inhibition of actions of glucagon in adipocytes by gastric inhibitory polypeptide. *Metabolism* **25**: 1197–1199.

Ebert R & Brown JC (1976) Effect of gastric inhibitory polypeptide (GIP) on lipolysis and cyclic AMP levels in isolated fat cells. *European Journal of Clinical Investigation* **6**: 327 (Abstract).

Ebert R, Frerichs H & Creutzfeldt W (1976) Serum gastric inhibitory polypeptide (GIP) response in patients with maturity onset diabetes and in juvenile diabetics. *Diabetologia* **12**: 388.

Elahi D, Andersen DK, Brown JC et al (1979) Pancreatic α- and β-cell responses to GIP infusion in normal man. *American Journal of Physiology* **237** (Endocrinology and Metabolism of Gastrointestinal Physiology 6): E185–E191.

Elrick ML, Stimmler L, Hlad CJ & Arai Y (1964) Plasma insulin response to oral and intravenous glucose administration. *Journal of Clinical Endocrinology and Metabolism* **24**: 1076–1082.

Falko JM, Crockett SE, Cataland S & Mazzaferri EL (1975) Gastric inhibitory polypeptide

(GIP) stimulated by fat ingestion in man. *Journal of Clinical Endocrinology and Metabolism* **41:** 260–265.

Jorde R, Burhol PG & Schulz TB (1983) Fasting and postprandial plasma GIP values in man measured with seven different antisera. *Regulatory Peptides* **7:** 87–94.

Jörnvall H, Carlquist M, Kwauk S et al (1981) Amino acid sequence and heterogeneity of gastric inhibitory polypeptide (GIP). *FEBS Letters* **123:** 205–210.

Konturek SJ, Tasler J & Obtuzowicz W (1972) Localization of cholecystokinin release in the intestine of dog. *American Journal of Physiology* **222:** 16–20.

Krarup T & Holst JJ (1984) The heterogeneity of gastric inhibitory polypeptide in porcine and human gastrointestinal mucosa evaluated with five different antisera. *Regulatory Peptides* **9:** 35–46.

Kuzio M, Dryburgh JR, Malloy KM & Brown JC (1974) Radio-immunoassay for gastric inhibitory polypeptide. *Gastroenterology* **66:** 357–364.

Labarre J (1932) Sur les possibilités d'un traitement du diabete par l'incrétine. *Bulletin Academie Royale Médicine Belgium* **12:** 620–634.

Labarre J & Still EV (1930) Studies on the physiology of secretin. *American Journal of Physiology* **91:** 649–653.

Laughton NM & Macallum AB (1932) The relation of duodenal mucosa to the internal secretion of the pancreas. *Proceedings of the Royal Society of London (Biology)* **111:** 37–46.

Lerner RL & Porte D Jr (1970) Uniphasic insulin responses to secretin stimulation in man. *Journal of Clinical Investigations* **49:** 2276–2280.

Loew ER, Gray JS & Ivy AC (1940) Is a duodenal hormone involved in carbohydrate metabolism? *American Journal of Physiology* **129:** 659–663.

McIntosh CHS, Pederson RA, Koop H & Brown JC (1979) Inhibition of GIP stimulated somatostatin-like immunoreactivity (SLI) by acetylcholine and vagal stimulation. In Miyoshi A (ed) *Gut Peptides: Secretion, Function and Clinical Aspects*, pp 100–104. Tokyo: Kodansha.

McIntyre N, Holdsworth CD & Turner DS (1964) New interpretation of oral glucose tolerance. *Lancet* **ii:** 20–21.

Maletti M, Amiranoff B, Laburthe M & Rosellin G (1983) Mise en évidence de Réceptors Spécifiques du inhibiteur gastrique (GIP). *Comptes Rendus de l'Academie des Sciences* **297:** 563–564.

Maletti M, Portha B, Carlquist M et al (1984) Evidence for and characterization of specific high affinity binding sites for the gastric inhibitory polypeptide in pancreatic β-cells. *Endocrinology* **115:** 1324–1331.

Marks V & Turner DS (1977) The gastrointestinal hormones with particular reference to their role in the regulation of insulin secretion. *Essays Medical Biochemistry* **3:** 109–152.

Meyer JH (1975) Release of secretin and cholecystokinin. In Thompson JC (ed) *Gastrointestinal hormones*, pp 475–489. Austin: University of Texas Press.

Moody AJ, Thim L & Valverde I (1984) The isolation and sequencing of human gastric inhibitory polypeptide (GIP). *FEBS Letters* **172:** 142–148.

Moore B, Edie ES & Abram JM (1906) On the treatment of diabetes mellitus by acid extract of duodenal mucous membrane. *Biochemical Journal* **1:** 28–38.

Morgan LM (1979) Immunoassayable gastric inhibitory polypeptide: investigations into its role in carbohydrate metabolism. *Annals of Clinical Biochemistry* **16:** 6–14.

Morgan LM, Wright JW & Marks V (1979) The effect of oral galactose on GIP and insulin secretion in man. *Diabetologia* **16:** 235–239.

O'Dorisio TM, Cataland S, Stevenson M & Mazzaferri EL (1976) Gastric inhibitory polypeptide (GIP). Intestinal distribution and stimulation by amino acids and medium-chain triglycerides. *American Journal of Digestive Disorders* **21:** 761–765.

Pederson RA & Brown JC (1976) The insulinotropic action of gastric inhibitory polypeptide in the perfused isolated rat pancreas. *Endocrinology* **99:** 780–785.

Pederson RA, Schubert HE & Brown JC (1975) Gastric inhibitory polypeptide. Its physiological release and insulinotropic action in the dog. *Diabetes* **24:** 1050–1056.

Perley MJ & Kipnis DM (1967) Plasma insulin responses to oral and intravenous glucose: studies in normal and diabetic subjects. *Journal of Clinical Investigation* **46:** 1954–1962.

Pfeiffer EF, Telib M, Ammon J, Melani F & Ditschuneit H (1965) Direkte Stimulierung der Insulinsekretion in vitro durch Sekretin. *Deutsches Medizinische Wochenschrift* **90:** 1663–1667.

Rabinovitch A & Dupré J (1972) Insulinotropic and glucagonotropic activities of crude preparation of cholecystokinin-pancreozymin. *Clinical Research* **20:** 945 (Abstract).

Ross SA, Brown JC & Dupré J (1977) Hypersecretion of gastric inhibitory polypeptide following oral glucose in diabetes mellitus. *Diabetes* **26:** 525–529.

Salera M, Giacomoni P, Pironi L et al (1982) Gastric inhibitory polypeptide release after oral glucose: relationship to glucose intolerance, diabetes mellitus, and obesity. *Journal of Clinical Endocrinology and Metabolism* **55:** 329–336.

Sykes S, Morgan LM, English J & Marks V (1980) Evidence of preferential stimulation of gastric inhibitory polypeptide secretion in the rat by actively transported carbohydrates and their analogues. *Journal of Endocrinology* **85:** 210–217.

Thomas FB, Sinar D, Mazzaferri EL et al (1978) Selective release of gastric inhibitory polypeptide by intraduodenal amino acid perfusion in man. *Gastroenterology* **74:** 1261–1265.

Unger RH & Eisentraut AM (1969) Entero-insular axis. *Archives of Internal Medicine* **123:** 261–266.

Unger RH, Ketterer H, Dupré J & Eisentraut AM (1967) The effects of secretin, pancreozymin and gastrin on insulin and glucagon secretion in anesthetized dogs. *Journal of Clinical Investigations* **46:** 630–645.

Wang CC & Grossman MI (1951) Physiological determination of release of secretin and pancreozymin from intestine of dog with transplanted pancreas. *American Journal of Physiology* **164:** 527–545.

Zunz E & Labarre J (1929) Contributions à l'étude des variations physiologiques de la sécrétion interne du pancréas: Relations entre les sécrétions externe et interne du pancréas. *Archives of International Physiology* **31:** 20–44.

6

Hypertension

P. L. DRURY

Hypertension in patients with non-insulin-dependent diabetes (NIDDM) has become a topic of great theoretical and practical interest over recent years (First International Symposium on Hypertension Associated with Diabetes, 1985). This chapter will try to put into context advances in the understanding of its pathogenesis as well as providing a practical approach to the investigation and management of the condition. There are, however, excellent comprehensive reviews of the epidemiology of hypertension in diabetes (Fuller, 1985; Pacy, 1987) and of the detailed use of individual groups of drugs in treatment of hypertension (Struthers, 1985; Peiris and Gustafson, 1986; Working Group on Hypertension in Diabetes, 1987; Kendall et al, 1988) which will not be covered in great detail here.

EPIDEMIOLOGY

General principles

It is a widely held view that there is a major association between hypertension and non-insulin-dependent diabetes, a contention supported by the everyday observation of those working in diabetic clinics that a very high proportion of such patients are frankly hypertensive by World Health Organization (WHO) criteria (Table 1), or are already receiving anti-hypertensive therapy.

Scientific proof for the assertion is more difficult to find and there remains continuing controversy as to whether it is entirely or partly a true association, or whether it can be explained by factors such as body weight, selection bias for hospital-based studies and possible variation of the blood pressure (BP) at or after diagnosis. Much of the early epidemiological work,

Table 1. WHO criteria for hypertension in adults.

	Systolic	Diastolic
Normotension	< 140	< 90
Borderline	140–160	90–95
Hypertension	≥ 160	≥ 95

All pressures are in mm Hg.

and some of that more recently published, has major flaws in the method-ology in factors such as choice of the control group, comparability of study methods for diabetic and control groups, use of the appropriate size cuffs for blood pressure measurement and correction of blood pressure for obesity (Table 2), (Fuller, 1985).

In contrast to the situation in insulin-dependent diabetes (IDDM), use of the WHO criteria for hypertension is reasonable in most patients with NIDDM since they are older, and since the definition is similar to the level at which benefit from treatment is claimed in more recent intervention studies in non-diabetics (Sleight, 1987).

The finding by Kelleher et al (1988) of an increased prevalence of hyper-tension among the siblings of patients with known NIDDM, again suggest-ing a link between the two conditions, is of some interest.

Table 2. Potential confounding issues in the apparent association between non-insulin-dependent diabetes and hypertension.

Obesity—The measurement error effect (inadequate cuff size etc)

The real effect of increasing BP with increasing body weight

Sampling bias of hospital study populations

Indirect association of diabetogenic action of some widely-used anti-hypertensive agents (e.g. thiazide/beta-blockers)

Detection bias—diabetics seen and BP measured more often

International epidemiology

The recent WHO multi-national study of vascular disease in diabetics aged between 35 and 54 (including insulin-dependent, insulin-treated and non-insulin-dependent patients) showed that 22–39% of men were hypertensive, with a mean of 32%, while the range in women was from 26–49% with a mean of 36% (WHO Multinational Study, 1985). While there is significant difference between the centres, there is a remarkable consistency overall in the figures.

Raw figures from several studies in Western Europe show the prevalence of measured hypertension in diabetic clinics is as high as 50% in patients under 65 years of age, the highest rates being seen in women and Afro-Caribbeans (Pacy et al, 1987).

Most would now agree that there is good evidence that systolic blood pressure is significantly higher in men and women with newly-detected and borderline diabetes, but that the difference is either absent or less marked in those with previously diagnosed diabetes. There may be also a significant excess of hypertension in the very elderly (Barrett-Connor et al, 1981).

For the interested reader, detailed reviews of this complex subject have recently been published (Fuller, 1985; Pacy, 1987). Whatever the argu-ments, all would agree with three simple statements: that hypertension is a common problem in patients with NIDDM by whatever criteria are used; that it frequently does not respond to non-pharmacological intervention; and that choice of appropriate therapy is often difficult.

The role of diabetic nephropathy

Unlike the situation in insulin-dependent diabetes (Mogensen, 1988a), only a small proportion of patients with NIDDM will have progressive diabetic nephropathy, if defined as falling glomerular filtration rate, as a cause of their hypertension. The duration of diabetes is a confounding factor here, as patients with NIDDM have a lesser life expectancy than those with IDDM and frequently die of ischaemic heart disease before they might be expected to develop progressive nephropathy. Persistent proteinuria appears to be at least as common in NIDDM as in IDDM, but less often progresses to renal failure (Fabre et al, 1982; Cooper et al, 1988). The issue, however, remains contentious.

It is vital to identify these patients since treatment of hypertension may slow the rate of deterioration as in IDDM (Drury, unpublished data). There are reports showing an increased prevalence of progressive nephropathy among non-white populations with NIDDM compared with local European populations, certainly for American Blacks and British Afro-Caribbean and Asian patients (Grenfell and Watkins, 1986; Grenfell et al, 1988).

The pathogenesis and treatment of nephropathy and hypertension are discussed in great detail in a recent comprehensive volume, though much of this refers to IDDM (Mogensen, 1988b).

MORTALITY AND HYPERTENSION IN NIDDM

In the non-diabetic population there is unequivocal and extensive data showing that blood pressure, both systolic and diastolic, is a major factor determining mean life expectancy and that this relationship extends throughout the range of blood pressure, lowest mortality being associated with lowest blood pressure (Society of Actuaries, 1980). Evidence from both cohort insurance and population studies in diabetes, mainly but not exclusively NIDDM, is entirely consistent with this, the major increase in cause of death being coronary heart disease with a smaller component from stroke. Despite these findings a large proportion of the excess mortality risk could not be explained by the non-cardiovascular risk factors of diabetes, hypertension, hyperlipidaemia and smoking (Kannel and McGee, 1979a, 1979b; Fuller et al, 1983).

The best known data are from the Framingham, Bedford and Whitehall studies, where there were stronger associations between BP, especially systolic, and cardiovascular mortality than were found with smoking, cholesterol and obesity. The relationship extended to those with impaired glucose tolerance. In the Whitehall study, the relative mortality risks for the top quintile of systolic BP compared with the lower four quintiles were 1.90 for normoglycaemia, 2.42 for glucose intolerance and 2.60 for diabetes

(Fuller et al, 1983). The mortality data are shown in Figure 1 taken from their paper.

Similar data have been reported in a much smaller study by Aromaa et al (1984) in Finland.

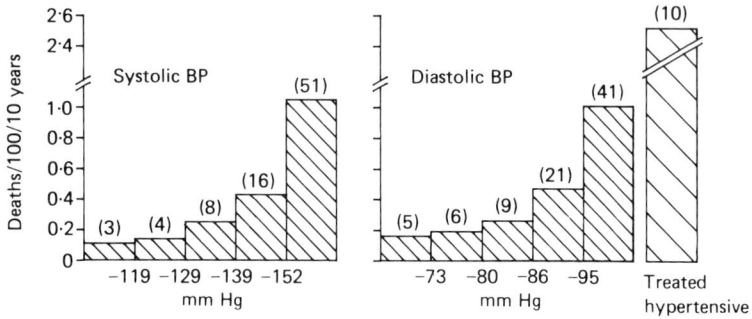

Figure 1. Relationship of 10 year stroke mortality to blood pressure in the Whitehall study. From Fuller et al (1983), with permission.

AETIOLOGY AND PATHOGENESIS

In the absence of better understanding of the pathogeneses of the condition involved, any classification of hypertension in diabetes is at present simply pragmatic. Table 3 is designed simply to aid sensible diagnosis and management.

The great majority of patients have apparent essential hypertension and, except where specifically stated, the following discussion refers to this combination. Two areas where there has been recent progress are discussed here; other possible pathogenetic factors including the role of the renin–

Table 3. A classification of hypertension in NIDDM.

Secondary diabetes and hypertension
  Acromegaly
  Phaeochromocytoma
  Cushing's syndrome
  Drug-induced (e.g. oestrogen/steroids)

Secondary hypertension and unrelated diabetes
  Primary renal disease (e.g. renal artery stenosis)
  Drug-induced (e.g. oestrogens/steroid)

Hypertension associated with progressive nephropathy

Coincident essential hypertension

Isolated systolic hypertension

angiotensin system and catecholamines have recently been reviewed in detail (Drury, 1985).

Hyperinsulinism and hypertension

There has been much interest in the relationship between blood pressure and insulin, especially in the obese (Reaven and Hoffman, 1987), though relatively little of the experimental work has directly concerned the hypertensive diabetic patient.

The complex initial evidence can be summarized as follows:

1. Patients with high BP are less glucose tolerant than matched patients with normal BP (Jarrett et al, 1978).
2. Patients with untreated hypertension have higher insulin levels than matched normotensive controls (Modan et al, 1985; Manicardi et al, 1986).
3. There is a very significant correlation between plasma insulin concentration and blood pressure (Lucas et al, 1985; Manicardi et al, 1986).
4. Fall in BP after exercise training programmes seems to be limited to those who are initially hyperinsulinaemic and whose plasma insulin levels fall most (Krotiewski et al, 1979).

More recent studies like those of Ferranini et al (1987) have measured insulin sensitivity, glucose turnover and whole body glucose oxidation in young patients with essential hypertension and in age- and weight-matched normal controls. They found total glucose uptake to be inversely related to both systolic and diastolic BP and evidence of insulin resistance involving glucose but not lipid or potassium metabolism. Mbanya and colleagues (1988), with rather small numbers in some groups and examining only the basal fasting state, studied control subjects, essential (non-diabetic) hypertensives and both normotensive and hypertensive patients with NIDDM, measuring fasting glucose, insulin and C–peptide. They found normal fasting insulin levels and normal glucose : insulin ratios in the patients with essential hypertension while the hypertensive NIDDM group had higher fasting insulin levels and lower glucose : insulin ratios than all other groups.

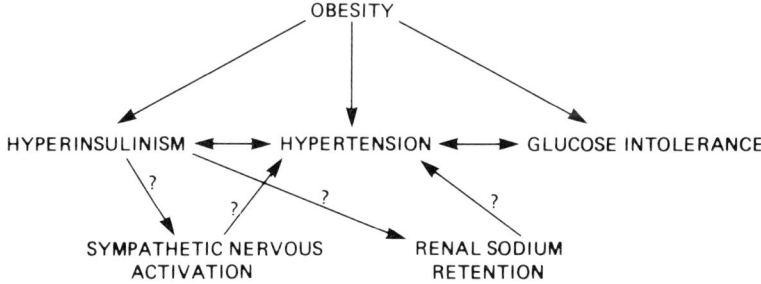

Figure 2. Possible relationships between insulin and hypertension.

The hypertensive diabetics had the highest insulin : C-peptide ratios suggesting that low hepatic extraction of insulin may play a role.

Explanations for the association include the effect of insulin on renal sodium retention demonstrated by DeFronzo (1981) and an effect on activation of the sympathetic nervous system. These and other possible mechanisms are discussed by Landsberg (1987).

No unified hypothesis is yet possible from this wealth of data with the many relationships involved. Figure 2 shows the well-recognized connections, though it should be emphasized that these are associations and that a causal link has not been proven.

Sodium

Exchangeable sodium is increased by about 10% in all untreated groups of NIDDM, whether hypertensive or not (Weidmann et al, 1985). The distribution of this additional 10% is unclear, though it is reduced to normal in hypertensive subjects with the use of thiazide diuretics. It only correlates with blood pressure in those subjects with NIDDM and diabetic nephropathy (O'Hare et al, 1985) suggesting that it may not be causally related to BP in those without renal involvement. The NIDDM patients with nephropathy appear to show similar pathophysiological changes to those with IDDM and nephropathy.

PRACTICAL INVESTIGATION

The first and essential requirement is that measurement of blood pressure should be accurately and reproducibly performed with reliable equipment; the British Hypertension Society has recently published simple guidelines (Petrie et al, 1987). Rarely should less than three sets of readings over a period of a month be used for diagnosis unless there is incontrovertible evidence of severe hypertension.

Investigation of hypertension in this situation is for four main purposes:

1. To exclude secondary causes of hypertension and/or diabetes.
2. To establish the degree of organ damage, especially to heart and kidneys.
3. To determine whether other risk factors are present, especially smoking and hyperlipidaemias.
4. To assist in choice of type, order or dosage of therapy.

Is secondary hypertension present?

Very little modern data is available for the prevalence of the secondary causes of hypertension among patients with NIDDM. All available information (and clinical common sense!) shows acromegaly, Cushing's syndrome and phaeochromocytoma to be very uncommon, yet when they do occur they are frequently missed for long periods. Few would consider that biochemical screening for these abnormalities on every patient is worthwhile, but the question should be asked each time, simple clinical histories taken and the relevant signs sought. Where there is a serious possibility, then full investigation should be undertaken.

A more difficult problem is that of other renal causes, especially renal artery stenosis. There is conflicting evidence as to whether it is truly commoner in diabetes, and this may well reflect the differing groups of patients studied (Munichoodappa et al, 1979). Where widespread vascular disease of the peripheral and coronary vasculature is present, then the possibility must be borne in mind. Routine investigation is not practically possible or justifiable, but significant renal dysfunction, a history of renal problems or haematuria warrant further studies. Careful follow-up of renal function after institution of hypotensive therapy is mandatory; any unexplained deterioration in renal function should alert the clinician to the possibility and provoke investigation, often requiring renal arteriography.

Is there evidence of end-organ damage?

In all but the very elderly the author believes, but cannot prove, that all diabetic hypertensive patients should have basic investigations including serum creatinine, urinalyis, electrocardiogram and chest X-ray.

In essential hypertension, the presence of end-organ damage is associated with a poorer outcome. Electrocardiographic (ECG) evidence of left ventricular hypertrophy (LVH) and/or evidence of ischaemic heart disease and cardiomegaly, implying ventricular dilatation, appear to carry the same associations in diabetes. In particular ECG evidence of LVH, an insensitive test, suggests long-standing significant hypertension. It is likely that echocardiographic assessment of LVH will be more widely used in the future.

Renal impairment may not result from hypertensive changes but warrants investigation as a possible cause of the hypertension. It may limit the use or dosage of some drugs e.g. calcium antagonists, ACE inhibitors, while proteinuria, even microalbuminuria, is associated with a worse prognosis in NIDDM particularly from ischaemic heart disease (Jarrett et al, 1984; Mogensen, 1986). The relationship also appears to be true in non-diabetic subjects, and appears to be a non-specific marker of widespread vascular disease (Yudkin et al, 1988). As such it appears that microalbuminuria carries different, though equally serious, implications in NIDDM compared with IDDM.

Are other risk factors present?

Hypertension should not be considered on its own. Other risk factors for mortality, morbidity and complications should be included in the overall assessment. Most important of these are smoking, hyperlipidaemia and diabetic control.

Do the results alter type or dosage of therapy?

Many of the implications of these investigations have already been discussed. Cardiomegaly or evidence of heart failure will militate against the use of negatively inotropic drugs (e.g. beta-blockers, nifedipine) and suggest the use of ACE inhibitors and/or diuretics, while evidence of ischaemic heart disease without failure would favour calcium antagonists and cardioselective beta-blockers. There is insufficient evidence as to which drugs are most effective but reasonable parallels with the MRC mild hypertension study would suggest that beta-blockers are better tolerated by men and diuretics by women (MRC Working Party, 1981).

Impaired renal function will reduce the required dosage of many of these drugs, and acute deterioration after institution or increase of therapy should prompt a reappraisal for renal artery stenosis.

TREATMENT

Non-pharmacological measures

Recent years have seen a welcome reappraisal of the role of non-drug therapy for hypertension (Table 4). While some measures, such as reducing smoking and caffeine intake, are simply good clinical practice, others remain highly controversial even in non-diabetic hypertension.

There are few data on the effect on these individual manoeuvres on blood pressure in NIDDM, though the effect of weight reduction alone is worthwhile and certain (Reisen et al, 1978). Dodson and colleagues (1984), in a series of well-controlled studies, used a high fibre, low fat and low sodium diet in patients with NIDDM and mild hypertension and found a useful significant reduction of BP from 181/97 to 165/88 mm Hg compared with changes of 170/97 to 164/95 mm Hg in the control group. Weight, urinary sodium, HbA1 and triglycerides all fell in the treated group, making it impossible to know which of the components were predominantly responsible for the improvement. In further studies the same group have shown that similar modified diets are as effective at reducing BP as metoprolol (Pacy et al, 1984a) and bendrofluazide (Pacy et al, 1984b) while only the diet-treated patients showed significant improvements in risk factors such as lipid profile and glycaemic control.

Table 4. Non-pharmacological measures for control of hypertension.

Weight loss
Alcohol reduction
Dietary sodium restriction
Dietary potassium increase
Dietary fibre increase
Reduction of simultaneous smoking/caffeine intake
Increased physical exercise
Relaxation

Pharmacological measures

The drugs currently available for hypertension in diabetes are legion and few have been subjected to comparative controlled trial in patients with NIDDM. The main groups are listed in Table 5, together with a single recent reference to the use of each major group in NIDDM.

There are, however, four main groups of agents currently used for institution of anti-hypertensive treatment in the UK (in alphabetical order) ACE inhibitors, beta-blockers, calcium antagonists and diuretics. Vasodilators, combined alpha-beta blockers and centrally acting agents are all used to a lesser extent.

Single-agent comparisons suggest that all these groups are effective as anti-hypertensive agents, while only Corcoran et al (1987) have studied combinations finding atenolol, nifedipine and captopril with bendrofluazide all more effective than bendrofluazide alone. There was no clear evidence of

Table 5. Major groups of anti-hypertensive drugs and side effects of particular relevance in diabetes.

ANGIOTENSIN-CONVERTING ENZYME INHIBITORS (Gambara et al, 1985) Captopril Enalapril Lisinopril	Renal impairment (rare) Hyperkalaemia
CALCIUM ANTAGONISTS (Abadie et al, 1985; Odigwe et al, 1986) Nifedipine (especially SR) Diltiazem Verapamil (especially SR)	Negative inotropic action Ankle oedema Some doubt on glucose tolerance
CARDIOSELECTIVE BETA-BLOCKERS (Ostman, 1983) Atenolol Bisoprolol Metoprolol	Impairment of glucose tolerance Worsened lipid profile Poor recovery from hypoglycaemia Sexual dysfunction Worsen peripheral vascular symptoms
DIURETICS (Houston, 1986; Berglund et al, 1986) Thiazides	Impairment of glucose tolerance Worsened lipid profile Sexual dysfunction Hypokalaemia May precipitate hyperosmolar state
Indapamide and frusemide have fewer problems (See Osei et al, 1986 for indapamide) *Combined alpha-beta blocker* Labetolol	Same as beta-blockade
Centrally acting agents Methyl dopa	Orthostatic hypotension Impotence
Vasodilators/α-adrenergic blockers Hydrallazine	Postural hypotension, impotence Tachycardia
Prazosin	First-dose syncope

SR = Sustained release. For more complete data see National High Blood Pressure Education Program (1988).

any superiority of any agent on blood pressure control, side effects or metabolic changes, although the numbers were too small to exclude this possibility.

Several suggested lines of pharmacological therapy for hypertensive diabetics have recently been published (Struthers, 1985; Peiris and Gustafson, 1986; Kaplan et al, 1987; Working Group on Hypertension in Diabetes, 1987; Kendall et al, 1988). These largely rework previous lines of discussion and reiterate the lack of true multiple-drug comparative studies as opposed to industry-funded single agent comparisons.

The US Working Group Report concentrated largely on the role of thiazides and beta-blockers, the latter endorsed by Kendall et al (1988) while the others emphasize the relative immediate safety of ACE inhibitors, calcium antagonists and prazosin (Struthers, 1985; Kaplan et al, 1987).

There is thus no widespread consensus of opinion on optimal drug therapy and insufficient data on which to base absolute guidelines—indeed the same can be said for essential hypertension. There is a welcome tendency to regard choice of an anti-hypertensive agent as an individual selection for each patient, taking into account age, sex and race as well as their own risk factors, complications and other medical problems. A valuable recent American report is worthy of study (National High Blood Pressure Education Program, 1988).

The suggestions given here are thus personal and based on my own interpretation of the relative importance of the efficacy, tolerability and long-term effects of the respective agents:

1. There is no place in NIDDM for the use of non-selective beta-blockers, especially propranolol. The effects on lipids and glucose tolerance are greater than those of the wide selection of selective agents now available.
2. Thiazide diuretics should only be used in the lowest of doses. While they are rational therapy for hypertension in this situation, their anti-hypertensive effect is little if any increased while the metabolic consequences on glucose tolerance and lipids appear to be dose-related, probably related in part to decreased body potassium. Chlorthalidone, which causes the worst hypokalaemia, should be avoided.
3. The combination of thiazides and beta-blockers should be avoided whenever possible as the metabolic disadvantages are at least additive (Bengsston et al, 1984), with a relative risk for diabetes of 14 for the combination compared with three and six for the individual components. If used at all, minimum doses should be employed and combinations including chlorthalidone (e.g. Tenoretic, Lopresoretic) eschewed.
4. While many of the metabolic consequences of diuretic therapy can be avoided by prevention of hypokalaemia (Helderman et al, 1983), potassium-sparing agents should be used with care as they can cause fatal hyperkalaemia in diabetes. Additionally spironolactone has recently been withdrawn for essential hypertension in the UK because of concerns over tumour development in rats.

Treatment of specific problems

Apparent hypertension in the newly-diagnosed

Unless pressure is dangerously high, perhaps above 180/110 mm Hg, drug therapy should await confirmation of BP levels after initial dietary management of diabetes, ideally with weight loss and adequate control of the diabetes.

Patients with claudication

There is clear evidence that all beta-blockers, including those with intrinsic sympathetic activity, reduce exercise tolerance compared with placebo or captopril in non-diabetic patients with claudication (Roberts et al, 1987). First-line therapy should therefore be chosen from ACE inhibitors, calcium antagonists or low-dose thiazide diuretics—particular attention needs to be paid to the patients' cardiac status.

Patients with ischaemic heart disease

Unfortunately there remains no convincing evidence of any primary 'cardio-protective' effect of beta-blockers, but they or calcium antagonists will often be used if angina is present or if the patient has already had an infarct. If there is evidence of left ventricular failure or significant cardiomegaly then diuretics and/or ACE inhibitors should be the preferred line of therapy, though the combination of beta-blockade and thiazide diuretic is best avoided in view of its metabolic effects (see above).

Patients with hypertension and heart failure

As implied above diuretics and/or ACE inhibitors are preferred first-line agents; care must be taken not to impair renal perfusion and regular creatinine and electrolyte measurements are mandatory.

Patients with impotence

Both beta-blockers and diuretics are associated with impotence, as are many of the older hypotensive agents (e.g. methyl dopa, guanethidine). While the problem is frequently multifactorial, with a vascular component in particular, these agents are best avoided and ACE inhibitors, calcium antagonists and prazosin (Lipson, 1984) used in preference.

Patients of Afro-Caribbean origin

These subjects usually respond poorly to beta-blockers and ACE inhibitors as single agents, while diuretics are especially effective. Calcium antagonists are equally effective as are diuretic + beta-blocker/ACE combinations. These differences probably reflect a genetically determined slower excretion of sodium in this racial group. There is little information on other racial groups.

Follow up, compliance and measures of success

There has been little recent work on the audit of anti-hypertensive therapy, and less still in diabetic hypertensives. Compliance appears to be less of a problem than previously, perhaps because of patient understanding of the aims of treatment, the use of drugs with fewer side effects and less frequent dosage regimes and increasing co-operation and communication between hospital physicians and GPs.

Many clinics now use a co-operation card carrying details of medication and BP readings for each patient, and some patients now measure their own BP or have it checked at the workplace. It can be easily combined as part of a diabetic shared care scheme.

Setting of a 'target' pressure is worthwhile, taking into account age and sex, while objective evidence of response may be obtained from loss of signs of left ventricular hypertrophy on ECG and reduction in cardiothoracic ratio on chest X-ray where these were abnormal. Renal function and plasma potassium should be checked regularly while on treatment.

Finally the physician must remain alert to the development of side-effects and check on the 'quality of life' while patients are taking these powerful agents.

SUMMARY

The awareness of hypertension as one of the major risk factors for mortality and morbidity in NIDDM has increased greatly in the past few years. It is now accepted practice to measure BP at least yearly in all such patients. Unfortunately, one cannot yet be sure to what extent diabetics benefit from anti-hypertensive therapy, and the simple assumption that treatment of the increased risk reduces that risk must be constantly questioned. No specific data are yet available for NIDDM, though it would be remarkable if the benefits of decreased cerebrovascular mortality and probable reduced total mortality (Sleight, 1987) did not apply to the higher-risk diabetic subject, at least at the higher levels of diastolic pressure (>105 mm Hg). There is, though, no evidence that mortality or morbidity of coronary artery disease, the major killer in NIDDM, is reduced even in non-diabetics and the present author does not consider there to be any evidence suggesting that thresholds for treatment of hypertension in uncomplicated patients with NIDDM should be lower than those for non-diabetics, unless progressive nephropathy is present. Current advice in the non-diabetic is that levels of blood pressure in adults consistently above 95 mm Hg warrant therapy, aiming to reduce it below 90 mm Hg (World Health Organization, 1986).

While the importance of hypertension should not be underestimated, it should not deflect attention from the other risk factors. Cessation of smoking, and by implication its reduction, will, for all smoking patients but the most hypertensive, produce a greater reduction in cardiovascular and total mortality risk than will anti-hypertensive therapy. There are also early signs that effective dietary and/or drug treatment of significant hyperlipidaemia lowers cardiovascular mortality.

Choice of anti-hypertensive therapy is especially important, not only for efficacy but also for quality of life, in patients who already suffer major restrictions on diet, freedom and life expectancy. While controlled trials in the subject are of immense importance in determining optimum therapy, there is currently no evidence to favour any particular group of drugs, and an individual patient's therapy should be decided on the basis of their own circumstances.

REFERENCES

Abadie E, Villette JM, Gauville C, Tabuteau F, Fiet J & Passa Ph (1985) Influence of nifedipine on carbohydrate metabolism of non-insulin dependent diabetics. *Diabete et Metabolisme* **11:** 141–146.

Aromaa A, Reunanen A & Pyorala K (1984) Hypertension and mortality in diabetic and non-diabetic Finnish men. *Journal of Hypertension* **2 (supplement 3):** 205–207.

Barrett-Connor E, Criqui MH, Klauber MR & Holdbrook M (1981) Diabetes and hypertension in a community of older adults. *American Journal of Epidemiology* **113:** 276–284.

Bengsston C, Bohlme G, Lapidus L et al (1984) Do antihypertensive drugs precipitate diabetes? *British Medical Journal* **289:** 1495–1497.

Berglund G, Andersson O & Widgren B (1986) Low-dose antihypertensive treatment with a thiazide diuretic is not diabetogenic. *Acta Medica Scandanavica* **220:** 419–424.

Cooper ME, Frauman A, O'Brien RC, Seeman E, Murray RML & Jerums G (1988) Progression of proteinuria in Type 1 and Type 2 diabetes. *Diabetic Medicine* **5:** 361–368.

Corcoran JS, Perkins JE, Hoffbrand BI & Yudkin JS (1987) Treating hypertension in non-insulin-dependent diabetes: a comparison of atenolol, nifedipine, and captopril combined with bendrofluazide. *Diabetic Medicine* **4:** 164–168.

DeFronzo RA (1981) The effect of insulin on renal sodium metabolism: a review with clinical implications. *Diabetologia* **21:** 165–171.

Dodson PM, Pacy PJ, Bal P, Kubicki AJ, Fletcher RF & Taylor KG (1984) A controlled trial of a high fibre, low fat and low sodium diet for mild hypertension in Type 2 (non-insulin-dependent) diabetes. *Diabetologia* **27:** 522–526.

Drury PL (1985) Hypertension in diabetes mellitus. In Edwards CRW & Carey RM (eds) *Essential hypertension as an endocrine disease*, pp 301–332. London: Butterworth.

Fabre J, Balant LP, Dayer PG, Fox HM & Vernet AT (1982) The kidney in maturity onset diabetes mellitus. A clinical study of 510 patients. *Kidney International* **21:** 730–738.

Ferranini E, Buzzigogli G, Bonadonna R et al (1987) Insulin resistance in essential hypertension. *New England Journal of Medicine* **317:** 350–357.

First International Symposium on Hypertension Associated with Diabetes (1985). *Hypertension* **7** (Part II): II-1—II-174.

Fuller JH (1985) Epidemiology of hypertension associated with diabetes mellitus. *Hypertension* **7** (part II): II-3—II-7.

Fuller JH, Shipley MJ, Rose G, Jarrett RJ & Keen H (1983) Coronary heart disease and stroke mortality by degree of glycaemia: the Whitehall study. *British Medical Journal* **287:** 867–870.

Gambara G, Moriato F, Cicerello E et al (1985) Captopril in the treatment of hypertension in Type 1 and Type 2 diabetic patients. *Journal of Hypertension* **3 (supplement 2):** S149–S151.

Grenfell A & Watkins PJ (1986) Clinical diabetic nephropathy: natural history and complications. *Clinics in Endocrinology and Metabolism* **15:** 783–806.

Grenfell A, Bewick M, Parsons V, Snowden S, Taube D & Watkins PJ (1988) Non-insulin-dependent diabetes renal replacement therapy. *Diabetic Medicine* **5:** 172–176.

Helderman JH, Elahi D, Andersen DK et al (1983) Prevention of the glucose intolerance of thiazide diuretics by maintence of body potassium. *Diabetes* **32:** 106–111.

Houston MC (1986) Adverse effects of antihypertensive drug therapy on glucose intolerance. *Cardiology Clinics* **4:** 117–135.

Jarrett RJ, Keen H, McCartney M et al (1978) Glucose tolerance and blood pressure in two population samples: their relation to diabetes mellitus and hypertension. *International Journal of Epidemiology* **7:** 15–24.

Jarrett RJ, Viberti GC, Argyropoulos A, Hill RD, Mahmud U & Murrells TJ (1984) Micro-albuminuria predicts mortality in non-insulin-dependent diabetes. *Diabetic Medicine* **1:** 17–19.

Kannel WB & McGee DL (1979a) Diabetes and cardiovascular disease. The Framingham study. *Journal of the American Medical Association* **241:** 1225–1229.

Kannel WB & McGee DL (1979b) Diabetes and glucose tolerance as risk factors for cardio-vascular disease. the Framingham study. *Diabetes Care* **2:** 120–126.

Kaplan NM, Rosenstock J & Raskin P (1987) A differing view of treatment of hypertension in patients with diabetes mellitus. *Archives of Internal Medicine* **147:** 1160–1162.

Kelleher C, Kingston SM, Barry DG et al (1988) Hypertension in diabetic clinic patients and their siblings. *Diabetologia* **31:** 76–81.

Kendall MJ, Lewis H, Griffith M & Barnett AH (1988) Drug treatment of the hypertensive diabetic. *Journal of Human Hypertension* **1:** 249–258.

Krotiewski M, Mandroukas K, Sjostrom L, Sullivan L, Wetterauist H & Bjorntorp P (1979) Effects of long-term physical training on body fat, metabolism and blood pressure in obesity. *Metabolism* **28:** 650–658.

Landsberg L (1987) Insulin and hypertension: lessons from obesity. *New England Journal of Medicine* **317:** 378–379.

Lipson LG (1984) Treatment of hypertension in diabetic men: problems with sexual dysfunc-tion. *American Journal of Cardiology* **53:** 46A–50A.

Lucas CP, Estigaribia JA, Darga LL & Reaven GM (1985) Insulin and blood pressure in obesity. *Hypertension* **7:** 702–706.

Manicardi V, Camellini L, Bellodi G, Coscelli C & Ferranini E (1986) Evidence for an association of high blood pressure and hyperinsulinaemia in obese man. *Journal of Clinical Endocrinology and Metabolism* **62:** 1302–1304.

Mbanya J-C, Thomas TH, Wilkinson R, Alberti KGMM & Taylor R (1988) Hypertension and hyperinsulinaemia: a relationship in diabetes but not in essential hypertension. *Lancet* **i:** 733–734.

Modan M, Halkin H, Almog G et al (1985) Hyperinsulinaemia: a link between hypertension, obesity and glucose tolerance. *Journal of Clinical Investigation* **75:** 809–815.

Mogensen CE (1986) Microalbuminuria predicts clinical proteinuria and early mortality in matuuity-onset diabetes. *New England Journal of Medicine* **310:** 356–360.

Mogensen CE (1988a) Management of diabetic renal involvement and disease. *Lancet* **i:** 867–870.

Mogensen CE (1988b) *The kidney and hypertension in diabetes mellitus*, 423pp. Amsterdam: Martinus Nijhoff.

MRC Working Party on Mild to Moderate Hypertension (1981) Adverse reactions to bendro-fluazide and propranolol for the treatment of mild hypertension. *Lancet* **ii:** 539–543.

Munichoodappa C, D'Elia JA, Libertino JA, Gleason RE & Christlieb AR (1979) Renal artery stenosis in hypertensive diabetics. *Journal of Urology* **121:** 555–558.

National High Blood Pressure Education Program (1988) The 1988 report of the Joint National Committee on detection, evaluation and treatment of high blood pressure. *Archives of Internal Medicine* **148:** 1023–1038.

Odigwe CO, McCulloch AJ, Williams DO & Tunbridge WMG (1986) A trial of the calcium antagonist Nisoldipine in hypertensive non-insulin-dependent diabetic patients. *Diabetic Medicine* **3:** 463–467.

O'Hare JA, Ferriss JB, Brady D, Twomey B & O'Sullivan DJ (1985) Exchangeable sodium and renin in hypertensive diabetic patients with and without nephropathy. *Hypertension* **7** (part II): II–43—II–48.

Osei K, Holland G & Falko JM (1986) Indapamide—effects on apoprotein, lipoprotein, and glucoregulation in ambulatory diabetic patients. *Archives of Internal Medicine* **146:** 1973–1977.

Ostman J (1983) Beta-adrenergic blockade and diabetes mellitus. A review. *Acta Medica Scandanavica* **Supplement 672:** 69–77.

Pacy PJ (1987) Hypertension and diabetes mellitus. In Taylor KG (ed.) *Diabetes and the Heart*, pp 42–60. Tunbridge Wells: Castle House Publications.

Pacy PJ, Dobson PM, Kubicki AJ, Fletcher RF & Taylor KG (1984a) Comparison of the hypertensive and metabolic effects of metoprolol therapy with a high fibre, low sodium, low fat diet in hypertensive Type 2 diabetic subjects. *Diabetes Research* **1:** 201–207.

Pacy PJ, Dodson PM, Kubicki AJ, Fletcher RF & Taylor KG (1984b) Comparison of the hypotensive and metabolic effects of bendrofluazide therapy with a high fibre, low sodium, low fat diet in diabetic subjects with mild hypertension. *Journal of Hypertension* **2:** 215–220.

Periris AN & Gustafson AB (1986) Current therapeutic concepts in diabetic hypertension. *Diabetes Care* **9:** 409–414.

Petrie JC, O'Brien ET, Littler WA & De Swiet M (1987) *Recommendations on blood pressure measurement*. London: BMJ publications.

Reaven GM & Hoffman BB (1987) A role for insulin in the aetiology and course of hypertension? *Lancet* **ii:** 435–437.

Reisen E, Abel R, Modam M, Silverberg DS, Eliahou HE & Modan B (1978) Effect of weight loss without salt restriction on reduction of blood pressure in overweight hypertensive patients. *New England Journal of Medicine* **289:** 1–6.

Roberts DH, Tsao Y, McLoughlin GA & Breckenridge A (1987) Placebo-controlled comparison of captopril, atenolol, labetolol and pindolol in hypertension complicated by intermittent claudication. *Lancet* **ii:** 650–653.

Sleight P (1987) Essential Hypertension. In Weatherall, Ledingham & Warrell (eds) *Oxford Textbook of Medicine*, pp 13.360–13.382. Second edition. Oxford: Oxford University Press.

Society of Actuaries (1980) *Blood Pressure Study, 1979*. Chicago: Society of Actuaries.

Struthers AD (1985) The choice of anti-hypertensive therapy in the diabetic patient. *Postgraduate Medical Journal* **61:** 563–569.

Weidmann P, Beretta-Piccoli C & Trost BN (1985) Pressor factors and responsiveness in hypertension accompanying diabetes mellitus. *Hypertension* **7 (supplement II):** II.33–42.

Working Group on Hypertension in Diabetes (1987) Statement on hypertension in diabetes. *Arch Intern Medicine* **147:** 830–842, 1165–1166.

World Health Organization Multinational Study (1985) Prevalence of small vessel and large vessel disease in diabetic patients from 14 centres. *Diabetologia* **28 (supplement):** 615–640.

World Health Organization (1986) 1986 guidelines for the treatment of mild hypertension: memorandum from the WHO/ISH. *Hypertension* **8:** 957–961.

Yudkin JS, Forrest RD & Jackson CA (1988) Microalbuminuria as predictor of vascular disease in non-diabetic subjects. *Lancet* **2:** 530–533.

7

Pathology of macrovascular disease

THOMAS LEDET
LENE HEICKENDORFF
LARS M. RASMUSSEN

Large vessel disease is a major threat to health in patients with diabetes mellitus. While the pathogenesis remains unresolved, it is generally considered to be of atherosclerotic origin (Ruderman and Haudenschild, 1983). It is important to realize that an alternative hypothesis exits to explain the large vessel damage with the proposal of a specific diabetic macroangiopathy in combination with the usual atherosclerosis (Ledet et al, 1984). In this chapter the development of large vessel damage in patients with diabetes mellitus will be discussed from these two points of view.

DIABETIC ANGIOPATHY—DIABETIC MACROANGIOPATHY

The concept of one generalized specific vascular disease, proposed more than 20 years ago as a working hypothesis for vascular damage in long-term diabetic patients (Lundbaek, 1954), has created extensive confusion due to misinterpretation. The word *specific* indicates an abnormality seen sooner or later in **all** patients. Diabetic retinopathy, for example, is considered a specific diabetic phenomenon but, except for the microaneurysm, the individual retinal lesions can be demonstrated in other diseases. Also, not all diabetic patients will develop retinopathy. Consequently, from a pedantic standpoint, diabetic retinopathy is not a specific diabetic feature. Nonetheless it must still be considered pathognomonic of diabetes since the disease can be diagnosed from the retinal appearance. Thus the specificity is derived from a characteristic constellation of retinal lesions. By analogy, a specific angiopathy implies a set of unique vessel changes, or constellation of abnormalities, seen in most patients with long-term diabetes mellitus.

A second important point in the hypothesis of a diabetic angiopathy is the *generalization* of the vessel lesions. The changes in the vessel wall may slowly pervade the total blood vessel system giving rise to a variety of pictures in various organs.

Furthermore the existence of a *causal* relationship between classical metabolic abnormalities of diabetes and the development of vessel damage is an essential third requirement of the hypothesis.

Finally, use of the term *complication* may cause confusion since, strictly, it describes a morbid event occurring during a disease which is not an essential part of the disease. By definition therefore, diabetic angiopathy is a long-term manifestation of diabetes rather than a complication.

Diabetic macroangiopathy

The term diabetic macroangiopathy was introduced to indicate the presence of non-atherosclerotic specific large vessel disease in diabetic patients (Lundbaek, 1971). As part of diabetic angiopathy it represents a constellation of changes seen in the entire large blood vessel system rather than early and severe atherosclerosis confined to particular vessels or territories.

VESSEL WALL CHANGES IN HUMAN ARTERIES

Many reports of the prevalence and severity of arterial disease in diabetic patients have emanated from studies carried out in the Tecumseh (Epstein et al, 1965) and Framingham (Kannel and McGee, 1979) communities in the USA, civil servants in the Whitehall study in Britain (Reid et al, 1974), and the WHO multinational study (WHO, 1985). They all reported an increased incidence of cardiac disease among diabetic patients compared with non-diabetic subjects. While information about the structural changes in the large vessel wall are of utmost importance, any attempt to separate diabetic macroangiopathy from atherosclerosis on a morphological basis has been so infrequent that the amount of available data is rather limited. Since most studies have beeen designed to describe aspects of the lipid-atherosclerosis hypothesis it is important to realise that atherosclerosis is commonly conceived as a disease which involves the appearance of spotty intima lesions as fatty streaks and fibrous plaques. In the opinion of most workers in the field, the disease pattern of atherosclerosis is, in one way or another, related to a lipoprotein alteration or an abnormal passage of lipoprotein into the vessel wall.

Morphology

Lefkovits (1937) analysed the histological picture of the coronary arteries from a group of 31 diabetic and 20 non-diabetic patients. The presence of well developed intima thickening in the arteries from diabetic patients was observed although quantification was not attempted. The next reasonable morphological investigation was published three decades later by Goodale et al (1962). In this analysis quantification was performed on a carefully selected group of coronary arteries obtained from maturity onset diabetics and non-diabetics matched for age and sex. The thickness of the wall of the extramural arteries was found to be greater in samples from diabetic compared to non-diabetic patients. It was pointed out that lumen narrowing of the extramural arteries was not able to account for the frequency of myocardial infarction although most of the diabetic patients were rather old.

In a histomorphometric study of immersion fixed hearts from 10 non-insulin-dependent diabetic and 10 non-diabetic patients the thickness of the tunica media measured by micrometer was significantly reduced in peripheral segments from the diabetic patients (Dybdahl and Ledet, 1987). More recently, a highly significant correlation between arterial wall thickness measured by ultrasound and duration of diabetes was observed in 19 insulin-dependent patients (Christensen and Neubauer, 1988a, b).

The extent of raised lesions in the aorta and coronary arteries has been examined in a large multinational study (Robertson and Strong, 1968). Large vessels from diabetic patients had larger lesions than vessels from non-diabetic patients although the investigation was by macroscopic inspection and a difference in the detailed appearance could not therefore be detected. In a semi-quantitative study of non-insulin-dependent and non-diabetic patients, Waller et al (1980) found the average number of coronary arteries with greater than 75% narrowing was almost identical (2.5 versus 3.0). Diabetic patients had more severe luminal narrowing when symptomatic heart disease was present and the degree of narrowing was the same in proximal and distal segments. No relationship was observed between duration of diabetes and lumen size but the frequency of retinopathy was increased in diabetic patients with heart disease.

An important study on young insulin-dependent patients, below the age when atherosclerosis usually develops, examined extramural coronary arteries using the same semi-quantitative analysis as above. Lumen size was decreased by 50% or more in about half of the length of the segments compared with only 1% severe narrowing in arteries from non-diabetic patients (Crall and Roberts, 1978).

The frequency of diffuse coronary artery disease, examined by a combination of post mortem arteriography and histology, was significantly greater in 185 patients with predominantly non-insulin-dependent diabetes and 185 sex-matched non-diabetic patients (Vigorita et al, 1980). In another study when diffuse arterial disease was diagnosed from in vivo coronary arteriograms no difference was observed although the 37 insulin-dependent and non-insulin-dependent patients and the 70 non-diabetic patients were carefully matched for age, sex, blood pressure and hyperlipidaemia (Dortimer et al, 1977).

Although there is a paucity of data on wall thickness and lumen size it seems that large arteries from diabetic patients develop thicker walls but thinner tunica media than non-diabetic individuals. The changes in the thickness of the wall appear to correlate with duration of diabetes. The arterial lumen is unchanged in young diabetic patients without manifestations and reduced in young diabetics with severe long-term manifestations and in non-insulin-dependent patients with heart disease. The frequency of diffuse arterial disease is increased and correlates with duration of diabetes.

Histochemistry and biochemistry

In recent years the arterial wall has been investigated using modern histochemical and biochemical techniques. When we examined the extramural coronary arteries from 20 elderly diabetic and 20 non-diabetic patients by semiquantitative histological and histochemical evaluation 20 years ago, the arterial changes obtained from the diabetic patients were particularly prominent in the peripheral segments with the presence of an accumulation of a periodic-acid-Schiff (PAS)-positive material and deposition of calcium (Ledet, 1968). Although no analysis was performed in detail the amount of fat was found to be increased as well. More recently we have extended our investigations of the wall of the coronary arteries from patients with non-insulin-dependent diabetes (Dybdahl and Ledet, 1987). Using a quantitative histochemical approach we found an accumulation of a PAS-positive (Figure 1) but alcian blue negative material (positive alcian blue = acid mucopoly-saccarides) together with an increase in the amount of connective tissue in tunica media from extramural coronary arteries (Figure 2). It is important to emphasize that these results were also seen in areas without evidence of atherosclerosis. Very recently quantitative immunohistochemical data have been obtained from a study we have performed on aortae from a series of insulin-dependent and non-insulin-dependent diabetic patients. The results indicate that part of the PAS-positive material seen in areas without athero-sclerosis may correspond to fibronectin (Rasmussen and Heickendorff, 1988a). Moreover, we were also able to demonstrate in tunica media of aorta, at the immunohistochemical level, that the amount of basement membrane components as type IV collagen and laminin was increased (Rasmussen and Heickendorff, 1988b) (Figure 3). An important feature is that the alterations in tunica media again were found to be diffuse and unrelated to intimal lesions.

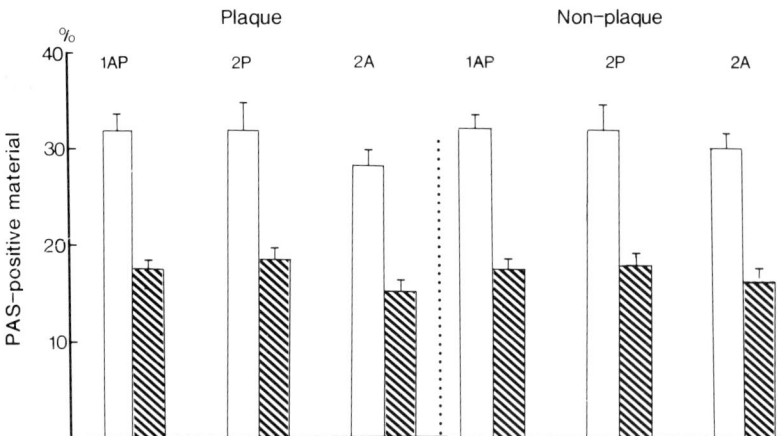

Figure 1. The amount of PAS-positive substance in tunica media from the extramural coronary arteries obtained from type II diabetic patients. 1AP = the average results from the first 3 centimetres of the anterior (A) and posterior (P) artery. 2A = peripheral segments of the anterior artery, 2P = peripheral segments of the posterior artery. The clear columns = diabetic patients and the hatched columns = non-diabetic patients.

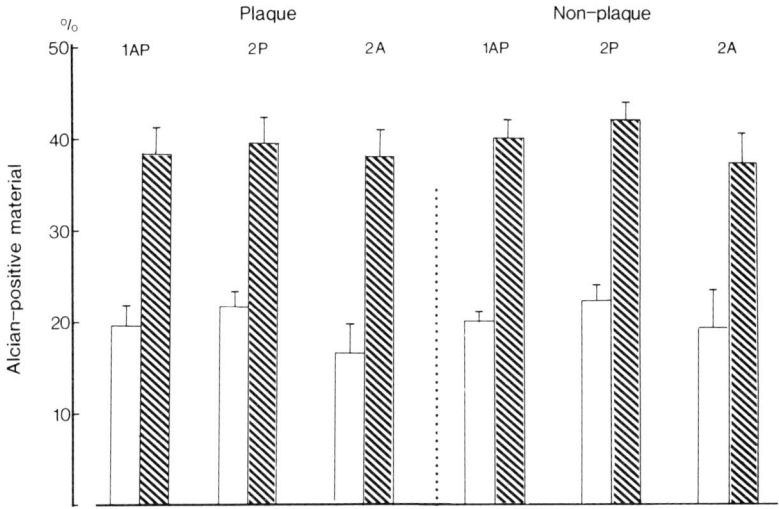

Figure 2. The amount of acid mucopolysaccharides (= alcian blue-positive material) substance in tunica media from extramural coronary arteries collected from type II diabetic individuals. 1AP = the average results from the first 3 cm of the anterior (A) and posterior (P) artery. 2A = peripheral segments of the anterior artery, 2P = peripheral segments of the posterior coronary artery. The clear columns = diabetic patients and the hatched columns = non-diabetic patients.

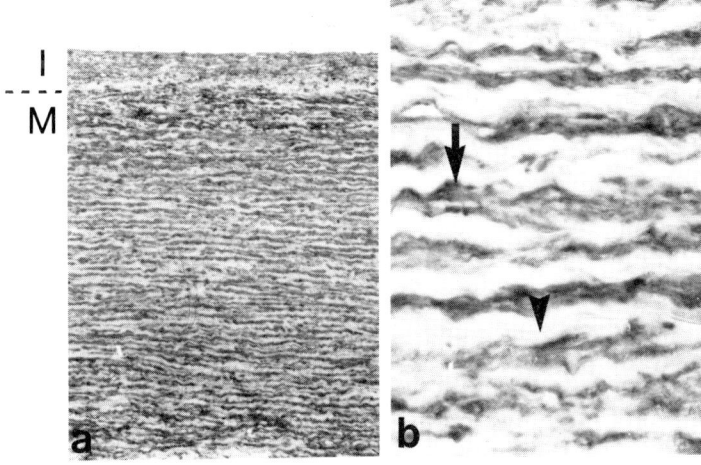

Figure 3. Human aorta stained with antibodies directed against type IV collagen, using a PAP-method. **(a)** Tunica intima (I) and tunica media (M) shown in 60 × magnification. **(b)** Section of tunica media shown in higher magnification (× 350). Arrow points at large amounts of stainable material, which is situated in the pericellular space between the elastic lamellae. Arrow head indicates elastic membrane.

Calcification

Arterial calcification was analysed by Root (1949) in 83 young diabetic patients (aged 25–34 years). He demonstrated a clearcut relationship between calcification and duration of diabetes. Ferrier (1964) obtained a series of data from low voltage roentgenograms of the large vessels of amputated limbs from diabetic and non-diabetic patients. A more pronounced media calcification and lumen reduction of the metatarsal arteries was found among the diabetic patients. Ferrier (1964) and later Christensen (1968) demonstrated that linear arterial calcification is a characteristic feature in diabetes, quite different from the spotty lesions usually seen in severe atherosclerosis. In an investigation published 15 years ago, the media calcification was found to be more extensive in the femoral artery and its tributaries among non-insulin-dependent diabetic compared to non-diabetic patients. Moreover, there was no difference in the amount of intima calcification, but the calcium deposition in tunica media was statistically correlated to a decrease in the glucose tolerance (Neubauer, 1971).

Conclusions

It is clear from the investigation of the morphological pattern in the arterial wall that a set of changes can be demonstrated in areas without the presence of classical atherosclerotic abnormalities. These consist of the accumulation of a PAS-positive substance, connective tissue, basement membrane components such as fibronectin, type IV collagen, laminin as well as calcium deposition combined with a reduction in acid mucopolysaccharides. It is of note that PAS-positive, but acid mucopolysaccharide negative deposits are usually considered to be the histopathological marker of diabetic microangiopathy (Ledet, 1975; Ledet et al, 1984).

EXPERIMENTAL DIABETES AND LARGE VESSEL DAMAGE

More information seems to have been acquired about the pathogenesis of diabetic large vessel disease from animal models of experimental or spontaneous diabetes. Duff and McMillan (1949) published a series of novel data which demonstrated that atherogenic diets given to alloxan diabetic rabbits may well increase the plasma cholesterol but the effect on the development of large vessel abnormalities was less than that in non-diabetic rabbits. Several years later these interesting findings were confirmed by Kloeze & Abdellatiff (1975).

Large vessel damage was studied in rabbits with alloxan diabetes given a small dose of cortisone together with a cholesterol-rich diet for 4 months. Plaque formation in the diabetic rabbits was pronounced in the medium sized coronary arteries and composed mainly of foam cells in the the tunica intima. Body weight was identical in normal and diabetic rabbits but blood cholesterol was higher in the diabetic rabbits (Wellman and Volk, 1970). Recently, morphological changes were analysed in aortae obtained from alloxan diabetic rabbits fed for up to 40 weeks on a low cholesterol diet. Micrometric measurements demonstrated that the intima thickness was significantly higher in the diabetic group. Also, macroscopic quantification of the area of sudanophilic material on the surface of aortae showed a significantly larger region in the diabetic animals, and that the majority of lesions were small raised plaques of collagen and smooth muscle cells (Miller and Wilson, 1984).

Diabetic rats given a high fat diet for 3–6 months also develop pronounced cardiovascular lesions (Kalant et al, 1964; Still et al, 1964; Wilson et al, 1967). In almost all studies the diabetic rats had high serum cholesterol concentrations. In one study however, advanced plaque, composed of foam cells in the tunica media of the large blood vessels, was seen in diabetic rats with a serum cholesterol concentration similar to the non-diabetic rats (Still et al, 1964). This investigation suggests the presence of an effect of diabetes independent of serum cholesterol. It has been demonstrated from our laboratory that the number of cells in the tunica media of the large coronary arteries is increased in rats with experimental diabetes for 9 months (Baandrup et al, 1981). Furthermore it was observed that insulin treatment resulting in almost normal glucose metabolism suppressed the development of these changes.

Squirrel monkeys with alloxan diabetes and increased serum cholesterol have also been used as models for the evaluation of the development of large vessel abnormalities (Lehner et al, 1971). The incidence of macroscopical lesions in large vessels was found to be higher among diabetic animals than among the controls. An important study by Howard (1979) demonstrated that monkeys with spontaneous diabetes, on a normal diet, develop larger plaques and more sudanophilia in the aorta than control animals. The analyses were performed as quantitative measurements and the serum cholesterol was normal in both groups. In addition a correlation between the incidence of aortic changes and the degree of abnormality of the intravenous glucose tolerance test was observed.

The development of large vessel abnormalities in animals with experimental diabetes mellitus is difficult to evaluate. In most studies, high fat diets or animals with high serum cholesterol concentrations have been used yet there are data which clearly indicate that lesions can develop in the large vessels without a concomitant increase in the serum cholesterol level. These results suggest that a factor(s) in the abnormal metabolism of diabetes may be of importance. The consequences of the changes in the vessel wall with experimental diabetes still remain to be elucidated. Two studies have been published estimating the biomechanical alterations after 30 and 95 days of diabetes, however, no influence on the biomechanical properties was detected (Andreassen et al, 1981; Andreassen and Oxlund, 1987).

Hyperinsulinaemia and large vessel disease

The 'insulin hypothesis', suggesting that inappropriately high circulating insulin concentrations may cause vessel damage was put forward nearly 20 years ago by Stout and Vallance-Owen (1969). It derived from a series of experiments with non-diabetic rats and chickens given large doses of insulin which showed enhanced synthesis of cholesterol in the aorta (Stout 1969, 1979). It has not been possible to confirm these findings in KK mice with elevated plasma insulin nor in diabetic rats treated with insulin (Chattopadhyay and Martin, 1969; Chobanian et al, 1974). Nor has it been possible to demonstrate an effect of insulin upon the transfer of cholesterol from plasma to arterial wall (Christensen and Jensen, 1975). It has been suggested that insulin causes increased proliferation of cells in tissue culture but cells needed to be starved, by serum deprivation for several days, before an insulin effect could be shown and then only at high insulin concentrations (200–2500 mU/l) (Pheifle et al, 1980; Stout et al, 1975; King et al, 1983). In one study combining in vitro and in vivo techniques insulin reduced thymidine incorporation (Capron et al, 1986). We, and others, have not been able to demonstrate an effect of insulin (Ledet, 1976b). Finally there was a growth-promoting effect of serum from recent onset insulin-dependent diabetics although serum insulin was only 0–6 µU/l (Ledet, 1976b). Also, against the hypothesis are our observations of a beneficial effect of insulin treatment on the development of lesions in large vessels from rats with experimental diabetes (Baandrup et al, 1981).

Growth hormone and large vessel disease

Important information has been obtained in recent years applying tissue culture techniques to the problem of atherosclerosis (Ross, 1971; Fischer-Dzoga et al, 1973). The cells have mainly been derived from either the tunica media or tunica intima from various arteries.

In our laboratory, increased outgrowth and proliferation of rabbit arterial smooth muscle cells was seen after exposure to normolipaemic serum from either insulin-dependent diabetic patients or alloxan diabetic rabbits (Ledet, 1976a; Ledet et al, 1976). Similar results were obtained using pooled serum from patients with non-insulin-dependent diabetes mellitus (NIDDM) (Koschinsky et al, 1979). Several attempts have been made to identify the factor(s) in diabetic serum responsible for the increased growth. Glucose added to serum from non-diabetic individuals did not reproduce the effect (Ledet et al, 1976; Koschinsky et al, 1979). In a series of experiments with serum from insulin-dependent males, however, ultrafiltration and dialysis indicated the presence of an active compound with a molecular weight between 3000 and 30 000 daltons (Ledet, 1976a). Recently serum from non-insulin-dependent diabetic patients was studied revealing that only a factor with a molecular weight of 3500 daltons increased the growth of human arterial smooth muscle cells (Koschinsky et al, 1985). This factor remained active after heating and was not affected by a lipid dissolving agent.

When the effect of endothelial denudation on growth of arterial smooth muscle cells was analysed in a combined in vitro and in vivo study, cell growth in intima-media preparations from rats with poorly controlled or adequately controlled experimental diabetes was identical (Capron et al, 1986).

The increased serum growth hormone seen in diabetic patients is an alternative causal factor for the development of diabetic angiopathy (Lundbaek et al, 1970). The frequency of small and large blood vessel disease is rather low among growth-hormone-deficient dwarfs with diabetes (Merimee et al, 1973). In a series of studies we have investigated the growth in tissue culture of arterial smooth muscle cells after addition of physiological amounts of human growth hormone (1 ng/ml). Growth hormone increased growth significantly, and anti-growth hormone serum was able to normalize the growth effect of serum from diabetic patients (Ledet, 1976c; 1981). Our results point to growth hormone as one possible factor in serum from diabetic patients responsible for the observed growth rate. It is therefore of considerable interest that Bettman et al (1981) have published data which showed reduced proliferation of intima smooth muscle cells after hypophysectomy in rats with vessel wall damage.

Recent studies have demonstrated that incubation of low-density lipoprotein (LDL) in vitro with glucose can result in glycosylation of lysine residues of LDL with a resultant decrease in the binding of LDL to receptors on cultured human fibroblasts (Gonen et al, 1981). The binding and degradation by normal fibroblasts of LDL obtained from seven non-insulin-dependent diabetic and 10 non-diabetic subjects has been examined by Kraemer et al (1982). The average glucose value was 12.6 mmol/l in the diabetic group, but the results revealed no difference between diabetic and non-diabetic LDL binding. A similar result was found when LDL was bound and degraded by mouse peritoneal macrophages. A small but significant increase in the cholesterylester synthesis and cholesterylester accumulation was seen in human monocyte-derived macrophages after incubation with LDL from insulin-dependent diabetic patients in whom the amount of non-enzymatically glycosylated LDL was higher than in the non-diabetic group (Lyons et al, 1987). In a recent study performed on a limited number of rabbits it was demonstrated that in the presence of antibodies against glycosylated LDL the clearance rate of glycosylated LDL was greatly accelerated (Wiklund et al, 1987). Moreover, it was also shown that the uptake into the aorta of glycosylated LDL was considerably lower than native LDL. It appears from these studies that no effects, or only a small influence, on fibroblasts and macrophages can be detected using non-enzymatic glycosylated LDL from insulin-dependent and non-insulin-dependent diabetic patients. Perhaps the presence of small amounts of antibodies against glycosylated LDL which can be predicted in diabetic patients facilitates the degradation of glycosylated LDL and reduces the uptake into the aorta. Consequently the importance of glycosylated LDL for the development of lesions in the larger blood vessels in diabetic patients still remains to be determined.

The secretion of procollagen type I and type III was estimated in the incubation medium from aortic smooth muscle cell cultures after addition of serum from diabetic patients (Ledet and Vuust, 1980). This study showed that serum from diabetic patients enhanced type I collagen production. Fibronectin is partly a component of the basement membrane-like material obtained from aortic smooth muscle cells and partly a component of the extracellular matrix of the arterial wall. Data from the same tissue culture study demonstrated an enhanced secretion of fibronectin in the presence of serum from diabetic patients. We were not able to change the production of collagen and fibronectin using high concentrations of glucose or ketones. Insulin (100 µU/l) however, reduced the secretion of collagens and fibronectin, whereas growth hormone augmented, as did serum from diabetic patients, the elaboration of type I collagen and fibronectin.

Biochemical investigations of the basement membrane-like material surrounding the individual smooth muscle cell in the arterial wall has been performed (Heickendorff and Ledet, 1983a, b) (Figure 4). Using serum from either insulin-dependent or non-insulin-dependent diabetic patients the accumulation of basement membrane-like material was found to be increased and this effect could not be attributed to either reduced removal of the basement membrane-like material or the presence of high concentrations of glucose in the incubation medium (Figure 5) (Rasmussen and Ledet, 1988). It has not been possible to change the deposition rate of basement membrane-like material using various concentrations of insulin, ketones or glucagon (Ledet and Heickendorff, 1987). However, human growth hormone (1 ng/ml) was able to enhance the accumulation of basement membrane-like material isolated from cultures of aortic smooth muscle cells

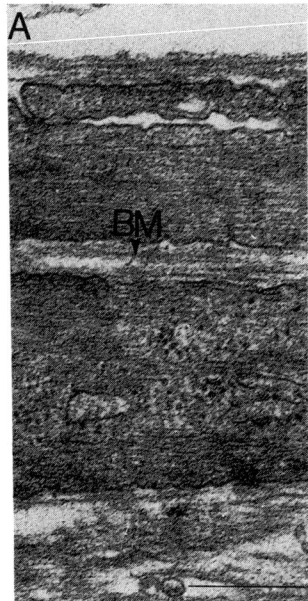
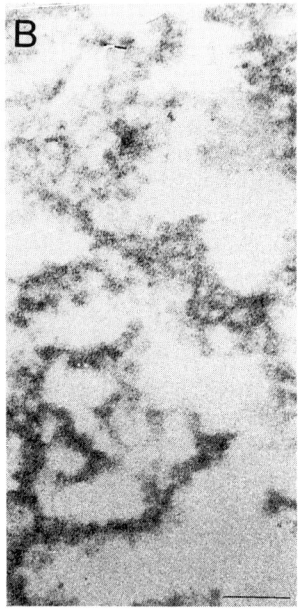

Figure 4. A: An electron micrograph of a 5-week-old primary culture of rabbit aorta smooth muscle cells. The cells are organized in multilayer with large amounts of basement membrane-like material (BM) covering the cell surfaces. Bar=1 um. **B:** Isolated BM material obtained from cultured smooth muscle cells by a sonication-differential centrifugation procedure. Bar=0.2 um.

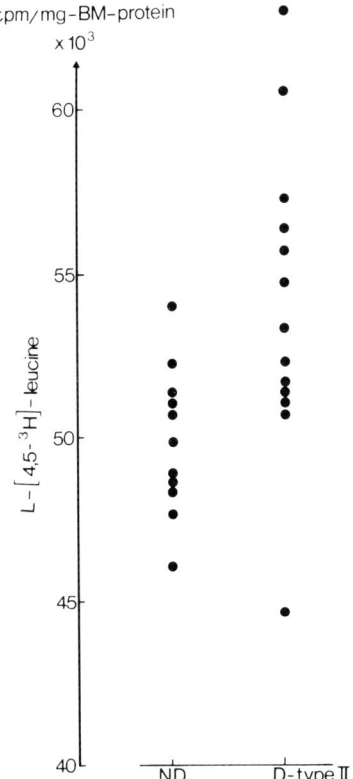

Figure 5. Effect of serum from type II diabetic patients on accumulation of basement membrane-like material (BM). Cultures of smooth muscle cells from rabbit aortae were incubated with 0.5 uCi/ml of ³H-leucine and test sera. A significantly higher incorporation of leucine into BM is seen in cultures incubated with sera from diabetic patients (D-type II) compared to sera from non-diabetic subjects (ND).

(Ledet and Heickendorff, 1985). It could also be demonstrated, using radioactive sulphate, that the amount of glycosaminoglycans was reduced.

The results from in vitro studies are compatible with the morphological observations demonstrating large amounts of PAS-positive material which exhibited reduced reaction for acid mucopolysaccharides in the extramural coronary arteries from patients with non-insulin-dependent diabetes. Moreover our in vitro results suggest, though do not prove, that part of the development of the diabetic macroangiopathy may be ascribed to a factor(s) present in normolipaemic serum from diabetic patients and that the increased growth hormone level may be of some importance.

SUMMARY

In this chapter we have presented information on the development of large vessel damage in diabetes mellitus. A series of changes occur independent of the presence of atherosclerosis. The abnormalities include accumulation of PAS-positive material, laminin, fibronectin, type IV collagen and connective tissue with lack of acid mucopolysaccharides, and deposition of calcium. It is of particular interest that accumulation of PAS-positive material and lack of acid mucopolysaccharides are recognized as the histological markers of diabetic microangiopathy. These changes are in agreement with the hypothesis of a non-atherosclerotic large vessel damage, that is, diabetic macroangiopathy. From this standpoint the working hypothesis of a specific diabetic macroangiopathy should generate new ways to study the mechanism of the large vessel disease of diabetes over and above the traditional concept of classical atherosclerosis.

REFERENCES

Andreassen TT & Oxlund H (1987) Changes in collagen and elastin of the rat aorta induced by experimental diabetes and food restriction. *Acta Endocrinologica (Copenhagen)* **115:** 338–344.

Andreassen TT, Seyer-Hansen K & Oxlund H (1981) Biomechanical changes in connective tissues induced by experimental diabetes. *Acta Endocrinologica (Copenhagen)* **98:** 432–436.

Baandrup U, Ledet T & Rasch R (1981) Experimental diabetic cardiopathy preventable by insulin treatment. *Laboratory Investigation* **45:** 169–173.

Bettmann MA, Stemerman MB & Ransil BJ (1981) The effect of hypophysectomy on experimental endothelial cell regrowth and intimal thickening in the rat. *Circulation Research* **48:** 907–912.

Capron L, Jarnet J, Kazandjian S & Housset E (1986) Growth promoting effect of diabetes and insulin on arteries. An in vitro study of rat aorta. *Diabetes* **35:** 973–978.

Chattopadhyay DP & Martin JM (1969) Effect of insulin on the in vitro synthesis of sterol and fatty acid by aorta and liver from diabetic rats. *Journal of Atherosclerosis Research* **10:** 131–134.

Chobanian AV, Gerritsen GC, McCombs L & Brecher PI (1974) Arterial lipid metabolism in diabetic animal models with reduced or elevated plasma insulin levels. In Schettler G & Weizel A (eds) *Atherosclerosis III, Proceedings of the Third International Symposium*, pp 114–117. Berlin, Heidelberg, New York: Springer Verlag.

Christensen NJ (1968) Muscle blood flow, measured by xenon[133] and vascular calcifications in diabetics. *Acta Medica Scandinavica* **183:** 449–454.

Christensen S & Jensen I (1975) Uptake of labelled cholesterol from plasma by aortic intima-media in control and insulin injected rabbits. *Journal of Atherosclerosis Research* **5:** 258–259.

Christensen T & Neubauer B (1988a) Internal diameter of common femoral artery in patients with insulin dependent diabetes mellitus. *Acta Radiologica Diagnosis* (in press).

Christensen T & Neubauer B (1988b) Increased arterial wall stiffness and thickness in medium sized arteries in patients with insulin dependent diabetes mellitus. *Acta Radiologica Diagnosis* (in press).

Crall FV & Roberts WC (1978) The extramural and intramural coronary arteries on juvenile diabetes mellitus. *American Journal of Medicine* **645:** 221–230.

Dortimer AC, Sahenoy PN, Shiroff RA et al (1977) Diffuse coronary artery disease in diabetic patients. Facts or fictions? *Circulation* **57:** 133–136.

Duff GL & McMillan (1949) The effect of alloxandiabetes on experimental cholesterol atherosclerosis in the rabbit. *Journal of Experimental Medicine* **82:** 611–630.

Dybdahl H & Ledet T (1987) Diabetic macroangiopathy. Quantitative histopathological studies of the extramural coronary arteries from type 2 (non-insulin dependent) diabetic patients. *Diabetologia* **30:** 882–886.

Epstein FH, Ostrander LD, Johnson BC et al (1965) Epidemiological studies of cardiovascular disease in a total community—Tecumseh, Michigan. *Annals of Internal Medicine* **62:** 1170–1187.

Ferrier TM (1964) Radiologically demonstrable arterial calcifications in diabetes mellitus. *Austrian Annals of Medicine* **13:** 222–228.

Fischer-Dzoga K, Jones K, Vesselinovitch D & Wissler RW (1973) Ultrastructural and immunohistochemical studies of primary cultures of aortic medial cells. *Experimental and Molecular Pathology* **18:** 162–176.

Gonen B, Jacobsen D, Farrar P & Schonfeld G (1918) In vitro glycosylation of low density and high density lipoproteins. *Diabetes* **30:** 875–878.

Goodale F, Daoud AS, Florentin R, Lee KT & Gittelsohn A (1962) Chemico-anatomic studies of arteriosclerosis and thrombosis in diabetics. 1: Coronary arterial wall thickness, thrombosis and myocardial infarcts in autopsied North Americans. *Experimental and Molecular Pathology* **1:** 353–363.

Heickendorff L & Ledet T (1983a) Arterial basement membrane-like material isolated and characterised from rabbit aortic myomedial cell cultures. *Biochemical Journal* **211:** 397–404.

Heickendorff L & Ledet T (1983b) The carbohydrate components of arterial basement membrane-like material. Studies on rabbit aortic myomedial cells in culture. *Biochemical Journal* **211:** 735–741.

Howard CF Jr (1979) Aortic atherosclerosis in normal and spontaneously diabetic Macaca nigra. *Atherosclerosis* **33:** 479–493.

Kalant N, Teitelbaum JI, Cooperberg AA & Harland WA (1964) Dietary atherogenesis in alloxan diabetes. *Journal of Laboratory and Clinical Medicine* **63:** 147–157.

Kannel WB & McGee DL (1979) Diabetes and glucose tolerance as risk factors for cardiovascular disease: The Framingham study. *Diabetes Care* **2:** 920–926.

King GL, Buzney SM, Kahn RC et al (1983) Different responsiveness to insulin of endothelial and support cells from micro and macrovessels. *Journal of Clinical Investigation* **71:** 974–979.

Kloeze J & Abdellatiff AMM (1975) Effects of palm-kernel oil and sunflower seed oil on serum lipids and atherogenesis in alloxan diabetic rabbits. *Atherosclerosis* **22:** 349–368.

Koschinsky T, Bunting CE, Rutter R & Gries FA (1985) Sera from type 2 (non-insulin dependent) diabetic and healthy subjects contain different amounts of a very low molecular weight growth peptide for vascular cells. *Diabetologia* **28:** 223–228.

Koschinsky T, Bunting CE, Schwippert B & Gries FA (1979) Increased growth of human fibroblasts and arterial smooth muscle cells from diabetic patients related to diabetic serum factors and cell origin. *Atherosclerosis* **33:** 245–252.

Kraemer FB, Chen YDI, Cheung RMC & Reaven GM (1982) Are the binding and degradation of low density lipoprotein altered in type 2 (non-insulin dependent) diabetes mellitus? *Diabetologia* **23:** 28–33.

Ledet T (1968) Histological and histochemical changes in the coronary arteries of old diabetic patients. *Diabetologia* **4:** 268–272.

Ledet T (1975) Diabetic cardiopathy. Quantitative histological studies of the heart from young juvenile diabetics. *Acta pathologica et microbiologica Scandinavica* Section A **84:** 421–454.

Ledet T (1976a) Growth of rabbit aortic smooth-muscle cells in serum patients with juvenile diabetes. *Acta pathologica et microbiologica Scandinavica* Section A **84:** 508–516.

Ledet T (1976b) Growth hormone stimulating the growth of arterial medial cells in vitro. Absence of effect of insulin. *Diabetes* **25:** 1011–1018.

Ledet T (1976c) Growth hormone antiserum suppresses the growth effect of diabetic serum. Studies on rabbit aortic medial cell cultures. *Diabetes* **26:** 798–803.

Ledet T (1981) Diabetic macroangiopathy and growth hormone. *Diabetes* **30 (supplement)** 14–17.

Ledet T & Heickendorff L (1985) Growth hormone effect on accumulation of arterial basement membrane-like material studied on rabbit aortic myomedial cell cultures. *Diabetologia* **28:** 922–927.

Ledet T & Heickendorff L (1987) Insulin, ketones, glucose and glucagon: Effects on the arterial basement membrane in vitro. *Acta Endocrinologica (Copenhagen)* **115:** 139–141.

Ledet T & Vuust J (1980) Arterial procollagen type I, type III, and fibronectin. Effects of diabetic serum, glucose, insulin, ketones and growth hormone studied on rabbit aortic myomedial cell cultures. *Diabetes* **29:** 964–970.

Ledet T, Fischer-Dzoga K & Wissler RW (1976) Growth of rabbit aortic smooth muscle cell cultured in media containing diabetic and hyperlipemic serum. *Diabetes* **25**: 207–215.

Ledet T, Gøtsche O & Heickendorff L (1984) The pathology of diabetic cardiopathy: Pathogenetic reflections. In Jarret RJ (ed) *Diabetes and Heart Disease*, pp 26–46. Amsterdam: Elsevier Science Publ. B.V.

Lefkovits AaM (1937) Coronary disease in diabetes mellitus. *Journal of Laboratory and Clinical Medicine* **23**: 354–357.

Lehner NDM, Clarkson TB & Lofland HB (1971) The effect of insulin deficiency, hypothyroidism, and hypertension on atherosclerosis in the Squirrel Monkey. *Experimental and Molecular Pathology* **15**: 230–244.

Lundbæk K (1954) Diabetic angiopathy—A specific vascular disease. *Lancet* **I**: 377–379.

Lundbæk K (1971) Blood vessel disease. In Lundbæk K & Keen H (eds) *Diabetes Mellitus. Acta Diabetologica Latina* **8 (supplement 1):** 34.

Lundbæk K, Christensen NJ, Jensen VA et al. (1970) Diabetes, diabetic angiopathy and growth hormone. *Lancet* **II**: 131–133.

Lyons TJ, Klein RL, Baynes JW, Stevenson HC & Lopes-Virella MS (1987) Stimulation of cholesterylester synthesis in human monocyte derived macrophages by low-density lipoproteins from type 1 (insulin dependent) diabetic patients: the influence of non-enzymatic glycosylation of low density lipoproteins. *Diabetologia* **30**: 916–923.

Merimee TJ, Fineberg ES & Hollander W (1973) Vascular disease in the chronic hGH-deficient state. *Diabetes* **22**: 813–819.

Miller RA & Wilson RB (1984) Atherosclerosis and myocardial ischemic lesions in alloxan-diabetic rabbits fed a low cholestoral diet. *Arteriosclerosis* **4**: 586–591.

Neubauer B (1971) A quantitative study of peripheral arterial calcification and glucose tolerance in elderly diabetics and nondiabetics. *Diabetologia* **7**: 409–413.

Pheifle B, Ditschuneit HH & Ditschuneit H (1980) Insulin as a cellular growth regulator of rat arterial smooth muscle cells in vitro. *Hormone and Metabolic Research* **12**: 381–385.

Rasmussen LM & Heickendorff L (1988a) Changes in fibronectin content in aortae from diabetic subject. An immunohistochemical and biochemical study. (submitted).

Rasmussen LM & Heickendorff L (1988b) Increased amount of BM components in aortae form diabetic subjects. An immunohistochemical investigation. (submitted).

Rasmussen LM & Ledet T (1988) Serum form diabetic patients enhances the synthesis of arterial basement membrane-like material studies on rabbit aortic myomedial cell culture. *Acta pathologica et microbiologica Scandinavica* **96**: 77–83.

Reid DD, Brett GZ, Hamilton PJS, Jarret RJ, Keen H & Rose R (1974) Cardiorespiratory disease and diabetes among middle aged male civil servants. *Lancet* **I**: 469–473.

Robertson WB & Strong JP (1968) Atherosclerosis in persons with hypertension and diabetes mellitus. *Laboratory Investigation* **18**: 78–91.

Root HF (1949) Diabetes and vascular disease in youth. *American Journal of Medical Science* **217**: 545–553.

Ross R (1971) The smooth muscle cell. II. Growth of smooth muscle in culture and formation of elastic fibres. *Journal of Cell Biology* **50**: 172–186.

Ruderman NB & Haudenschild C (1983) Diabetes as a atherogenic factor. *Progress in Cardiovascular Disease* **26**: 373–412.

Still WJS, Martin JM & Gregor WH (1964) The effect of alloxan diabetes on experimental atherosclerosis in the rat. *Experimental and Molecular Pathology* **3**: 141–147.

Stout RW (1969) Insulin stimulation of cholesterol synthesis by arterial tissue. *Lancet* **II**: 476–478.

Stout RW (1979) The effect of insulin on the incorporation of sodium (1 ^{14}C) acetate into lipids of the rat aorta. *Diabetologia* **7**: 367–372.

Stout RW & Vallance-Owen J (1969) Insulin and atheroma. *Lancet* **I**: 1078–1080.

Stout RW, Bierman EL & Ross R (1975) Effect of insulin on the proliferation of cultured primate arterial smooth muscle cell. *Circulation Research* **36**: 319–327.

Turner IL & Bierman EL (1978) Effects of glucose and sorbitol on proliferation of cultured human skin fibroblasts and arterial smooth muscle cells. *Diabetes* **27**: 583–588.

Vigorita VJ, Moore GW & Hutschins GM (1980) Absence of correlation between coronary arterial atherosclerosis and severity or duration diabetes of adult onset. *American Journal of Cardiology* **46**: 535–542.

Waller BRF, Palumbo PJ & Roberts WC (1980) Status of the coronary arteries at necropsy in diabetes mellitus with onset after age 30 years. *American Journal of Medicine* **69**: 498–506.

Wellmann KF & Volk VWV (1970) Experimental atherosclerosis in normal and subdiabetic rabbits. I. Short-term studies. *Archives of Pathology* **90**: 206–217.

WHO (1985) Multinational study of vascular disease in diabetics. Prevalence of small vessel and large vessel disease in diabetic patients from 14 centres. *Diabetologia* **28**: 615–640.

Wiklund O, Witztum JL, Carew TE, Pittman RC, Elam RL & Steinberg D (1987) Turnover and tissue sites of degradation of glucosylated low density lipoprotein in normal and immunized rabbits. *Journal of Lipid Research* **28**: 1098–1109.

Wilson RB, Martin JM & Hartoft WS (1967) Evaluation of the relative pathogenic roles of diabetes and serum cholesterol levels in the development of cardiovascular lesions in rats. *Diabetes* **16**: 71–82.

8

Macrovascular disease and hyperinsulinaemia

D. A. ROBERTSON
P. J. HALE
M. NATTRASS

The main cause of early deaths and increased morbidity in diabetes is an excess of large vessel disease presenting as coronary arterial, peripheral vascular and cerebrovascular occlusion (Entmacher et al, 1964). It is widely held that the development of the microvascular complications characteristic of, although not absolutely specific for diabetes, is influenced by the degree of elevation of blood glucose and duration of the disease (Pirart, 1978; Nielsen and Ditzel, 1985). The evidence for a comparable specific diabetic macroangiopathy, which is favoured by some (Lundbaek, 1973), is not universally accepted. There can be little doubt that macrovascular disease in diabetes is atherosclerotic in nature (Jarrett et al, 1982a). The histopathology of the atherosclerotic lesion is the same in non-diabetic and diabetic patients regardless of the degree of glucose intolerance in the latter group (Strandness et al, 1964). The epidemiological risk factors which influence the prevalence of atherosclerosis in the non-diabetic population are also apparent in the diabetic population (Jarrett, 1984; Pyörälä et al, 1987). Any differences between the diabetic and non-diabetic populations lie in the extent of the atherosclerosis. Atherosclerotic vascular disease in the diabetic population is more severe and more widespread in the vascular tree (Robertson and Strong, 1968) and there is a loss of the relative protection normally enjoyed by women of childbearing age (Kannel and McGee, 1979a). The distribution differs with a predilection for the coronary arteries (Vigorita et al, 1980) and the distal vessels of the lower limb (Strandness et al, 1964).

A change in emphasis of theories of atherosclerosis has occurred in the last two decades. A proliferative response of the arterial wall is generally considered necessary for atherogenesis. The main cell type of the developing atherosclerotic lesion is thought to be the vascular smooth muscle cell which alters to become a sessile cell capable of synthesis of intracellular matrix and possibly other substances (Schwartz et al, 1986).

The growth of vascular smooth muscle in culture has allowed hypotheses of atherogenesis to be tested. One of these proposes a proliferative response to unspecified injury to the arterial endothelium (Ross and Glomset, 1976; Ross, 1986). This may be mediated by platelet interaction with damaged endothelial cells releasing substances which stimulate smooth muscle cells to migrate into the intima, proliferate and become increasingly metabolically active. Monocytes invade the new lesion while cells derived from both smooth muscle and macrophage lines acquire intracellular lipid droplets to form foam cells. This hypertrophic intimal lesion with intra- and extra-cellular droplets of cholesteryl esters and newly synthesized extracellular matrix forms a fatty streak. The lipids are believed to derive mainly from serum lipoproteins although they are taken up, modified and esterified intracellularly (Small, 1977). The lesion may regress at this stage or progress to a mature fibrous plaque of predominantly smooth muscle cells surrounding a necrotic lipid core (Ross and Glomset, 1976; Ross, 1986). Ultimately a denuded raised lesion develops which may ulcerate, generate mural thrombus and is potentially occlusive.

Many factors, both intrinsic and extrinsic, will act on the arterial plaque to influence its progression or resolution. These will presumably include the risk factors determined from large prospective population studies amongst which are recognized smoking, hypertension, abnormal serum lipoproteins, obesity, lack of exercise, male sex and presence of diabetes (Kannel and McGee, 1979b; Pyörälä, 1979; Ducimetiere et al, 1980; Fuller et al, 1983; Pyörälä et al, 1987).

INCREASED RISK

The relationship between non-insulin-dependent diabetes and athero-sclerotic vascular complications is somewhat confused. Population studies, on the whole, have not distinguished between insulin-dependent and non-insulin-dependent diabetes, but because of the ages of the cohorts the great majority of diabetic patients followed were probably non-insulin-dependent.

The best estimates for the additional relative cardiovascular risk attribu-table to diabetes when correction is made for all other risk factors are two to three fold for men and possibly as much as five fold for women (Kannel and McGee, 1979b; Jarrett, 1984; Pyörälä et al, 1987). In addition, diabetic patients demonstrate a higher prevalence of other independent risk factors such as hypertension and obesity (Wingard et al, 1983; Reaven and Hoffman, 1987). The nature of this additional risk was not determined in these studies.

The lack of a well-documented effect of duration of non-insulin-dependent diabetes on prevalence of atherosclerosis is difficult to explain. Patients often present with macrovascular disease well before diabetes is diagnosed and the relative cardiovascular risk attributable to impaired glucose toler-ance appears to be very close to that for diabetes (Fuller et al, 1983; Jarrett, 1984; Pyörälä et al, 1987).

Specific risk factors in non-insulin-dependent diabetes

Two potentially relevant features of a non-insulin-dependent population are an elevated blood glucose and an elevated fasting plasma insulin. In addition, in less hyperglycaemic diabetic patients and in those with impaired glucose tolerance, postprandial plasma insulins are often elevated (Reaven et al, 1976; Reaven and Olefsky, 1977; Ganda et al, 1985).

Glucose

It has been suggested that hyperglycaemia may influence atherogenesis by non-enzymatic glycosylation of lipoproteins or by the accumulation of advanced glycosylation end-products over many years in the structural proteins of the arterial wall (Kennedy and Baynes, 1984).

Certainly glycosylated proteins in diabetes include the lipoproteins and their function can be demonstrated to be abnormal under certain conditions (Colwell et al, 1983). Despite this the epidemiological evidence that long-term hyperglycaemia is a contributor to atherosclerosis risk in diabetes is poor, and the threshold at which blood glucose after oral glucose is a predictor for additional risk is around the 95th centile in population studies (Fuller et al, 1983; Jarrett, 1984). It seems unlikely that this degree of hyperglycaemia would be sufficient to produce a significant excess of glycosylated proteins even over many years.

Although glucose metabolism through the polyol pathway is a serious contender for a mechanism to mediate the effect of hyperglycaemia on microvascular disease there is little evidence to suggest that this is important in macrovascular disease (Brownlee et al, 1984).

Insulin

The possibility that circulating insulin levels have a role in the development of atherosclerosis in both diabetic and non-diabetic patients has been discussed for many years and extensively reviewed recently (Janka and Standl, 1987; Stout, 1987; Jarrett, 1988; Stolar, 1988).

Early work with animal models of atherogenesis documented effects of insulin lack and insulin treatment. Cholesterol feeding of rabbits produces lesions of the arterial wall which resemble atherosclerotic plaques but which resolve promptly after a normal diet is resumed. Alloxan treatment giving rise to insulin deficient diabetes appeared to prevent plaque formation (Duff et al, 1954). Exogenous insulin in both diabetic and non-diabetic rabbits accelerates the development of these lesions and inhibits their regression (Marquieé, 1978).

HYPERINSULINAEMIA

The development of a specific immunoassay for insulin allowed the observation that atherosclerotic vascular disease was associated with hyperinsulinaemia even when glucose tolerance was normal. This was demonstrated in coronary artery disease (Peters and Hales, 1965), in patients with peripheral vascular disease (Welborn et al, 1966) and for stroke (Gertler et al, 1972). The observation of hyperinsulinaemia in impaired glucose tolerance and basal hyperinsulinaemia in most patients with non-insulin-dependent diabetes was extended to insulin-treated insulin-dependent diabetic patients for peripheral blood, if not for the portal circulation (Hayford and Thompson, 1982).

Close relatives of non-insulin-dependent diabetic patients have an exaggerated insulin response to oral glucose (Leslie et al, 1986) as do populations in which a high incidence of non-insulin-dependent diabetes occurs (Haffner et al, 1986). Longitudinal studies suggest a biphasic insulin response in the evolution of diabetes in these populations. A strong insulin response to oral glucose in a normal subject predicts development of impaired glucose tolerance in Nauruans, but subsequent progression to diabetes is associated with impairment of this insulin response (Sicree et al, 1987). The exact level of hyperglycaemia at which the insulin response is attenuated varies between studies and for some lies within the diabetic range (Reaven et al, 1976).

Spontaneous diabetes in the obese rhesus monkey shows many features similar to human non-insulin-dependent diabetes. In this disorder obesity develops in middle life and is accompanied by marked fasting and stimulated hyperinsulinaemia but normal blood glucose. After several years relatively rapid deterioration of glucose tolerance and development of fasting hyperglycaemia occurs. During this brief phase, fasting plasma insulin returns to the normal range and insulin response to glucose is much reduced (Hansen and Bodkin, 1986).

A temporal relationship

A prolonged period with hyperinsulinaemia but normal glucose tolerance may account for the lack of obvious relationship between cardiovascular risk and duration of non-insulin-dependent diabetes after diagnosis. The patient may have been exposed to increased atherosclerotic risk for many years, yet at diagnosis this might not be apparent.

Three large prospective population studies on the middle-aged examining cardiovascular risk and measuring circulating insulin were started in the 1960s and reported at much the same time. Their results have been extensively discussed, since in each a predictive effect of circulating insulin concentration was seen for various aspects of coronary heart disease. They are summarized in Table 1 together with results from two prospective studies of non-insulin-dependent diabetes and a study of patients with impaired glucose tolerance. The predictive associations are strong using univariate analyses, but taking into account the intercorrelations of obesity, hypertension, serum lipids and insulin in multivariate analysis the relationships between plasma insulin and cardiovascular end-points were weakened. More importantly, inconsistencies arose. In the Paris study, fasting insulin retained significant predictive power, whereas in the Helsinki study it was the post-glucose insulin values at one hour and two hours which remained significant and for the Busselton population significant relationships were lost.

A recent review of these data (Jarrett, 1988) expresses the view that the

Table 1. Prospective studies of insulin levels and cardiovascular risk.

Population	n	Insulin measured	Results of studies (by univariate analysis)	Reference
NON-DIABETIC				
Helsinki (men)	982	1) Fasting 2) 1 + 2 h post oral glucose	Insulin at each time point positively associated with myocardial infarction, coronary heart disease, mortality and incidence of new coronary heart disease at 5 years	(Pyörälä, 1979)
Paris (men)	6439	1) Fasting 2) 2 h post oral glucose	Insulin/glucose ratios positively associated with myocardial infarction and new coronary heart disease at 5 years	(Ducimetiere et al, 1980)
Busselton, W. Australia (men and women)	3390	1 h after non-fasted oral glucose	Positively associated with incidence of coronary heart disease in elderly men only	(Welborn and Wearne, 1979)
GLUCOSE INTOLERANT				
Bedford (men and women)	241	2 h post oral glucose	No association seen	(Jarrett et al, 1982b)
NIDDM				
Schwabing (men and women)	501	1) Fasting free insulin 2) Fasting C-peptide 3) Insulin dose	All measures associated with increased incidence of stroke, coronary heart disease and peripheral vascular disease	(Standl and Janka, 1985)
Oxford (men and women)	247	1) Fasting insulin 2) Insulin following intravenous glucose	Log insulin/body mass index and post-glucose insulin area positively associated with new electrocardiographic abnormalities at 5 years	(Hillson et al, 1984)

inconsistencies might have arisen because of confounding factors related to insulin levels but not measured in these studies (such as high density lipoprotein cholesterol concentrations, altered haemostasis and possibly body fat distribution) or because of differential interaction between risk factors at differing insulin levels. This last is also suggested by more recent data from the Paris study (Fontbonne and Eschwege, 1987).

POSSIBLE MECHANISMS OF AN INSULIN EFFECT ON ATHEROSCLEROSIS RISK

Clearly a more detailed examination of insulin's possible causal role as a risk factor for atherogenesis is required. This possible effect of hyperinsulin-aemia on atherosclerosis may be acting directly on the arterial wall, or it may be mediated indirectly through other means. It has long been recognized that in non-insulin-dependent diabetes there are abnormalities of haemo-stasis, blood pressure and serum lipids. The relationship of each of these to plasma insulin deserves consideration in turn.

Possible direct mechanisms

Despite the possibility that insulin might influence atherogenesis by effects on conventionally measured cardiovascular risk factors, population studies cannot adequately explain the degree of relative risk for atherosclerotic vascular disease from these risk factors alone (Kannel and McGee, 1979c; Fuller et al, 1983; Pyörälä et al, 1987). There is no simple explanation for this discrepancy but the relatively small number of diabetic patients in large population studies results in wide confidence intervals for relative risk. Even so, there may be differential effects of risk factors in diabetes and multi-variate modelling techniques may not deal adequately with the clustering of interrelated risk factors seen in diabetic patients (Wingard et al, 1983; Pyörälä et al, 1987; Reaven and Hoffman, 1987; Jarrett, 1988). We may simply not be measuring all relevant risk factors or our understanding of the underlying mechanisms may be flawed, such that glycosylation or some other specifically diabetic mechanism alters protein function in ways we do not yet suspect. There is a possibility that atherosclerosis is mainly geneti-cally determined and many risk factors are merely associated markers for the underlying disorder. This allows us to speculate that diabetes and atherosclerosis are genetically linked but not causally related (Jarrett, 1984).

Nevertheless it is still attractive to postulate a direct effect of insulin on the arterial wall. Insulin has long been recognized to have growth promoting and lipogenic effects in diabetic patients and it would not be unreasonable to seek local effects on vascular smooth muscle (Stout, 1987).

Proliferative effects

1) In vitro. Vascular smooth muscle cells do not replicate if grown in medium without added serum. This inhibition can be overcome by added insulin, at least in part, and has been demonstrated in cell cultures derived from animals including monkeys (Stout et al, 1975) and from man (Pfeifle and Distchuneit, 1981). Although maximal stimulation is only approached at concentrations of 10 000 mU/l, a modest effect is seen at physiological insulin concentrations. Other workers have not found this effect in media with a greater concentration of added serum (Ledet, 1976). Smooth muscle cell DNA synthesis as measured by 3H-thymidine incorporation is probably more sensitive to insulin, although the concentrations required are still high (King et al, 1983).

2) In vivo. It is questionable how important the growth promoting effects of insulin are in vivo, particularly since the proliferative effect depends on its ability to stimulate the receptor for an insulin-like growth factor (IGF-1) (King et al, 1980). Some workers suggest that serum growth factors, which are present in greater concentrations in diabetes, might act synergistically with insulin (Kochinsky et al, 1985). Attempts to demonstrate growth promoting effects of exogenous insulin on the arterial wall in animals have been disappointing, perhaps because of inability to prevent chronic hypo-glycaemia which appears to suppress cell mitosis (Capron et al, 1986).

Lipogenic effects

The metabolic effects of insulin mediated by its sensitive and specific receptor include suppression of triglyceride hydrolysis (lipolysis) and stimu-lation of fatty acid synthesis. Insulin receptors are found on arterial smooth muscle cells (King et al, 1983) and these effects of insulin may explain earlier work in which alloxan diabetes suppresses lipid synthesis in arterial wall and intra-arterial injection of insulin overcomes this locally (Cruz et al, 1961).

1) Fatty acid synthesis. More recent work has confirmed that high circu-lating insulin levels can stimulate arterial wall fatty acid synthesis acutely in rats (Stout, 1975). Animal models of chronic peripheral hyperinsulinaemia demonstrate increased fatty acid synthetic activity and triglyceride content in arterial smooth muscle (Falholt et al, 1985) which is also seen in hyper-insulinaemic patients with coronary artery disease and impaired glucose tolerance (Falholt et al, 1987).

2) Cholesterol synthesis. Insulin stimulates the uptake of acetate and glucose into sterols in the arterial wall in rats (Stout, 1977). It also increases the activity of hydroxymethylglutaryl CoA dehydrogenase (HMG CoA reductase), the rate limiting enzyme of cholesterol synthesis (Bhathena et al, 1974), whose activity is also regulated by low density lipoprotein (Goldstein and Brown, 1977).

Lipoprotein metabolism

The mechanisms whereby lipids, predominantly cholesteryl esters, are deposited in the developing plaque are incompletely understood. Low density lipoprotein (LDL) particles are taken up by a specific receptor, then endocytosed and degraded in lysozomes to release free cholesterol and cholesteryl esters (Goldstein and Brown, 1977). The free cholesterol inhibits intracellular cholesterol synthesis but the cholesteryl esters must be hydrolysed before they can leave the cell in the nascent high-density lipoprotein (HDL) particle (Small, 1977).

It has been demonstrated that insulin stimulates the uptake and degradation of LDL particles in fibroblasts from diabetic and non-diabetic tissues (Chait et al, 1979). This is also believed to occur in the smooth muscle cell (Janka and Standl, 1987).

It has also been postulated that deposition of the relatively insoluble cholesteryl esters is favoured both by stimulation of the re-esterification of free cholesterol by the microsomal acetyl CoA:cholesterol acyl transferase system (ACAT) (Goldstein and Brown, 1977) and by inhibition of their hydrolysis (Grant, 1979). There is evidence which suggests that this latter action might be influenced by insulin. There are two enzyme activities recognized which might be regulators of cholesteryl ester hydrolysis in the smooth muscle cell. The first is a neutral cytoplasmic hydrolase which may be identical to the hormone sensitive lipase of adipose tissue (Khoo et al, 1976), which activity is inhibited by insulin. The second is a lysosomal hydrolase most active under acid conditions which demonstrates product inhibition by free fatty acids (Sakurada et al, 1976), and possibly by free intracellular cholesterol (Grant, 1979). The increased synthesis of fatty acids and cholesterol induced by hyperinsulinaemia may therefore favour deposition of cholesteryl esters in intracellular droplets in the cells of a developing atherosclerotic plaque.

Studies in animals with streptozotocin diabetes on the other hand demonstrate reduction in acid hydrolase activity which is returned to normal after prolonged insulin treatment (Wolinksy et al, 1978). The interpretation of these results is again obscured by the development of chronic hypoglycaemia in the insulin treated group.

Possible indirect mechanisms

Haemostasis

The proposal that an increased thrombotic tendency might contribute to atherosclerosis has been accepted to a greater or lesser extent for many years. In current theories of atherogenesis interest has concentrated on the interaction of platelets with vascular endothelium and subsequent release of growth factors in the initiation of the lesions (Ross and Glomset, 1976; Ross, 1986). The endothelium produces two substances which are postulated to influence this process: von Willebrand factor which stimulates platelet adherence and prostacyclin which inhibits it. In addition the endothelium produces plasminogen activator, important in the stimulation of fibrinolysis (Colwell et al, 1983).

Abnormalities of platelet function, clotting factors and various measures of clot lysis have been described in non-insulin-dependent diabetes. The general finding is of increased platelet aggregation, increased tendency to clot and impaired fibrinolysis (Table 2). This is somewhat obscured by difficulties in standardizing techniques and in the selection of patients and controls (Colwell et al, 1983).

Very little work has been done which examines plasma insulin in relation to haemostasis. However two studies have produced intriguing results for platelet aggregation. One study (Sagel et al, 1975) demonstrated that increased aggregation in diabetic patients did not correlate with blood glucose levels, and could also be demonstrated in impaired glucose tolerance and in some offspring of non-insulin-dependent diabetic parents with reportedly normal glucose tolerance. Another study confirmed this (Gensini et al, 1979) and also demonstrated increased von Willebrand factor activity in these groups. In neither study was insulin measured or patient characteristics clearly defined, but it is possible that hyperinsulinaemia or an associated metabolic abnormality was responsible for these results.

Table 2. Possible effects of hyperinsulinaemia on haemostasis.

1. Increased platelet reactivity in impaired glucose tolerance and diabetes. (Sagel et al, 1975)

2. Increased von Willebrand factor activity in impaired glucose tolerance and diabetes. (Gensini et al, 1979)

3. Decreased production of prostacyclin by arterial wall in vitro. (Lasche and Larsen 1982; Jeremy et al, 1983)

4. Fibrinolytic activity in normal subjects is negatively correlated with insulin concentrations. (Vague et al, 1986)

5. Fibrinolytic activity is reduced by increased insulin dose in diabetes. (Juhan-Vague et al, 1984)

Most studies in animal models of diabetes and diabetic patients have shown inhibition of the production of prostacyclin. A concentration dependent inhibition of prostacyclin release by insulin from rat aorta in vitro has been demonstrated (Lasché and Larsen, 1982; Jeremy et al, 1983). This effect was seen even at the lowest insulin concentration used (250 mU/l) which is supraphysiological, but may be of relevance to postprandial insulin levels in some patients with obesity or impaired glucose tolerance.

Measures of fibrinolysis in subjects with normal glucose tolerance are inversely correlated with overnight fasting insulin levels. As insulin levels decline further during a 24 h fast, fibrinolysis can be demonstrated to increase in individual subjects. Plasminogen activator inhibitor concentrations in these subjects behave in a complementary fashion (Vague et al, 1986). The same workers have demonstrated that intensive treatment of poorly controlled, insulin deficient diabetic patients by an artificial pancreas increases peripheral insulin concentrations and decreases measured fibrinolysis (Juhan-Vague et al, 1984).

Although none of these studies is particularly persuasive, it may be worth investigating whether euglycaemic changes in plasma insulin influence haemostasis either acutely or in the longer term.

Blood pressure

The increased prevalence of hypertension in diabetes is demonstrated in most population studies (Jarrett, 1984). A proportion is associated with diabetic nephropathy but much of the hypertension of the non-insulin-dependent patient is not clearly separable from essential hypertension (Drury, 1983). Raised blood pressure, abnormal serum lipids and obesity appear to cluster in non-insulin-dependent diabetes. Impaired glucose tolerance and abnormal lipids are more common in newly diagnosed hypertensive patients than in the general population (MacMahon et al, 1985; Modan et al, 1985).

There is evidence that hyperinsulinaemia, both fasting and stimulated, is associated with hypertension even when allowance is made for degree of obesity. This has been reported for newly diagnosed non-insulin-dependent diabetes (Lowenthal et al, 1985), patients with impaired glucose tolerance (Christlieb et al, 1985), and in the obese (Lucas et al, 1985). This has also been observed in newly diagnosed hypertensive patients (Modan et al, 1985; Singer et al, 1985), and in normal populations a modest association between blood pressure and fasting insulin concentrations has been demonstrated across the normal range (Fournier et al, 1986).

Two plausible mechanisms whereby insulin might induce blood pressure changes have been suggested.

1. Insulin has been shown to have a direct effect on the kidney. Plasma insulin increments under euglycaemic conditions stimulate renal sodium reabsorption at the proximal convoluted tubule in normal subjects (DeFronzo, 1981). Hypertensive non-insulin-dependent diabetic patients have a 10% excess of total exchangeable sodium. Reduction of this excess by diuretic treatment is associated with marked improvement in blood pressure (Weidmann et al, 1979).
2. There is also evidence for an effect of insulin on sympathetic nervous activity and thereby on vasomotor tone. Euglycaemic insulin infusion increases sympathetic nervous activity as measured by plasma noradrenaline release (Rowe et al, 1981), while fasting in hyperinsulinaemic obese patients leads to a reduction in concentrations of plasma insulin and noradrenaline and an associated fall in blood pressure well before significant weight loss occurs (Landsberg, 1986).

If, as suggested previously, predisposed individuals are exposed to hyperinsulinaemia over many years before diabetes is diagnosed sufficient time will elapse for the hypertension to become self-sustaining, even if subsequently insulin levels fall. Thus the relationship of blood pressure to plasma insulin may become weaker when non-insulin-dependent diabetes is established (Lowenthal et al, 1985). A recent review (Reaven and Hoffman, 1987) has postulated that clustering of impaired glucose tolerance, obesity and abnormal serum lipoproteins with hypertension may explain why treating blood pressure alone has produced relatively disappointing results in terms of prevention of cardiovascular disease in the general population.

The commonly used drugs of the thiazide and beta-adrenergic antagonist groups have been demonstrated to impair glucose tolerance and worsen lipoprotein profiles (Struthers et al, 1985; Rohlfing and Brunzell, 1986). It is not entirely clear how these agents affect glucose tolerance but the most likely mechanism is by an impairment of insulin release. In the case of thiazide diuretics this appears to be related to potassium depletion and may be prevented by potassium supplementation (Helderman et al, 1983). Beta-blockers do not alter daily insulin profiles in non-insulin-dependent diabetic patients despite an elevation of blood glucose, which also suggests an attenuated insulin response (Wright et al, 1979). There is also some evidence for peripheral insulin resistance with thiazide diuretics (Hicks et al, 1973) although this was not substantiated by 'glucose clamp' studies (Helderman et al, 1983).

Lipids

The lipoprotein abnormalities described in non-insulin-dependent diabetes include decreased high density lipoprotein cholesterol (HDL–C), elevated very low density lipoprotein triglycerides (VLDL–TG) and to a lesser degree elevation of low density lipoprotein cholesterol (LDL–C) (Nikkilä, 1984). These are thought to contribute to the development of athero-sclerosis in diabetes by extension of the relationships seen in normogly-caemic populations although not all workers have confirmed this (Reckless et al, 1978). Many of these lipoprotein abnormalities are present at diagnosis and in the Framingham study they were demonstrable in women ten years before diabetes was diagnosed (Kannel and McGee, 1979c).

A study of subjects both of whose parents suffered from non-insulin-dependent diabetes defined a group of women with these lipoprotein abnormalities, fasting and stimulated hyperinsulinaemia but very mild impairment of glucose tolerance (Ganda et al, 1985).

Studies which have examined the relationship between serum lipo-proteins and insulin levels are summarized in Table 3. In normal subjects, obese patients and patients with non-insulin-dependent diabetes, a consis-tent positive association is seen between plasma insulin and triglycerides (as VLDL–TG) and a negative association is seen with HDL–C concentrations. There is evidence for a weaker positive association with LDL–C in some studies.

It seems possible that some of the apparent association betwen plasma insulin and cardiovascular risk in the Paris, Helsinki and Busselton studies may have been related to unmeasured HDL–C concentrations.

SUMMARY

The evidence that hyperinsulinaemia represents an independent risk factor for cardiovascular disease is tantalizing but the hypothesis cannot be said to be proven. The inconsistencies arising from the major prospective studies require that further work be done. Hyperinsulinaemia may not carry the same implications in all subjects and its interactions with other risk factors

Table 3. Correlations between serum lipoprotein fractions and insulin concentrations.

Population	No.	Insulin measured (corrections made)	HDL–C	LDL–C	VLDC–TG	Total Triglyceride	Total Cholesterol	Reference
NORMOGLYCAEMIC								
Children and adults	323	1) Fasting (Obesity/age) 2) Post oral glucose (Obesity/age)	Neg	Pos	–	Pos	Pos	(Orchard et al, 1983)
Adolescents	817	Fasting (Obesity/age)	Neg	Pos	Pos	Pos	NS	(Burke et al, 1986)
Adult men	94	1) Fasting 2) Post intravenous glucose	Neg	NS	NS	NS	NS	(Stalder et al, 1981)
Adults	927	Fasting (Obesity/age)	Neg	–	–	Pos	–	(Garcia-Webb et al, 1983)
Obese adults	122	Fasting (Obesity)	Neg	–	–	–	–	(Hornick and Felmeth, 1981)
HYPERGLYCAEMIC								
Selected atherosclerotic patients	33	Postprandial	–	–	–	Pos	–	(Reaven et al, 1967)
NIDDM and controls	349	Fasting (Obesity)	Neg	NS	Pos	Pos	NS	(Laakso et al, 1987)
NIDDM and controls	501	Fasting C-peptide (age)	Neg	–	–	Pos	–	(Standl and Janka, 1985)

(Neg, significant negative correlation; Pos, significan: positive correlation; NS, not significant; – not reported) and with blood glucose are not well described. Possible further research has been discussed and outlined at a recent meeting (Colwell, 1985). The suggestions include delineating the action of growth factors and insulin in defined serum-free tissue culture, and the use of more sophisticated culture models, such as smooth muscle covered by vascular endothelium. The choice of human or primate tissue is desirable because of the species specificity of the atherosclerotic lesions.

Prospective trials of modifying peripheral insulin levels in treated diabetic patients are probably still impracticable. The case for attempting to achieve normoglycaemia in diabetes to avoid microvascular complications is strong, and current insulin treatment regimens accept peripheral hyperinsulinaemia as a consequence of achieving portal insulin concentrations sufficient to suppress hepatic glucose output. It is hard to envisage a trial to examine reduced peripheral insulin concentrations which would not give unacceptably poor blood glucose control. Current studies of different methods and degrees of control of blood glucose might be used to provide some indication of whether such a trial could ever be justified.

The Diabetes Control and Complication Trial (DCCT) is a prospective multicentre study of intensive versus conventional insulin treatment in insulin-dependent diabetic patients in the USA, and the UK Prospective Study of therapies of maturity onset diabetes (UKPS) is following patients not satisfactorily controlled on diet, randomized to different treatment modalities. These may produce some evidence within the next few years, on insulin concentrations and complications (Tattersall and Scott, 1987).

Should any of this change current management of non-insulin-dependent diabetes? Despite claims of enthusiasts, special treatment regimens with intensive exercise, a particular oral agent or the addition of sulphonylureas to insulin therapy are either not generally applicable or have little theoretical basis (Martin, 1986).

Current 'good practice' in Europe as put forth in a consensus document (Alberti and Gries, 1988), recognizes the need to address risk factors other than diabetes in the management of the non-insulin-dependent diabetic patient. In addition to the conventional use of oral agents and insulin (with realistic treatment goals for the elderly and infirm) it is suggested that appropriate exercise, diet, weight reduction and treatment of hypertension and abnormal lipids be undertaken. Much of this intervention will reduce insulin resistance and circulating insulin concentrations whether or not insulin is given to control blood glucose. At the moment one cannot advise any different approach to treatment.

In the future it may become practicable to treat hyperglycaemia without peripheral hyperinsulinaemia either by portal delivery of insulin or by use of insulin analogues which exert a preferential effect on hepatic rather than peripheral metabolism. This useful property has been demonstrated for chemically modified porcine insulins in dogs (Tompkins et al, 1981) and for biosynthetic human proinsulin in non-insulin-dependent diabetic patients (Glauber et al, 1987). As yet, there are no reliable means by which one can estimate the effects of these agents on the arterial wall compared with native insulin. More studies into the specific effect of insulin on atherogenesis must be done before any recommendation can be made on the preferred agent for the long-term treatment of non-insulin-dependent diabetes.

REFERENCES

Alberti KGMM & Gries FA (1988) Management of non-insulin-dependent diabetes mellitus in Europe: a consensus view. *Diabetic Medicine* **5:** 275–281.

Bhathena SJ, Avigan J & Schreiner ME (1974) Effect of insulin on sterol and fatty acid synthesis and hydroxymethyl glutaryl CoA reductase in mammalian cells grown in culture. *Proceedings of the National Academy of Science, USA* **71:** 2174–2178.

Brownlee M, Vlassara H & Cerami A (1984) Non-enzymatic glycosylation and the pathogenesis of diabetic complications. *Annals of Internal Medicine* **101:** 527–537.

Burke GL, Webber LS, Srinavasan SR et al (1986) Fasting plasma glucose and insulin levels and their relationship to cardiovascular risk factors in children: Bogalusa heart study. *Metabolism* **35:** 441–446.

Capron L, Jarnet J, Kazandjian S & Housset E (1986) Growth-promoting effects of diabetes and insulin on arteries. An in vivo study of rat aorta. *Diabetes* **35:** 973–978.

Chait A, Bierman EL & Albers JJ (1979) Low density lipoprotein receptor activity in fibroblasts cultured from diabetic donors. *Diabetes* **28:** 914–918.

Christlieb AR, Krolewski AS, Warram JH & Soeldner JS (1985) Is insulin the link between hypertension and obesity? *Hypertension* **7 (supplement II):** 54–57.

Colwell JA (1985) Workshop on insulin and atherogenesis. *Metabolism* **34 (supplement I):** 91 pp.

Colwell JA, Winocour PD, Lopes-Virella ML & Halushka PV (1983) New concepts about the pathogenesis of atherosclerosis in diabetes mellitus. *American Journal of Medicine* **75 (supplement):** 67–80.

Cruz AB, Amatuzio DS, Grande F & Hay LJ (1961) Effect of intra-arterial insulin on tissue cholesterol and fatty acids in alloxan-diabetic dogs. *Circulation Research* **9:** 39–43.

DeFronzo RA (1981) The effect of insulin on renal sodium metabolism. A review with clinical implications. *Diabetologia* **21:** 165–171.

Drury PL (1983) Diabetes and arterial hypertension. *Diabetologia* **24:** 1–9.

Ducimetiere P, Eschwege E, Papoz L et al (1980) Relationship of plasma insulin levels to the incidence of myocardial infarction of coronary heart disease mortality in a middle-aged population. *Diabetologia* **19:** 205–210.

Duff GL, Brechin DJH & Finkelstein WE (1954) Effect of alloxan diabetes on experimental atherosclerosis in the rabbit. *Journal of Experimental Medicine* **100:** 371–380.

Entmacher PS, Root HF & Marks HH (1964) Longevity of diabetic patients in recent years. *Diabetes* **13:** 373–377.

Falholt K, Cutfield R, Alejandro R, Heding L & Mintz D (1985) The effects of hyperinsulinaemia on arterial wall and peripheral muscle metabolism in dogs. *Metabolism* **34:** 1146–1149.

Falholt K, Hjelms E, Jensen I et al (1987) Intracellular metabolism in biopsies from the aorta in patients undergoing coronary bypass surgery. *Diabete et Metabolisme* **13:** 312–317.

Fontbonne A & Eschwege E (1987) Diabetes, hyperglycaemia, hyperinsulinaemia and atherosclerosis: Epidemiological data. *Diabete et Metabolisme* **13:** 350–353.

Fournier AM, Gadia MT, Kubrusly DB, Skyler JS & Sosenko JM (1986) Blood pressure, insulin and glycemia in non-diabetic subjects. *American Journal of Medicine* **80:** 861–864.

Fuller JH, Shipley MJ, Rose G, Jarrett RJ & Keen H (1983) Mortality from coronary heart disease and stroke in relation to degree of glycaemia: the Whitehall Study. *British Medical Journal* **287:** 867–870.

Ganda OP, Soeldner JS & Gleason RE (1985) Alterations in plasma lipids in the presence of mild glucose intolerance in the offspring of two Type II diabetic parents. *Diabetes Care* **8:** 254–260.

Garcia-Webb P, Bonser AM, Whiting D & Masarei JRL (1983) Insulin resistance—a risk factor for coronary heart disease? *Scandinavian Journal of Clinical Laboratory Investigation* **43:** 677–685.

Gensini GF, Abbate R, Favilla S & Neri Serneri GG (1979) Changes of platelet function and blood clotting in diabetes mellitus. *Thrombosis and Haemostasis* **42:** 983–993.

Gertler MM, Leetma HE, Saluste E, Covalt DA & Rosenberger JL (1972) Covert diabetes mellitus in ischaemic heart and cerebrovascular disease. *Geriatrics* **27:** 105–120.

Glauber HS, Henry RR, Wallace P et al (1987) The effects of biosynthetic human proinsulin on carbohydrate matabolism in non-insulin-dependent diabetes mellitus. *New England Journal of Medicine* **316:** 443–446.

Goldstein JL & Brown MS (1977) The low-density lipoprotein pathway and its relation to atherosclerosis. *Annual Review of Biochemistry* **46:** 897–930.

Grant N (1979) Insulin and atherosclerosis. *New England Journal of Medicine* **300:** 679–680.

Haffner SM, Stern MP, Hazuda HP, Pugh JA & Patterson JK (1986) Hyperinsulinemia in a population at high risk for non-insulin-dependent diabetes mellitus. *New England Journal of Medicine* **315:** 220–224.

Hansen BC & Bodkin NL (1986) Heterogeneity of insulin responses: phases leading to Type 2 (non-insulin-dependent) diabetes mellitus in the rhesus monkey. *Diabetologia* **29:** 713–719.

Hayford JT & Thompson RG (1982) Free and total insulin integrated concentrations in insulin-dependent diabetes. *Metabolism* **31:** 387–397.

Helderman JH, Elahi D, Andersen DK et al (1983) Prevention of the glucose intolerance of thiazide diuretics by maintenance of body potassium. *Diabetes* **32:** 106–111.

Hicks BH, Ward JD, Jarrett RJ, Keen H & Wise P (1973) A controlled study of clopamide, clorexolone and hydrochlorothiazide in diabetics. *Metabolism* **22:** 101–109.

Hillson RM, Hockday TDR, Mann JI & Newton DJ (1984) Hyperinsulinaemia is associated with development of electrocardiographic abnormalities in diabetes. *Diabetes Research* **1:** 143–149.

Hornick CA & Fellmeth BD (1981) High density lipoprotein cholesterol insulin and obesity in Samoans. *Atherosclerosis* **39:** 321–328.

Janka HU & Standl E (1987) Hyperinsulinaemia as a possible risk factor of macrovascular disease in diabetes mellitus. An overview. *Diabete et Metabolisme* **13:** 279–283.

Jarrett RJ (1984) The epidemiology of coronary heart disease and related factors in the context of diabetes mellitus and impaired glucose tolerance. In Jarrett RJ (ed) *Diabetes and heart disease* (Metabolic aspects of cardiovascular disease Vol 2), pp 1–23. Amsterdam: Elsevier.

Jarrett RJ (1988) Is insulin atherogenic? *Diabetologia* **31:** 71–75.

Jarrett RJ, Keen H & Chakrabarti R (1982a) Diabetes, hyperglycaemia and arterial disease. In Keen H & Jarrett RJ (eds) *Complications of diabetes*, pp 179–203. London: Edward Arnold.

Jarrett RJ, McCartney P & Keen H (1982b) The Bedford survey: Ten year mortality rates in newly diagnosed diabetics and normoglycaemic controls and risk indices for coronary heart disease in borderline diabetics. *Diabetologia* **22:** 79–84.

Jeremy JY, Mikhailidis DP & Dandona P (1983) Simulating the diabetic environment modifies in vitro prostacyclin synthesis. *Diabetes* **32:** 217–221.

Juhan-Vague I, Vague P, Poisson C et al (1984) Effect of 24 hours of normoglycaemia on tissue-type plasminogen activator plasma levels in insulin-dependent diabetes. *Thrombosis and Haemostasis* **51:** 97–98.

Kannel WB & McGee DL (1979a) Diabetes and cardiovascular disease: the Framingham Study. *Journal of the American Medical Association* **241:** 2035–2038.

Kannel WB & McGee DL (1979b) Diabetes and cardiovascular risk factors: the Framingham Study. *Circulation* **59:** 8–13.

Kannel WB & McGee DL (1979c) Diabetes and glucose tolerance as risk factors for cardiovascular disease: the Framingham Study. *Diabetes Care* **2:** 120–126.

Kennedy L & Baynes JW (1984) Non-enzymatic glycosylation and the chronic complication of diabetes: an overview. *Diabetologia* **26:** 93–98.

Khoo JC, Steinberg C, Huang JJ & Vagelos PR (1976) Triglyceride, diglyceride, monoglyceride and cholesterol ester hydrolases in chicken adipose tissue activated by adenosine 3′:5′-monophosphate-dependent protein kinase. *Journal of Biological Chemistry* **251:** 2882–2890.

King GL, Kahn CR, Rechler MM & Nissley SP (1980) Direct demonstration of separate receptors for growth and metabolic activities of insulin and multiplication-stimulating activity (an insulin like growth factor) using antibodies to the insulin receptor. *Journal of Clinical Investigation* **66**: 130–140.

King GL, Buzney SM, Kahn CR et al (1983) Differential responsiveness to insulin of endothelial and support cells from micro- and macrovessels. *Journal of Clinical Investigation* **71**: 974–979.

Kochinsky T, Bünting CE, Rütter R & Gries FA (1985) Vascular growth factors and the development of macrovascular disease in diabetes mellitus. *Hormone and Metabolic Research* **(supplement)** **17**: 23–27.

Laakso M, Pyörälä K, Voutilainen E & Marniemi J (1987) Plasma insulin and serum lipids and lipoproteins in middle-aged non-insulin-dependent diabetic and non-diabetic subjects. *American Journal of Epidemiology* **125**: 611–621.

Landsberg L (1986) Diet, obesity and hypertension: An hypothesis involving insulin, the sympathetic nervous system and adaptive thermogenesis. *Quarterly Journal of Medicine* **61**: 1081–1090.

Lasché EM & Larsen RE (1982) Interaction of insulin and prostacyclin production in the rat. *Diabetes* **31**: 454–458.

Ledet T (1976) Growth hormone stimulating the growth of arterial medical cells in vitro. Absence of effect of insulin. *Diabetes* **25**: 1011–1017.

Leslie RDG, Volkmann HP, Poncher M et al (1986) Metabolic abnormalities in children of non-insulin-dependent diabetics. *British Medical Journal* **293**: 840–842.

Lowenthal LM, Pim B, Hillson RM, Dhar H & Hockaday TDR (1985) Blood pressure at diagnosis of Type 2 diabetes correlates with plasma insulin concentration but not during the next five years. *Diabetes Research* **2**: 65–69.

Lucas CP, Estigarribia JA, Darga LL & Reaven GM (1985) Insulin and blood pressure in obesity. *Hypertension* **7**: 702–706.

Lundbaek K (1973) Diabetic angiopathy. *Acta Diabetologica Latina* **10**: 183–207.

MacMahon SW, Macdonald GL & Blacket RB (1985) Plasma lipoprotein levels in treated and untreated hypertensive men and women. *Arteriosclerosis* **5**: 391–396.

Marquié G (1978) Effect of insulin in the induction and regression of experimental cholesterol atherosclerosis in the rabbit. *Postgraduate Medical Journal* **54**: 80–85.

Martin DB (1986) Type II diabetes. Insulin versus oral agents. *New England Journal of Medicine* **314**: 1314–1315.

Modan M, Halkin H, Almog S et al (1985) Hyperinsulinemia. A link between hypertension, obesity and glucose intolerance. *Journal of Clinical Investigation* **75**: 809–817.

Nielsen NV & Ditzel J (1985) Prevalence of macro- and microvascular disease as related to glycosylated haemoglobin in type I and type II diabetic subjects. *Hormone and Metabolic Research* **(supplement series)** **17**: 19–22.

Nikkilä EA (1984) Plasma lipid and lipoprotein abnormalities in diabetes. In Jarrett RJ (ed) *Diabetes and heart disease* (Metablic aspects of cardiovascular disease Vol 2), pp 133–167. Amsterdam: Elsevier.

Orchard TJ, Becker DJ, Bates M, Kuller LH & Drash AL (1983) Plasma insulin and lipoprotein concentrations: An atherogenic association? *American Journal of Epidemiology* **118**: 326–337.

Peters N & Hales CN (1965) Plasma-insulin concentrations after myocardial infarction. *Lancet* **1**: 1144–1145.

Pfeifle B & Ditschuneit H (1981) Effect of insulin on growth of cultured human arterial smooth muscle cells. *Diabetologia* **20**: 155–158.

Pirart J (1978) Diabetes mellitus and its degenerative complications: A prospective study of 4,400 patients observed between 1947 and 1973. *Diabetes Care* **1**: 168–188, 252–263.

Pyörälä K (1979) Relationship of glucose tolerance and plasma insulin to the incidence of coronary heart disease: Results from two population studies in Finland. *Diabetes Care* **2**: 131–141.

Pyörälä K, Laakso M & Uusitupa M (1987) Diabetes and atherosclerosis: an epidemiologic view. *Diabetes/Metabolism Reviews* **3**: 463–524.

Reaven GM & Olefsky JM (1977) Relationship between heterogeneity of insulin responses and insulin resistance in normal subjects and patients with chemical diabetes. *Diabetologia* **13**: 201–206.

Reaven GM & Hoffman BB (1987) A role for insulin in the aetiology and course of hypertension? *Lancet* **2**: 435–437.

Reaven GM, Lerner RL, Stern MP & Farquhar JW (1967) Role of insulin in endogenous hypertriglyceridemia. *Journal of Clinical Investigation* **46:** 1756–1767.

Reaven GM, Bernstein R, Davis B & Olefsky JM (1976) Non ketotic diabetes mellitus: insulin deficiency or insulin resistance? *American Journal of Medicine* **60:** 80–88.

Reckless JPD, Betteridge DJ, Wu P, Payne B & Galton DJ (1978) High-density and low-density lipoproteins and prevalence of vascular disease in diabetes mellitus. *British Medical Journal* **1:** 883–886.

Robertson WB & Strong JP (1986) Atherosclerosis in persons with hypertension and diabetes mellitus. *Laboratory Investigation* **18:** 538–551.

Rohlfing JJ & Brunzell JD (1986) The effects of diuretics and adrenergic-blocking agents on plasma lipids. *Western Journal of Medicine* **145:** 210–218.

Ross R (1986) The pathogenesis of atherosclerosis—An update. *New England Journal of Medicine* **314:** 488–500.

Ross R & Glomset JA (1976) The pathogenesis of atherosclerosis. *New England Journal of Medicine* **295:** 369–377, 420–425.

Rowe JW, Young JB, Minaker KC et al (1981) Effect of insulin and glucose infusions on sympathetic nervous system activity in normal man. *Diabetes* **30:** 219–225.

Sagel J, Colwell JA, Crook L & Laimins M (1975) Increased platelet aggregation in early diabetes mellitus. *Annals of Internal Medicine* **82:** 733–738.

Sakurada T, Orimo H, Okabe H, Noma A & Murakami M (1976) Purification and properties of cholesterol ester hydrolase from human aortic intima and media. *Biochimica et Biophysica Acta* **424:** 204–212.

Schwartz SM, Campbell GR & Campbell JH (1986) Replication of smooth muscle cells in vascular disease. *Circulation Research* **58:** 427–444.

Sicree RA, Zimmet PZ, King HOM & Coventry JS (1987) Plasma insulin response among Nauruans. Prediction of deterioration of glucose tolerance over 6 yr. *Diabetes* **36:** 179–186.

Singer P, Gödicke W, Voigt S, Hajdu I & Weiss M (1985) Post prandial hyperinsulinemia in patients with mild essential hypertension. *Hypertension* **7:** 182–186.

Small DM (1977) Cellular mechanisms for lipid deposition in atherosclerosis. *New England Journal of Medicine* **297:** 873–879, 924–929.

Stalder M, Pometta D & Sueram A (1981) Relationship between plasma insulin levels and high density lipoprotein cholesterol levels in healthy men. *Diabetologia* **21:** 544–548.

Standl E & Janka HU (1985) High serum insulin concentrations in relation to other cardiovascular risk factors in macrovascular disease of type 2 diabetes. *Hormone and Metabolic Research* **(supplement) 17:** 46–51.

Stolar MW (1988) Atherosclerosis in diabetes: The role of hyperinsulinemia. *Metabolism* **37 (supplement 1):** 1–9.

Stout RW (1975) The effect of insulin on the incorporation of D-glucose $U^{14}C$ into the lipids of the rat aorta in vivo. *Hormone and Metabolic Research* **7:** 31–34.

Stout RW (1977) The effect of insulin and glucose on sterol synthesis in cultured rat arterial smooth muscle cells. *Arteriosclerosis* **27:** 271–288.

Stout RW (1987) Insulin and atheroma—an update. *Lancet* **1:** 1077–1079.

Stout RW, Bierman EL & Ross R (1975) Effect of insulin on the proliferation of cultured primate arterial smooth muscle cells. *Circulation Research* **36:** 319–327.

Strandness DE, Priest RE & Gibbons EE (1964) Combined clinical and pathological study of diabetic and non-diabetic peripheral arterial disease. *Diabetes* **13:** 366–372.

Struthers AD, Murphy MB & Dollery CT (1985) Glucose tolerance during antihypertensive therapy in patients with diabetes mellitus. *Hypertension* **7: (supplement II)** 95–101.

Tattersall RB & Scott AR (1987) When to use insulin in the maturity onset diabetic. *Postgraduate Medical Journal* **63:** 859–864.

Tompkins CV, Brandenburg D, Jones RH & Sönksen PH (1981) Mechanism of action of insulin and insulin analogues. A comparison of the hepatic and peripheral effects on glucose turnover of insulin, proinsulin and three insulin analogues modified at positions A1 and B29. *Diabetologia* **20:** 94–101.

Vague P, Juhan-Vague I, Aillaud MF et al (1986) Correlation between blood fibrinolytic activity, plasminogen activator inhibitor level, plasma insulin level and relative body weight in normal and obese subjects. *Metabolism* **35:** 250–253.

Vigorita VJ, Moore GW & Hutchins GM (1980) Absence of correlation between coronary arterial atherosclerosis and severity or duration of diabetes mellitus of adult onset. *American Journal of Cardiology* **46:** 535–542.

Weidmann P, Beretta-Piccoli C, Keusch G et al (1979) Sodium-volume factor, cardiovascular reactivity and hypotensive mechanism of diuretic therapy in mild hypertension associated with diabetes mellitus. *American Journal of Medicine* **67:** 779–784.

Welborn TA & Wearne K (1979) Coronary heart disease incidence and cardiovascular mortality in Busselton with reference to glucose and insulin concentrations. *Diabetes Care* **2:** 154–160.

Welborn TA, Breckenridge A, Rubinstein AH, Dollery CT & Russel Fraser T (1966) Serum-insulin in essential hypertension and in peripheral vascular disease. *Lancet* **1:** 1336–1337.

Wingard DL, Barrett-Connor E, Criqui MH & Suarez L (1983) Clustering of heart disease risk factors in diabetic compared to non-diabetic adults. *American Journal of Epidemiology* **117:** 19–26.

Wolinsky H, Goldfischer S, Capron L et al (1978) Hydrolase activities in the rat aorta. 1. Effects of diabetes mellitus and insulin treatment. *Circulation Research* **42:** 821–831.

Wright AD, Barber SG, Kendall MJ & Poole PH (1979) Beta-adrenoceptor-blocking drugs and blood sugar control in diabetes mellitus. *British Medical Journal* **1:** 159–164.

9

Dietary therapy in NIDDM

GILLIAN C. PEARSON
JOHN K. WALES

The definitive dietary treatment of diabetes began at the end of the 18th century with John Rollo but the need for dietary advice for diabetic patients was known to both Ancient Greek and Indian physicians. Rollo's unpalatable diets were carbohydrate restricted but improved symptoms in the short term. They were further developed by Bouchardat based on his observations during the seige of Paris in 1870. The principle of undernutrition was taken to extreme by Catani and Allen just before the introduction of insulin therapy often with carbohydrate intakes as low as 10–30 g per day.

Following the introduction of insulin it became clear that food intake could be expanded but the degree and mode of this expansion was not clear. The concept of 'exchange' diets became established in which all foods were related to some standard which was either a food itself (e.g. a slice of bread) or an arbitrary number of calories from different sources, such as in the Lawrence Line Ration Scheme (Lawrence 1955) where one Black Line (10 g carbohydrate) and one Red Line (7.5 g protein + 9 g fat) were balanced in the diet assuming a daily requirement of 25 kcal/kg body weight. These diets which were both practical and relatively easy for the patient to use applied to both IDDM and NIDDM patients of average weight although it was always accepted that obese diabetic patients needed hypocaloric diets and weight loss.

In recent years there has been a refreshing re-examination of the dietary needs for diabetic patients to achieve good glycaemic control in both the USA (NIH Consensus Statement, 1987) and UK (British Diabetic Association, 1982) with specific recommendations being suggested in the former (Table 1). There is, as yet, a dearth of long-term studies on the effects of both 'older' and 'newer' dietary regimens on diabetic complications. A major problem in such studies and in clinical practice is patient compliance. Eating has psychological, social and economic overtones which cannot be ignored when considering the prescription of a diet for an individual patient.

Figure 1 shows the distribution of age and weight (BMI = weight kg/ (height m)^2 in 442 untreated NIDDM patients using WHO diagnostic criteria (1980), seen consecutively over a five year period. There was a slight excess of men over women but the women were older with 54% women over 65 years but only 33% men. This difference in age at presentation is in part

Table 1. Nutritional recommendations for NIDDM patients in US. Sources: National Institutes of Health Consensus statement, (1987); American Diabetes Association, (1979).

Intake	Recommendation
Calorie	1. to achieve and maintain desirable body weight 2. if weight reduction required, restrict intake to 500–1000 kcal below requirements
Carbohydrate	1. should be liberalized to 55–60% total calorie intake but individualized dependent on the impact on blood glucose and lipid profiles 2. unrefined carbohydrate and foods with high fibre content should be included in high % carbohydrate diets. 3. sucrose (table sugar) and unrefined carbohydrate may be acceptable in some patients upto 5% of carbohydrate calorie intake if patients are lean and do not have CHO induced hyperlipidaemia
Protein	0.8 g/Kg body weight or 12–20% calorie content of diet although the elderly may need more and patients with renal failure less.
Fat	1. Total fat restricted to <30% total calorie intake 2. Cholesterol <300 mg/day 3. Unsaturated fat > saturated
Salt	1 g/1000 kcal intake maximum 3 g/day reduced in hypertensive NIDDM patients
Alcohol	limited as in nondiabetic patients

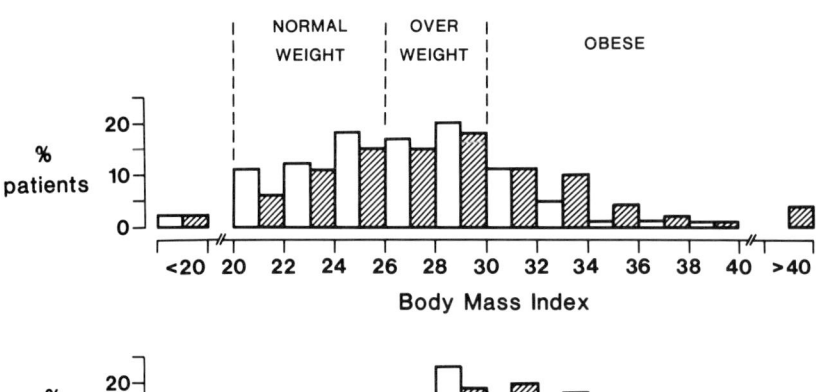

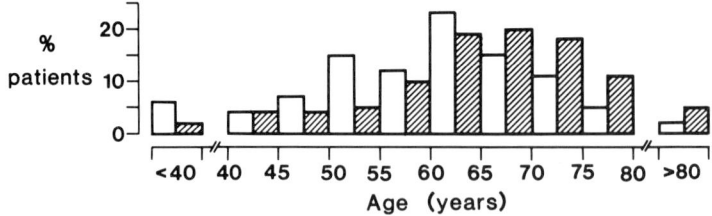

Figure 1. The distribution of body weight (expressed as body mass index) and age in 442 newly diagnosed, untreated NIDDM patients. Men (open columns) women (hatched columns).

due to 31% men presenting to their doctors without any substantive diabetic symptoms, glycosuria having been detected at routine employment or insurance medical examination or routine urine tests at other clinics, such as the hypertension clinic. Only 13% women presented in this way. A lack of symptoms may reduce a patient's motivation to keep to any therapy, including diet, however, the finding of diabetic retinopathy in 10% of these 442 patients does demonstrate the need for effective antidiabetic therapy in most patients and this does include diet.

Half the men were overweight (BMI >25) and 11% obese (BMI ⩾31) whereas 66% women were overweight and 25% obese. Therefore the importance of weight loss by energy controlled diets would seem to be clear. Indeed there are some physicians who assert that calorie restriction is the only requirement for a NIDDM diet (NIH Consensus Statement, 1987). Another important socio-economic factor in achieving dietary compliance is family support. A proportion of both women (24%) and men (11%) lived alone and presumably, in the main, cooked for themselves and lacked this type of family support.

These findings have been confirmed by the UK Prospective Diabetes Study (1988) although only new diabetic patients under the age of 65 years were studied. It is therefore to this group of diabetic patients that the dietary prescription is given as initial treatment, i.e. to older, overweight men and women, many of whom have no diabetic symptoms and many of whom have little family support at home.

THE DIETARY PRESCRIPTION

The most important dietary treatment for NIDDM patients is energy restriction resulting in a reduction of weight to normal. This can be problematical: the first obstacle being to decide what is a normal weight. As it is now fairly well recognized that there is no such thing as an ideal body weight for an individual (Jarrett, 1986) it is hard to give a target weight to a NIDDM patient. Studies indicate that weight losses of 10–16% of initial body weight lead to improved diabetic control (Hadden et al, 1975; Reaven et al, 1985; Henry et al, 1986a). This could therefore be used as a guideline. Alternatively, to aim for a BMI of at least less than 30 is a reasonable aim while 20–26 is regarded as the 'normal range'. Many diabetic patients find this degree of weight loss extremely difficult although there are some additional dietary strategies which will benefit them even without weight loss. These can also be recommended for non-obese NIDDM patients and are discussed below.

The major source of energy in the diet of the diabetic patient has altered over the years. Until recently fat supplied more than half the total energy intake. The rationale for this high fat intake was that carbohydrate had to be restricted in order to control blood glucose levels. Studies have shown however that high carbohydrate diets do not lead to worsening blood glucose control and in some cases lead to an improvement. It is now suggested that the diabetic diet should contain at least 50% energy intake in carbohydrate form. This means a reduced contribution to the diet from fat (ideally less than 30% of total energy intake) and it is hoped that this may reduce the incidence of coronary heart disease (CHD). A reduction in CHD by low fat diets might be mediated through a reduction in blood cholesterol levels although longer term studies will have to be carried out to see if this leads to an actual reduction in mortality from CHD in diabetes.

The potential disadvantage of increasing carbohydrate intake in a diet is the induction of hypertriglyceridaemia. To what extent this is a transient effect, and can be controlled by altering the type of carbohydrate consumed, is far from clear. At present the potential advantages of decreasing plasma cholesterol levels are thought to outweigh this disadvantage.

The reduction in fat intake should be achieved mainly by reducing saturated fat sources in the diet. When fat is used in cooking, a poly-unsaturated vegetable oil can be recommended.

Can a NIDDM patient eat sugar?

It is widely believed that short chain length carbohydrates (sugars), such as glucose, sucrose and lactose, are more rapidly digested and absorbed than longer chain complex carbohydrates such as starch. If foods containing short chain carbohydrates such as sweet foods are consumed, this leads to a more rapid rise in blood glucose levels. Foods containing complex carbohydrates, such as bread and potatoes, do not cause such a rapid rise.

For this reason it has been common practice to restrict, and in some cases eliminate, sucrose in the diabetic patient's diet yet other sources of simple carbohydrates, such as milk and fruit, have always been recommended. The rationale for this is not clear. A number of studies have indicated that the addition of sucrose to the diet of NIDDM patients does not worsen diabetic control. This has been shown in both single meal (Bantle et al, 1986; Vorster et al, 1987) and longer term studies (Jellish et al, 1984; Peterson et al, 1986b).

Another argument against permitting sucrose in the diabetic diet is that it will lead to more marked hypertriglyceridaemia than if complex carbo-hydrates are consumed (Albrink and Ullrich, 1986). If moderate amounts are allowed, however, this does not appear to be true. In the study of Jellish et al (1984) only high levels of sucrose intake, (220 g of sucrose or 40% of total energy intake per day) led to an increase in fasting plasma triglyceride levels. Intermediate (120 g or 20% total energy as sucrose) intake did not lead to increases in either fasting or postprandial triglyceride levels. The high sucrose diets contained more carbohydrate than the other diets and this may explain the effects on triglyceride levels. Peterson et al (1986b) did not show an increase in fasting plasma triglyceride levels after the six weeks on the added sucrose diet. Indeed in the study of Albrink and Ullrich (1986) the addition of up to 8% of the energy intake as sucrose did not increase plasma triglyceride levels. It is clear however that longer term studies are necessary.

One of the main practical problems of following the new recom-mendations to eat a diet high in complex carbohydrate is the large bulk of food that must be consumed. The replacement of some complex carbohydrate with sucrose may enable a diabetic patient to comply more easily with the dietary prescription. It would appear reasonable that amounts of up to 50 g sucrose per day could be allowed in a variety of forms, for example sugar on high fibre cereal; marmalade or jam on wholemeal bread.

Another reason often given for a restriction of sucrose in the diet is the argument that if small amounts are permitted this may lead to consumption of much larger amounts. This idea has never been tested, but since the evidence is that diabetic patients do not comply with the current dietary advice, if diets are more 'lenient', compliance may then actually improve, thus improving control. Additionally greater flexibility and taking individual dietary habits into account should lead to better compliance. Attempting to gain co-operation from a patient by engendering anxiety about dietary indiscretions does not appear to improve motivation or compliance.

For the obese subject, the situation is different. Sugar is definitely not advisable. A non-nutritive sweetener should be used.

Glycaemic indices

The glycaemic index of a food is a relatively new idea. A number of researchers have found that carbohydrate from different sources has a variable effect on postprandial blood glucose levels (Crapo et al, 1976; Jenkins et al, 1981). Jenkins et al (1981) first described this response as the glycaemic index of a food calculated from:

$$\frac{\text{Area under 2 hour blood glucose response curve for the test food}}{\text{Area under 2 hour blood glucose response curve for glucose}} \times 100$$

A summary of some glycaemic indices is shown in Table 2. It can be seen that the glycaemic index of a food is not related to either the chain length of the carbohydrate or to the fibre content of the food.

Some of the work on glycaemic indices has been criticized because it has been carried out using a small number of subjects, not all the subjects being diabetic, and the foods have been tested in isolation rather than when incorporated in meals. Preliminary work with diabetic patients however has indicated that not only are the differences between carbohydrate sources evident but that they may be more pronounced (Crapo et al, 1980). Studies which have included the carbohydrate as part of a meal have shown differing results. Coulston et al (1987) and Laine et al (1987) were unable to show that low glycaemic index foods led to significant differences in either blood glucose or insulin responses when incorporated into a meal, but Bornet et al (1987) and Collier et al (1986) were able to demonstrate a difference. The reason for these conflicting results could be due to the size of the meal and the proportion of carbohydrate consumed. In the studies of Coulston et al (1987) and Laine et al (1987), the meals supplied at least 40% of the total daily energy requirement for the subject. Both Bornet et al (1987) and Collier et al (1986) used meals of lower energy intake, which could be thought to represent a more realistic situation.

More research is required in this area as, at present, there is insufficient

Table 2. Glycaemic index: the area under the blood glucose response curve for each food expressed as a percentage of the area after taking the same amount of carbohydrate as glucose. Based on the work of Jenkins et al, 1981.

Glycaemic Index	Food
100	Glucose
80–99	Cornflakes Honey
70–79	Bread (wholemeal) Rice (white) Weetabix Broad beans Potato
60–69	Bread (white) Rice (brown) Shredded Wheat Banana Raisins Mars Bar
50–59	Spaghetti (white) Sweetcorn Digestive biscuits Sucrose Crisps
40–49	Spaghetti (wholemeal) Sponge cake Baked beans Oranges
30–39	Butter beans Haricot beans Chick peas Apples Ice Cream Yoghurt Tomato Soup
20–29	Kidney beans Lentils

and conflicting information available to predict accurately the glycaemic effect of a food within a complex meal and it is not yet possible to categorize sources of carbohydrate in food. In the future, dietitians may be able to concentrate on giving advice to patients on carbohydrate sources rather than amounts. The current recommendations to use lentils and beans as sources of complex carbohydrates would appear to be sound advice and quite widely used in the UK.

At present, most dietitians advise diabetics to consume a certain amount of carbohydrate, distributed throughout the day by using an exchange system. One carbohydrate exchange meal is equal to 10 grammes of carbo-hydrate. The British Diabetic Association (1982) in their recommendations state that carbohydrate exchanges are an essential part of the dietary management of the insulin-dependent diabetic. The use of carbohydrate exchanges does allow some degree of flexibility in the diet which is understood by the patient while still ensuring a regular and even distribution of carbohydrate throughout the day. However, when more information becomes available about the glycaemic effect of different carbohydrates, dietitians may be able to give more advice about the carbohydrate sources and exchanges could be discontinued. For NIDDM patients this may already be the case. Simple advice on regular meals and avoiding binging is more appropriate than an estimate of carbohydrate intake at each meal. However in the obese NIDDM patient a dietary strategy leading to weight loss is of the greatest importance.

Fibre

Studies have shown that pectin reduces postprandial blood glucose rise (Jenkins et al, 1976). There are few studies, however, which have shown cereal sources of fibre to be as effective in lowering postprandial blood glucose levels. Increasing dietary fibre by two and a half times, mainly from cereal soures, had no effect on blood glucose control in NIDDM patients (Hollenbeck et al, 1986), but Rivellese et al (1980) found that increasing dietary fibre did improve glycaemic control. However in their study 45% of the fibre was supplied by peas, beans and lentils, which are known to have a low glycaemic index. In practice the main sources in the diabetic diet of increased fibre intake are from cereals, such as wholemeal bread and high fibre breakfast cereals. It is therefore debatable whether this increase in fibre intake will improve blood glucose control although it has been shown that a long term increase in cereal fibre intake leads to improved glucose tolerance (Villaume et al, 1984).

It has also been suggested that increasing dietary fibre intake may prevent the increase in serum triglyceride levels associated with increased carbohydrate intake (Riccardi et al, 1984). However the sources of fibre in this study were again predominantly from beans, peas and lentils. Lousley et al (1984) also found reduced serum triglyceride levels in NIDDM patients on a high carbohydrate diet containing a high percentage of low glycaemic index carbohydrate. A number of bodies currently recommend to the general public dietary fibre intake from all sources (National Advisory Committee on Nutrition Education, 1983; Committee on Medical Aspects of Food Policy, 1984). There may be therefore additional health advantages for increasing fibre intake not specific to diabetic patients.

Alcohol

Ethanol inhibits gluconeogenesis thus having a hypoglycaemic effect. This effect is particularly apparent in people on very low carbohydrate diets, who have depleted glycogen stores (McLaughlin et al, 1973). The higher carbohydrate diet now recommended for diabetic patients should be protective against ethanol-induced hypoglycaemia.

In moderation ethanol does not have a deleterious effect on blood glucose control. Up to three alcoholic drinks per day is a reasonable allowance for NIDDM patients of average weight. This is a similar level to that recommended for non-diabetic subjects. One drink is equivalent to one glass of wine, half a pint of beer or one measure of spirits. It is not advisable to reduce food intake prior to alcohol, because of the possible hypoglycaemic effect. Alcohol combined with chlorpropamide can lead to facial flushes; these are less severe when alcohol is taken with a meal (Lolli et al, 1963). Overweight diabetic patients should avoid alcohol altogether since it is a concentrated source of energy.

Very low calorie diets

Very low calorie diets (VLCD) have been used to promote weight loss in NIDDM patients with some success (Henry et al, 1986b), but a recent report has highlighted reservations about such diets (Committee on Medical Aspects of Food Policy, 1987). NIDDM patients on oral hypoglycaemic agents should be supervized carefully because of the risk of hypoglycaemia if drug treatment is not adjusted when this diet is begun. There is also little evidence that the weight loss achieved by using VLCD is maintained. This is, to some extent, true for all weight-reducing regimes, but very rapid weight loss may be regained more quickly, particularly when no overall changes in eating habits have been acquired.

Sweeteners

There are a number of sweeteners available for use by diabetics. They can be broadly divided into non-nutritive and nutritive sweeteners. The non-nutritive sweeteners include saccharin, aspartame and acesulfame K and can be used freely by all NIDDM patients. The nutritive sweeteners such as sorbitol and fructose contain the same number of calories as sugar and therefore can only be used by normal weight diabetic patients. Fructose results in improved glycaemic control compared with other sources of carbohydrate including glucose (Bantle et al, 1986). It and products made with fructose are considerably more expensive than sucrose. It should be borne in mind when recommending fructose or sorbitol-containing products that there is a limit to the amount that can be consumed, the BDA recommend a maximum of 50 g per day.

COMPLIANCE WITH DIETARY ADVICE

Compliance with medical advice is known to be poor and reported to be in the region of 50% non-compliance (Ley, 1982). Therefore not surprisingly the compliance levels for dietary advice are also poor. If patients are unable to comply with apparently straightforward advice on taking medication, altering the eating habits of a lifetime must be a very daunting prospect. For example, figures reported for the success rate of treating obesity with diet vary from 7–50%; or conversely 50–93% patients on weight-reducing diets do not comply with dietary advice.

There has been little work reported on how successful NIDDM patients are at losing weight. Hadden et al (1975) do report good weight loss in their subjects. Seaton and Rose (1965) also reported that diabetic patients were less likely to default from treatment than other overweight subjects. Female subjects with a BMI of less than 35, over 40 years old and with a medical condition which will benefit from weight loss, have also been shown to respond well to one-to-one dietetic consultations (Pearson, 1987). Thus it could be anticipated that overweight diabetic patients should do better than other overweight non-diabetic subjects.

Compliance by NIDDM patients to other aspects of dietary advice is also poor. Only one third are described as being good compliers (Thomas, 1981; Wilson et al, 1986), and Kendall et al (1987) have suggested that only 47% of NIDDM patients questioned were following their diet. Various methods have been explored for improving dietary compliance. The first step may be to improve the education of NIDDM patients so that they have an understanding of both the reasons for their diet prescription and of the diet itself. Knowledge alone does not necessarily lead to compliance, however, a patient cannot comply with a diet without the knowledge of 'how' and 'why'. Reports show that 39% of NIDDM patients have no knowledge of their diet and 24% have only poor knowledge (Thomas, 1981). Kendall et al (1987) showed that 25% of diabetic patients had no dietary knowledge at all. The situation does not appear to have materially altered since West (1973) described the abject failure of dietary therapy in diabetic patients of all types.

The reasons for this failure may be poor communication between the dietitian and the patient. McNeal et al (1984) found that there was a significant mismatch between the reading and comprehension level of diabetic patients and the level of oral and printed materials. It is true that current methods of giving dietary advice to diabetics do not appear to be very effective (Page et al, 1981; McCulloch et al, 1983). Dietitians and other health professionals fail to take into account the cognitive ability of the patients. The information given is often complex, too much is presented at once, and is often given at a time of anxiety. Simply controlling the amount of information given at one interview and presenting it in a logical order could improve understanding.

The following factors should also be borne in mind when advising patients about diet.

1. Individualizing dietary advice is thought to be beneficial (Weinsier et al, 1974).
2. Involving the diabetic patient in the decision-making process and involving other family members in the treatment are other useful strategies (Weinsier et al, 1974; Sulway et al; 1980, McManus et al, 1986).
3. Sulway et al (1980) reported that 50% of patients had emotional difficulties due to their diabetes which required counselling. Regular follow up both to reinforce the advice given and to explore any difficulties is

therefore important. Many dietitians are now receiving training in counselling and communication skills and greater use should be made of these (Davidson et al, 1987).
4. McCulloch et al (1983) found that imaginative teaching methods, such as the use of videos, improved knowledge, compliance and control in IDDM patients. This approach could also be used for NIDDM patients.
5. Continuity of care by the same therapist is important in subjects who wish to lose weight (Hall et al, 1975; Stuart and Guire, 1978) and may well improve compliance with other dietary changes.
6. Group work may also be beneficial (Weinsier et al, 1974; Sulway et al, 1980).

ETHNIC GROUPS

Diabetes mellitus is more common in the Asian than the European community (Mather and Keen, 1985). Asians are estimated to make up about 4.5% of the total diabetic population attending British diabetic clinics, although it will vary considerably from one area of the country to another (Goodwin et al, 1987). The eating habits of the Asian community tend to be very different from the indigenous population and will vary within the Asian community depending upon religion and tradition. The diet overall tends to be high in fat, since most food is fried in oil, butter or ghee, and high in sugar, fizzy drinks being particularly popular (Wharton and Eaton, 1983). Diabetic Asians have been found to consume a high fat, high sugar, low fibre diet (Peterson et al, 1986; Samanta et al, 1987). Dietary knowledge appears to be poor. In one study 86% of patients had no dietary knowledge (Thomas, 1981).

There seems little point in advising that traditional foods be cooked other than in fat, but the type and amount of fat could be altered, for example switching to a polyunsaturated cooking oil, such as corn oil or groundnut oil, would be beneficial.

Communication is often a major problem with ethnic groups. There may be language barriers to be overcome, and patients may not be literate in either their own language or English. Education aids must be produced specifically for each group. The dietitian must acquire a good knowledge of both the cultural beliefs relating to food and the eating habits of the patient to provide relevant dietary advice.

THE EXTENT OF DIETARY MANIPULATION

It is claimed that in order to implement the modern dietary recommendations for diabetic patients, such major changes have to be made in food intake that these diets are short lived and unacceptable to the majority of patients. Table 3 shows the changes that need to be made in the diet of a 65 year old NIDDM patient of average weight and intelligence, using a computer aided diet assessment of daily food records designed by Jane

Close, a Research Dietitian in Leeds General Infirmary. Note the reduction in calorie, fat and sodium intake and the increase in carbohydrate, fibre and polyunsaturated fat intake contrasted with the modest changes in the type and quantities of food eaten.

ADJUVANTS TO DIETARY THERAPY

As compliance with diabetic diets is such a problem it is not surprising that physicians have turned to various drugs to enhance the effects of incomplete diet therapy.

Guar

Guar gum (Peterson and Mann, 1985) is an unabsorbable long chain poly-saccharide and is the ground endosperm of the seeds of *Cyanopsis tetragonolobus*, the cluster bean. Its effect is probably based on the delayed absorption of carbohydrate from the intestine and a reduction in post-prandial blood glucose and plasma insulin levels. Guar also has a hypo-cholesterolaemic activity thought to be due in part to an effect on bile salt binding in the gut. The optimal dose would appear to be 15 g/day in divided doses. It is not an easy substance to formulate and may initially have unpleasant gastrointestinal symptoms (diarrhoea and flatulence) which may deter patients. It has been incorporated into food. Its long term success in achieving improved glycaemic control and retardation of diabetic complications has not yet been determined.

α-glucosidase inhibitors

Another approach to reduce the postprandial blood glucose rise in NIDDM patients is by the competitive inhibition of the enzyme α-glucosidase in the intestine. The first drug in this field was acarbose, which is a pseudo-oligosaccharide obtained from cultures of Actinomycetales. These drugs delay the breakdown of poly- and oligo-saccharides contained in the diet and the absorption of mono- and di-saccharides thus reducing postprandial hyperglycaemia, although carbohydrate absorption overall is not reduced (Scott and Tattersall, 1988). Some newer drugs of this group are absorbed, unlike acarbose. The major side effects are again gastrointestinal.

Antiobesity drugs

As obesity would appear to play such an important role in the pathogenesis of NIDDM it would seem logical that antiobesity agents might also be effective. It is difficult to be sure whether these drugs have any intrinsic antidiabetic action outside their effect upon appetite and body weight. There is some evidence that fenfluramine, an intra-cerebral serotonin releasing agent, does have some intrinsic antidiabetic activity, but it is not great (Wales, 1979). However this drug and its metabolite, d-fenfluramine are

Table 3. A representative day's diet taken from a seven day food diary of a 65 year old white Caucasian NIDDM patient (weight—84 Kg: height 167 cm) with a previously prescribed diabetic diet of 1500 kCals (40% carbohydrate).

Food	Amt	kCals	Prot g	Fat g	CHO g	Alc g	Sugar g	Stch g	Fibre g
Breakfast									
White Bread	32 g	74	2	0.5	15.9	0	0.5	15.3	0.8
Margarine (animal									
and vegetable oils)	7 g	51	0	5.6	0	0	0	0	0
Subtotal		125	2	6.1	15.9	0	0.5	15.3	0.8
Mid-morning									
Currant bread	56 g	140	4	1.9	29	0	7.2	21.7	0.9
Margarine soft	10 g	73	0	8.1	0	0	0	0	0
Shortbread	14 g	70	0.8	3.6	9.1	0	2.4	6.7	0.2
Subtotal		283	5	13.6	38.1	0	9.6	28.4	1.1
Lunch									
White bread	56 g	130	4.3	0.9	27.8	0	1	26.8	1.5
Margarine (soft)	10 g	73	0	8.1	0	0	0	0	0
Tomato	60 g	8	0.5	0	1.6	0	1.6	0	0.9
Tongue	56 g	119	8.9	9.2	0	0	0	0	0
Chocolate biscuit	20 g	104	1.1	5.5	13.4	0	8.6	4.8	0.6
Subtotal		434	14.8	23.7	42.8	0	11.2	31.6	3
Mid-afternoon									
No food taken	0 g	0	0	0	0	0	0	0	0
Subtotal	0 g	0	0	0	0	0	0	0	0
Evening meal									
Roast chicken	112 g	173	25.8	7.7	0	0	0	0	0
Lettuce	20 g	2	0.2	0	0.2	0	0.2	0	0.3
Tomato	60 g	8	0.5	0	1.6	0	1.6	0	0.9
Cucumber	20 g	2	0.1	0	0.3	0	0.3	0	0
Salad cream (1 tbsp)									
low calorie	7 g	21	0.1	1.9	1	0	0.9	0.1	0
Brown bread	56 g	124	4.9	1.2	25	0	1	24	2.8
Margarine soft	14 g	102	0	11.3	0	0	0	0	0
Subtotal		342	31.6	22.1	28.1	0	4	24.1	4
Supper									
Diabetic lager	330 g	135	1.4	0	3.3	16.1	3.3	0	0
Apples whole	112 g	39	0.2	0	10.3	0	10.1	0.1	1.6
Roasted salted nuts	56 g	319	13.6	27.4	4.8	0	1.7	3	4.5
Semi-sweet biscuit	28 g	127	1.8	4.6	20.9	0	6.2	14.7	0.6
Subtotal		620	17	32	39.3	16.1	21.3	17.8	6.7
Daily allowance									
Skimmed milk	112 g	36	3.8	0.1	5.6	0	5.6	0	0
Milk	196 g	127	6.4	7.4	9.2	0	9.2	0	0
Subtotal		163	10.2	7.5	14.8	0	14.8	0	0
Totals		2057	80.3	105	179	16.1	61.4	117.2	15.6
Percentages			15.6%	46%	32.7%	5.4%			

Starch: Sugar ratio   =   1.9
Daily Fat intake
    Saturated   =   25.1 g
    Monounsaturated   =   37.3 g
    Polyunsaturated   =   17.1 g
    P/S ratio   =   0.68
Daily Sodium intake   =   2561.2 mg

Table 3. (cont'd) A diet for the same patient constructed so as to make as little impact on his eating habits and patterns; yet to approach the current dietary recommendations for such a patient. Note the reduction in Calorie, salt, % overall fat and saturated fat intakes and the increase in % carbohydrate and fibre intakes and P/S ratio (courtesy of Mrs Jane Close, Dietitian, Leeds General Infirmary.

Food	Amt	kCals	Prot g	Fat g	CHO g	Alc g	Sugar g	Stch g	Fibre g
Breakfast									
Sultana bran	56 g	170	4.3	0.7	39.2	0	8.4	30.8	7.3
Skimmed milk	112 g	36	3.8	0.1	5.6	0	5.6	0	0
Subtotal		206	8.1	0.8	44.8	0	14	30.8	7.3
Mid-morning									
Wholemeal bread	56 g	120	4.9	1.5	23.4	0	1.1	22.2	4.7
Margarine (Flora)	10 g	73	0	8.1	0	0	0	0	0
Digestive biscuit	14 g	65	1.3	2.8	9.2	0	2.2	6.9	0.7
Subtotal		258	6.2	12.4	32.6	0	3.3	29.1	5.4
Lunch									
Wholemeal bread	56 g	120	4.9	1.5	23.4	0	1.1	22.2	4.7
Margarine (Flora)	10 g	73	0	8.1	0	0	0	0	0
Tomato	60 g	8	0.5	0	1.6	0	1.6	0	0.9
Mackerel	56 g	124	10.6	9.1	0	0	0	0	0
Chocolate biscuit	20 g	104	1.1	5.5	13.4	0	8.6	4.8	0.6
Subtotal		429	17.1	24.2	38.4	0	11.3	27	6
Mid-afternoon									
Apples whole	112 g	39	0.2	0	10.3	0	10.1	0.1	1.6
Subtotal		39	0.2	0	10.3	0	10.1	0.1	1.6
Evening meal									
Roast chicken	56 g	86	12.9	3.9	0	0	0	0	0
Lettuce	20 g	2	0.2	0	0.2	0	0.2	0	0.3
Tomato	50 g	7	0.4	0	1.4	0	1.4	0	0.7
Cucumber	20 g	2	0.1	0	0.3	0	0.3	0	0
Frozen peas boiled	50 g	20	2.7	0.2	2.1	0	0.5	1.6	6
Salad cream (1 tbsp)	7 g	21	0.1	1.9	1	0	0.9	0.1	0
Boiled pots	168 g	134	2.3	0.1	33	0	0.6	32.4	1.6
Subtotal		272	18.7	6	38	0	3.9	34.1	8.6
Supper									
Diabetic lager	330 g	135	1.4	0	3.3	16.1	3.3	0	0
Apples whole	112 g	39	0.2	0	10.3	0	10.1	0.1	1.6
Digestive biscuit	14 g	65	1.3	2.8	9.2	0	2.2	6.9	0.7
Subtotal		239	2.9	2.8	22.8	16.1	15.6	7	2.3
Daily allowance									
Skimmed milk	300 g	99	10.2	0.3	15	0	15	0	0
Subtotal		99	10.2	0.3	15	0	15	0	0
Totals		1542	63.4	46.5	201.9	16.1	73.2	128.1	31.4
Percentages			16.4%	27.1%	49.1%	7.3%			

Starch: Sugar ratio	=	1.75
Daily Fat intake		
Saturated	=	7.8 g
Monounsaturated	=	9.2 g
Polyunsaturated	=	11.6 g
P/S ratio	=	1.48
Daily Sodium intake	=	2147.3 mg

known to reduce carbohydrate intake in animals, which would be expected to improve carbohydrate tolerance. Other drugs, such as fluoxamine, femoxetine and fluoxetine, may reduce non-protein calorie intake to a more marked degree (Blundell, 1984). The ability to manipulate the hunger and satiety centres of the brain is, perhaps, one of the most exciting areas of clinical research at present, in attempts to produce significant weight loss in obesity and perhaps also to improve glycaemia and reduce morbidity and mortality in NIDDM patients.

The obese diabetic patient, like the non-diabetic obese patient, is often regarded by doctors and nurses to be suffering from a self-inflicted disorder which does not need drugs and from which they can escape if they have the willpower. As there is no evidence that antiobesity drugs adversely affect glucose tolerance, such drugs may have a beneficial effect in combination with dietary advice, to reduce weight and thus glycaemia.

DIETARY FAILURE

In clinical practice NIDDM patients are usually only given dietary therapy for some weeks. This frequently improves symptoms often before weight loss but the improvement in glycaemia may not be sufficient. In the elderly patient (over 75 years), without significant diabetic complications no further therapy is indicated as it is unlikely the patients will survive to develop significant complications. In the majority of patients, drug therapy is then considered, either dietary adjuvants or specific antidiabetic therapy, such as insulin or oral hypoglycaemic agents. Often the diet is then relaxed by the patient in the belief that 'the tablets' are now the specific antidiabetic treatment and dieting is less important. This relaxation may give rise in turn to a poor response to such added therapy. In the obese patient, a biguanide would seem to be the drug of choice as sulphonylureas appear to slow down weight loss or even reverse it. If a sulphonylurea is used, a modification in the timing and amount of food taken may be required to avoid hypo-glycaemia, particularly in the older patient at night.

There is evidence to suggest that diet will only reverse a certain degree of glucose intolerance and, above this, drug or insulin therapy is required to achieve normoglycaemia (Wales, 1982). This is hardly diet failure, more inappropriate diet therapy. Some NIDDM patients, who initially are successfully treated by diet alone, slowly become less well controlled despite further advice and require the addition of other drug therapy. It is difficult to be sure whether this is true B cell exhaustion or merely boredom with diet and reducing compliance.

THE EFFICACY OF DIETARY THERAPY IN NIDDM PATIENTS

There are few studies from British Diabetic Clinics which are able to discuss the long term efficacy of diet therapy in NIDDM to achieve glycaemic control and none which can measure the ability of such therapy to prevent or reverse diabetic complications. In a study from Birmingham (Horrocks et al, 1987) using 'newer' dietary advice 23 out of 65 NIDDM patients remained well controlled on diet alone for three years. However after this period only 14% patients were still taking 50% calories as carbohydrate, fibre intake had only doubled whereas the initial advice was to increase intake 3–4 times, and there was no reduction in fat intake.

In Belfast (Hadden et al, 1986) of 233 NIDDM patients aged at diagnosis 40–69 and followed for six years, 80% remained well controlled on diet alone and what is more significant, the mortality from all causes was not greater in these diet-treated diabetic patients than for the general population in Northern Ireland. The diet used in this study could be regarded as an 'old type' (1500 cal, 150 g CHO—40% total calories; 70 g protein—20%; 60 g fat—38% with 500 g cholesterol; 13 g fibre and excluding sucrose with simple clear instruction). Attendance at the clinic was frequent being every three months including visits to both the doctor *and* the dietitian. The authors point out that their style of didactic care perhaps fits in better with the Ulster philosophy rather than elsewhere, and we are inclined to agree.

Comparisons with results obtained in other socio-economic groups or countries are particularly poor with regard to food intake, but the UGDP study (1970) showed after 13 years there were no differences in morbidity and mortality in those NIDDM patients treated with either diet alone or diet plus insulin therapy. Both did better than diet plus tolbutamide therapy with regard to cardiovascular mortality after 8.5 years therapy.

The studies of new dietary strategies in NIDDM, such as high fibre, high unrefined CHO, and the like, have been largely assessed in short term research studies in selected patients lasting weeks and months, rarely years. Some recommendations for NIDDM patients have been extended from work in insulin treated patients and even non-diabetic subjects. This has led to the present disarray in dietary advice given to patients as evidenced by a survey of European Diabetic Clinics (Toeller and Lion, 1987) where the only two recommendations for NIDDM patients which were common to all clinics were (a) to increase fibre intake and (b) the restriction and calculation of energy intake for the overweight patient.

SUMMARY

Clearly the dietary treatment of the NIDDM patient remains an act of faith bearing in mind the poor compliance of the patient to dietary advice, and the lack of long-term studies confirming the efficacy of diets (old or new) in the prevention of diabetic vascular complications. Few of the newer recommended diets seem to have been tested in the hurly-burly of the busy, understaffed diabetic clinic.

Perhaps another major hurdle has been the attitude of patients and doctors in failing to regard diet therapy as a form of treatment, akin to tablets. The phrase 'I eat my diet, doctor, then I have my usual meal' sums up the problem. There needs to be a change in attitude to diet by both doctors and patients so that the dietary changes suggested should be eating habits which would become second nature to patients—the so called 'healthy eating'—more fibre, less refined carbohydrate, less total and saturated fat and more polyunsaturated fats.

It seems difficult for a majority of NIDDM patients to add onto 'healthy eating' calorie restriction to achieve weight loss. This difficulty also applies to non-diabetic obese subjects with similar poor results. One cannot help but feel that NIDDM patients should benefit from the general change in attitude of the general population towards nutrition, but reinforced education concerning diet goals for NIDDM patients is an urgent requirement and needs closer examination by the diabetic health care team as to how it may be delivered to the individual NIDDM patients. Perhaps dietitians in particular should become more critical in their approach to diet strategies and should investigate and report on the results of this treatment.

REFERENCES

Albrink, MJ & Ullrich IH (1986) Interaction of dietary sucrose and fiber on serum lipids in healthy young men fed high carbohydrate diets. *American Journal of Clinical Nutrition* **43:** 419–428.

American Diabetes Association: Special Report (1979) Principles of nutrition and dietary recommendations for individuals with diabetes mellitus. *Diabetes* **28:** 1027–1030.

Bantle JP, Laine DC & Thomas JW (1986) Metabolic effects of dietary fructose and sucrose in types I and II diabetic subjects. *Journal of the American Medical Association* **256:** 3241–3246.

Blundell JE (1984) Serotonin and appetite. *Neuropharmacology* **23:** 1537–1551.

Bornet FRJ, Costagliola D, Rizkall SW et al (1987) Insulinaemic and glycaemic indexes of six starch-rich foods taken alone and in a mixed meat by type 2 diabetics. *American Journal of Clinical Nutrition* **45:** 588–595.

British Diabetic Association Medical Advisory Committee (1982) Dietary recommendations for diabetes for the 1980's—a policy statement by the British Diabetic Association. *Human Nutrition: Applied Nutrition* **36A:** 378–394.

Collier GR, Wolever TMS, Wong GS & Josse RG (1986) Prediction of glycaemic response to mixed meals in non-insulin-dependent diabetic subjects. *American Journal of Clinical Nutrition* **44:** 349–352.

Committee on Medical Aspects of Food Policy (1984) *Diet and Cardiovascular Disease. DHSS.* London: HMSO.

Committee on Medical Aspects of Food Policy (1987) *The use of very low calorie diets in obesity. DHSS.* London: HMSO.

Coulston AM, Hollenbeck CB, Swislocki ALM & Reaven GM (1987) Effect of source of dietary carbohydrate on plasma glucose and insulin responses to mixed meals in subjects with NIDDM. *Diabetes Care* **10:** 395–400.

Crapo PA, Reaven G & Olefsky J (1976) Plasma, glucose and insulin responses to orally administered simple and complex carbohydrates. *Diabetes* **25:** 741–747.

Crapo PA, Orville RD, Kolterman G, Waldeck N, Reaven GM & Olefsky JM (1980) Postprandial hormonal responses to different types to complex carbohydrate in individuals with impaired glucose tolerance. *American Journal of Clinical Nutrition* **33:** 1723–1728.

Davidson C, Kowalska AZ, Nutman PNS & Pearson GC (1987) Dietitian-Patient Communication: A critical appraisal and approach to training. *Human Nutrition: Applied Nutrition* **41A:** 381–389.

Goodwin AM, Keen H & Mather HM (1987) Ethnic minorities in British Diabetic Clinics: A questionnaire survey. *Diabetic Medicine* **4:** 266–269.

Hadden DR, Montgomery DAD, Skelly RJ et al (1975) Maturity onset diabetes mellitus:

response to intensive dietary management. *British Medical Journal* **3**: 276–278.

Hadden DR, Blair ALT, Wilson EA et al (1986) Natural history of diabetes presenting at age 40–69 years: a prospective study of the influence of intensive dietary treatment. *Quarterly Journal of Medicine* **59**: 579–598.

Hall SM, Hall RG, Borden BL & Hanson RW (1975) Follow up strategies in the behavioural treatment of the overweight. *Behavioural Research and Therapy* **13**: 167–172.

Henry RR, Wallace P & Olefsky JM (1986a) Effects of weight loss on mechanisms of hyperglycaemia in obese non-insulin-dependent-diabetes mellitus. *Diabetes* **35**: 990–998.

Henry RR, Wiest-Kent TA, Scheaffer L, Kolterman OG & Olefsky JM (1986b) Metabolic consequences of very-low-calorie-diet therapy in obese non-insulin-dependent diabetic and non-diabetic subjects. *Diabetes* **35**: 155–164.

Hollenbeck CB, Coulston AM & Reaven GM (1986) To what extent does increased dietary fibre improve glucose and lipid metabolism in patients with non-insulin-dependent diabetes mellitus. *American Journal of Clinical Nutrition* **43**: 16–24.

Horrocks PM, Blackmore R & Wright AD (1987) Long-term follow-up of dietary advice in maturity-onset diabetes. The experience of one centre in the U.K. Prospective Study. *Diabetic Medicine* **4**: 241–244.

Jarrett RJ (1986) Is there an ideal body weight? *British Medical Journal* **293**: 493–495.

Jellish WS, Emanuele MA & Abraira C (1984) Graded sucrose/carbohydrate diets in overtly hypertriglyceridemic diabetic patients. *American Journal of Medicine* **77**: 1015–1022.

Jenkins DJA, Goff DV, Leeds AR et al (1976) Unabsorbable carbohydrates and diabetes: decreased postprandial hyperglycaemia. *Lancet* **ii**: 172–174.

Jenkins DJA, Wolever TMS, Taylor RH et al (1981) Glycaemic index of foods: a physiological basis for carbohydrate exchange. *American Journal of Clinical Nutrition* **34**: 362–366.

Kendall PA, Janson CM, Sjogren DD & Jansen GR (1987) A comparison of nutrient-based and exchange group methods of diet instruction for patients with non insulin dependent diabetes. *American Journal of Clinical Nutrition* **45**: 625–637.

Laine DC, Thomas W, Levitt MD & Bantle JP (1987) Comparison of predictive capabilities of diabetic exchange lists and glycemic index of foods. *Diabetes Care* **10**: 387.

Lawrence RD (1985) *The Diabetic Life*. London: H K Lewis.

Ley P (1982) Satisfaction, compliance and communication. *British Journal of Clinical Psychology* **21**: 241–254.

Lolli G, Balboni C, Ballatore C et al (1963) Wine in the diets of diabetic patients. *Quarterly Journal on Studies with Alcohol* **24**: 412–416.

Lousely SE, Jones DB, Slaughter P, Carter RD, Jelfs R & Mann JI (1984) High carbohydrate high fibre diets in poorly controlled diabetes. *Diabetic Medicine* **1**: 21–25.

McCulloch DK, Mitchell RD, Ambler J & Tattersall RB (1983) Influence of imaginative teaching of diet on compliance and metabolic control in insulin dependent diabetes. *British Medical Journal* **287**: 1858–1861.

McLoughlin JM, Noel FJ & Moodie CA (1973) Hypoglycaemia in humans induced by alcohol and a low carbohydrate diet. *Nutrition Reports International* **8**: 331–336.

McManus H, Wales JK, Stickland MH & Pearson GC (1986) *A study of dietary knowledge and compliance in diabetic patients instructed by a family orientated teaching programme* pp 10. The British Dietetic Association International Symposium Abstracts: London.

McNeal B, Salisbury Z, Baumgardner P & Wheeler FC (1984) Comprehension assessment of diabetes education program participants. *Diabetes Care* **7**: 232–235.

Mather HM & Keen H (1985) The Southall Diabetes Survey: prevalence of known diabetes in Asians and Europeans. *British Medical Journal* **291**: 1081–1084.

National Advisory Committee on Nutrition Education (1983) *A discussion paper on proposals for nutritional guidelines for health education in Britain*. London: Health Education Council.

National Institutes of Health (1987) Consensus development conference on diet and exercise in non-insulin dependent diabetes mellitus. *Diabetes Care* **10**: 639–644.

Page PDG, Verstraete JR, Robb JR & Etzwiler DD (1981) Patient recall or self care recommendations in diabetes. *Diabetes Care* **4**: 96–98.

Pearson GC (1987) *The dietetic treatment of obesity in hospital and community clinics*. MPhil Thesis, CNAA Leeds Polytechnic.

Peterson DB & Mann JI (1985) Guar: Pharmacological fibre or food fibre. *Diabetic Medicine* **2**: 345–347.

Peterson DB, Dattari JT, Baylis JM & Jepson EM (1986a) Dietary practices of Asian diabetics. *British Medical Journal* **292:** 170–171.

Peterson DB, Lambert J, Gerring S et al (1986b) Sucrose in the diet of diabetic patients—just another carbohydrate? *Diabetologia* **29:** 216–220.

Reaven GM (1985) Beneficial effect of moderate weight loss in older patients with non-insulin-dependent diabetes mellitus poorly controlled with insulin. *Journal of the American Geriatric Society* **33:** 93–95.

Riccardi G, Rivellese A, Pacioni D Genovese S, Mastranzo P & Mancini M (1984) Separate influence of dietary carbohydrate and fibre on the metabolic control in diabetes. *Diabetologia* **26:** 116–121.

Rivellese A, Riccardi G, Giaco A et al (1980) Effect of dietary fibre on glucose control and serum lipoproteins in diabetic patients. *Lancet* **ii:** 447–450.

Samanta A, Campbell JE, Spalding DL, Parja KK, Neogi SK & Burden AC (1987) Dietary habits of Asian diabetics in a general practice clinic. *Human Nutrition: Applied Nutrition* **41A:** 160–163.

Scott AR & Tattersall RB (1988) Alpha-glucosidase inhibition in the treatment of non-insulin dependent diabetes mellitus. *Diabetic Medicine* **5:** 42–46.

Seaton DA & Rose K (1965) Defaulters from a weight reduction clinic. *Journal of Chronic Disease* **18:** 1007–1011.

Stuart RB & Guire K (1978) Some correlations of the maintenance of weight loss through behaviour modification. *International Journal of Obesity* **2:** 225–235.

Sulway M, Tupling H, Webb K & Harris G (1980) New techniques for changing compliance in diabetes. *Diabetes Care* **3:** 108–111.

Thomas BJ (1981) How successful are we at persuading diabetics to follow their diet—and why do sometimes fail? In Turner M & Thomas B (eds) *Nutrition and Diabetes*. London: John Libbey.

Toeller M & Lion S (1987) Survey of the management of diet in 26 Diabetes Centres in Europe. *Diabetic Medicine* **4:** 129–134.

UK Prospective Diabetes Study (1988) IV Characteristics of newly presenting Type 2 diabetic patients: Male pre-ponderance and obesity at different ages. *Diabetic Medicine* **5:** 154–159.

University Group Diabetes Program (1970) A study of the effects of hypoglycaemic agents on vascular complications in patients with adult-onset diabetes. II Mortality results. *Diabetes* **19:(supplement 2)** 785–830.

Villaume C, Beck B, Gariot P, Desalme A & Debry G (1984) Long term evolution of the effect of bran ingestion on meal-induced glucose and insulin responses in healthy men. *American Journal of Clinical Nutrition* **40:** 1023–1026.

Vorster HH, Van Tonder E, Kotze JP & Walker ARP (1987) Effects of graded sucrose additions on taste preference, acceptability, glycaemic index, and insulin response to butter beans. *American Journal of Clinical Nutrition* **45:** 575–579.

Wales JK (1979) The effect of fenfluramine on obese: maturity-onset diabetic patients. *Acta Endocrinologica* **90:** 616–623.

Wales JK (1982) Treatment of Type II (non-insulin dependent) diabetic patients with diet alone. *Diabetologia* **23:** 240–245.

Weinsier RL, Seeman A, Herrera MG, Simmons JJ & Collins ME (1974) Description of a successful methodologic approach to gaining diet adherence. *Diabetes* **23:** 669–673.

West KM (1973) Diet therapy of diabetes: an analysis of failure. *Annals of Internal Medicine* **79:** 425–434.

Wharton PA & Eaton PM (1983) Sorrento Asian Food Tables: Food tables; recipes and customs of mothers attending Sorrento Maternity Hospital, Birmingham, England. *Human Nutrition: Applied Nutrition* **37A:** 378–402.

WHO Expert Committee on Diabetes mellitus. (1980) *WHO Technical Report Series* 646, Geneva: WHO.

Wilson W, Ory DV, Biglan A, Glasgow RE, Toobert DJ & Campbell DR (1986) Psychosocial predictors of self care behaviours (compliance) and glycaemic control in non-insulin-dependent diabetes mellitus. *Diabetes Care* **9:** 614–622.

10

Sulphonylureas in the treatment of non-insulin-dependent diabetes

ARNE MELANDER

A common, but not well founded, opinion is that sulphonylureas have very limited therapeutic value. Another unjustified view is to regard sulphonylureas as potentially harmful. They have been ascribed an increased risk of cardiovascular mortality, and it is often claimed that sulphonylurea treatment is counterproductive because it can lead to chronic hyperinsulinaemia and weight gain. It has also been argued that sulphonylurea treatment could cause exhaustion of the insulin-producing cells. These criticisms are either scientifically incorrect or based upon inappropriate use of sulphonylureas. As will be described in this chapter these drugs can be highly beneficial in the treatment of non-insulin-dependent diabetes mellitus (NIDDM).

THE THERAPEUTIC AIM: EUGLYCAEMIA

The major aims in the treatment of NIDDM are:

1. amelioration of symptoms
2. prevention or minimization of diabetic complications.

Not only classical symptoms, e.g. thirst and polyuria, but also the complications, myocardial infarction, intermittent claudication, renal impairment, neuropathy and retinopathy, are at least partially related to the chronic hyperglycaemia that is the main characteristic of the disease. While thirst and polyuria result from marked hyperglycaemia, complications may occur at marginal elevations of blood glucose. The risk of cardiovascular complications is already increased in early NIDDM and even in impaired glucose tolerance (IGT) or 'borderline diabetes' which in some patients may be a pre-NIDDM phase (Persson, 1977; Fuller et al, 1980; Jarrett et al, 1982; Donahue et al, 1987). Therefore, since untreated hyperglycaemia is a self-perpetuating disorder leading to progressive impairment of both insulin secretion and insulin action (Unger and Grundy, 1985), therapeutic intervention should be initiated as early as possible, and should aim at complete normalization of blood glucose (euglycaemia).

Rationale for sulphonylurea therapy

Although hypocaloric dietary regulation can be very effective in reducing fasting hyperglycaemia (Liu et al, 1985; Bitzén et al, 1988a), it rarely suffices to reach or maintain fasting euglycaemia (UK Prospective Study, 1983; Hadden et al, 1986; Bitzén et al, 1988a). Moreover, dietary regulation does not improve the impaired acute insulin release in response to meals which helps to explain the prolonged elevation of postprandial blood glucose and the subsequent hyperinsulinaemia (Turtle, 1970; Cerasi et al, 1973; DeFronzo et al, 1983; O'Rahilly et al, 1986; Bitzén et al, 1988a). In contrast (rapid-acting) sulphonylureas can restore the acute insulin release (Bitzén et al, 1988b, 1988c; Melander et al, 1988). Accordingly, hypocaloric dietary regulation and sulphonylurea therapy are complementary treatments, both of which are needed to attain euglycaemia (Melander et al, 1988). In support of this view, the combination of hypocaloric dietary regulation and a rapid- and short-acting sulphonylurea has been shown to promote normalization of blood glucose and to keep glucose levels close to normal for several years in NIDDM patients detected by screening (Bitzén et al, 1988c).

Early treatment may prevent complications

The importance of early detection and intervention is further emphasized by the results of a long-term study using sulphonylurea treatment and dietary advice in patients with impaired glucose tolerance. Ten to twelve years treatment with this combination postponed the progression of IGT to manifest NIDDM (Sartor et al, 1980) and reduced not only the blood lipids and blood pressure (Sartor et al, 1980) but also the increased cardiovascular morbidity (Persson, 1977) and mortality (Knowler et al, 1987) in such subjects.

STRUCTURE–FUNCTION RELATIONSHIPS OF SULPHONYLUREAS

Sulphonylureas were detected by serendipity during a search for more effective antibacterial sulphonamides (Janbon et al, 1942). However, their effect and mechanism of action are quite physiological. They promote the release of insulin from the B cells, possibly by involving receptors on these cells (see below). Linkage of different radicals to the sulphonylurea nucleus provides a large variation in the potency, onset of action and effect duration of different sulphonylureas (Table 1). The temporal aspects may be particularly important from the clinical point of view, as discussed later.

Mechanisms of action

Insulin release

Sulphonylureas enhance the release of insulin from the pancreatic B cells (Jackson and Bressler, 1981). Possibly the release of insulin is evoked by

Table 1. Examples of sulphonylurea structure-activity relations

$$R_1-SO_2-NH-\underset{\underset{O}{\|}}{C}-NH-R_2$$

Compound	R_1	R_2	Onset and duration	B cell binding	Potency
tolbutamide	CH_3—⟨O⟩—	$-CH_2-CH_2-CH_2-CH_3$	rapid- and short-acting	low	low
chlorpropamide	Cl—⟨O⟩—	$-CH_2-CH_2-CH_3$	slow- and long-acting	low	low
glibenclamide	CH_2—⟨O⟩— $CH_2-NH-\underset{\underset{O}{\|}}{C}$—⟨O⟩ with Cl and OCH_3	⟨H⟩	slow- and long-acting	high	high
glipizide	CH_2—⟨O⟩— $CH_2-NH-\underset{\underset{O}{\|}}{C}$—⟨pyrazine CH_3⟩	⟨H⟩	rapid- and short-acting	high	high

sulphonylurea binding to, and activation of, receptors on the B cell surface. The drugs may mimic the action of some endogenous agonist, e.g. a gastrointestinal insulin-releasing peptide (Siconolfi-Baez and Lebovitz, 1985). The much higher B cell binding of 'second-generation' sulphonylureas such as glibenclamide and glipizide, as compared with that of 'first-generation' sulphonylureas such as tolbutamide and chlorpropamide, may explain the higher activity of the former (Siconolfi-Baez and Lebovitz, 1985; Melander et al, 1988).

An early defect in subjects with IGT or NIDDM is the delay of the acute insulin release in response to meals or glucose, which partially explains the prolonged elevation of postpradial glucose and the subsequent hyperinsulinaemia (Turtle, 1970; Cerasi et al, 1973; DeFronzo et al, 1983; O'Rahilly et al, 1986). Rapid- and short-acting sulphonylureas are able to enhance the acute insulin release and thereby improve postprandial glucose control (Bitzén et al, 1988b; 1988c). The reduction of postprandial glucose can reduce the prolonged hyperinsulinaemia seen in early NIDDM, and is of importance since chronic hyperinsulinaemia may be atherogenic and promote hypertension (Reaven and Hoffmann, 1987).

In addition to its direct insulin-releasing effect, sulphonylurea therapy improves B cell function secondarily as a consequence of reduced hyperglycaemia (Ferner et al, 1987).

Insulin action

In addition to impaired insulin release, subjects with IGT or NIDDM have a reduced tissue sensitivity to insulin (reduced insulin action). Like hypocaloric dietary regulation (Bitzén et al, 1988a) sulphonylurea treatment may improve insulin action (Lebovitz et al, 1977; Greenfield et al, 1982; Simonson et al, 1984). This improvement occurs both in the liver and in extrahepatic tissues and probably results from a postreceptor effect (Simonson et al, 1984). While sulphonylureas are able to enhance insulin action by a direct effect experimentally, the improved insulin action seen during sulphonylurea therapy is probably secondary to the enhanced secretion of insulin and the subsequent reduction of hyperglycaemia. Enhanced insulin action during sulphonylurea therapy has only been observed in NIDDM patients with residual B cell function (Melander et al, 1988).

Hepatic extraction of insulin

Some of the insulin secreted from the pancreatic B cells is bound to receptors in the liver and then extracted and cleared by this organ. Therefore, the systemic availability of insulin is determined not only by the amount secreted from the pancreas but also by the proportion that escapes hepatic extraction. Recent studies indicate that glipizide and glibenclamide not only increase the secretion of insulin but also reduce its hepatic extraction. The reduced hepatic extraction could be a secondary effect due to the increased rate of insulin secretion (Melander et al, 1988).

Other effects of sulphonylureas

Blood lipids

Numerous studies have dealt with the possible influence of sulphonylurea therapy on the hyperlipidaemia of NIDDM, and both positive and negative effects have been reported. Overall, it seems most likely that there are no direct effects of sulphonylureas on plasma lipids, but that any effects are secondary to changes in the degree of glucose control (Melander et al, 1988).

Platelets

Anti-platelet effects of sulphonylureas, particularly with gliclazide, have been described. However, the anti-platelet effects are probably secondary to the improved glucose control following sulphonylurea treatment, and there is no convincing evidence that gliclazide is superior to any other sulphonylurea in this respect (Melander et al, 1988).

Differences between sulphonylureas

Potency

As pointed out above and in Table 1, the mechanism(s) of action of sulphonylureas may be similar, but there are pronounced differences in their potencies (intrinsic molar activities) which may reflect differences in binding to B cell receptors. Glibenclamide and glipizide have the highest binding and are the most potent sulphonylureas (Siconolfi-Baez and Lebovitz, 1985; Melander et al, 1988). Acetohexamide and tolazamide seem to be equipotent with tolbutamide and chlorpropamide, while gliquidone, glibornuride and gliclazide are somewhat less potent than glipizide and glibenclamide (Ferner and Chaplin, 1987; Melander et al, 1988).

Although the difference in intrinsic activity is pronounced, there is no evidence for a corresponding difference in clinical efficacy. There are few controlled prospective studies comparing the long-term efficacy of newer and older sulphonylureas (Ferner and Chaplin, 1987).

Onset and duration of effect

In contrast to the potency differences, variations in sulphonylurea pharmacokinetics, i.e. in the rate of absorption and the rate and extent of distribution, metabolism and excretion, have clinical importance because they lead to clinically relevant differences in the rate of onset and in the duration of effect.

The rate of onset of the sulphonylurea effect is important as it relates to the capacity to reduce the delay in acute insulin release. The effect duration is also important as it relates to the issues of discontinuous sulphonylurea exposure, chronic hyperinsulinaemia and prolonged hyperglycaemia (see below).

The most rapid- and short-acting sulphonylurea available is glipizide, probably because it has the most rapid absorption, distribution and elimination (Melander et al, 1988). Glipizide can also restore the acute insulin release and improve postprandial glucose control without causing chronic hyperinsulinaemia (Bitzén et al, 1988b, 1988c).

The most slow- and long-acting sulphonylurea is chlorpropamide (Melander et al, 1988), and it is more liable to promote chronic hyperinsulinaemia and prolonged hypoglycaemia than most other sulphonylureas (see below).

Glibenclamide is slower in onset than glipizide, particularly when administered in the non-micronized formulation that is still being marketed in many countries. However, glibenclamide is more slow-acting than glipizide even when these two sulphonylureas are infused at equal rates and to similar plasma levels (Groop et al, 1987). A possible pharmacokinetic explanation of the slower onset of action could be a slower distribution, and the longer duration could be due to a slower distribution, longer elimination half-life, accumulation of an active metabolite, and/or to the fact that glibenclamide, in contrast to other sulphonylureas, may accumulate within B cells (Hellman et al, 1984; Melander et al, 1988).

A comprehensive review of the kinetic-dynamic relationships of sulphonylureas has been published recently (Ferner and Chaplin, 1987).

Desensitization of B cells by continuous exposure to sulphonylureas

It has been shown that the insulin–releasing effect of a single sulphonylurea dose (tolbutamide) may vanish during chronic treatment with (another) sulphonylurea (tolazamide) and may reappear after withdrawal of the chronic treatment (Karam et al, 1986). This implies that chronic, continuous exposure to sulphonylurea may desensitize the B cell to this stimulus, in analogy with the receptor down-regulation that occurs in any cell continuously stimulated by an endogenous or exogenous receptor agonist. It is of interest in this context that high concentrations of sulphonylureas inhibit insulin biosynthesis in vitro (Andersson and Borg, 1980). The findings also imply that the insulinotropic effect of sulphonylureas might be best maintained during long-term therapy if the dosage permits a discontinuous exposure to the drug i.e. so that the plasma and tissue concentrations of the drug would fall below the critical level sometime during the night.

In support of this assumption it has been observed that the improved acute insulin release that is promoted by a single dose of glipizide may be maintained for several years if the exposure is discontinuous ($\leqslant 10$ mg once daily) and may be attenuated by continuous exposure ($\leqslant 20$ mg in divided dosage) (Bitzén et al, 1988c). Furthermore, there is evidence that continuous glipizide exposure at a high level (25 mg/day) may impair rather than improve glucose control (Wåhlin-Boll et al, 1982).

It would thus appear that long-term sulphonylurea treatment may be most efficacious if performed with a rapid- and short-acting sulphonylurea in low and/or once-daily dosage (Table 2). If high dosage has been necessary to obtain euglycaemia initially, dose reduction should be considered as soon as euglycaemia has been established. Maintenance of high and divided dosage could promote a secondary failure (see below).

ADVERSE EFFECTS OF SULPHONYLUREAS

The overall frequency of adverse effects is low, and they are usually mild and reversible. Among these are nausea, dizziness, headache and skin reactions. Rare cases of agranulocytosis, thrombocytopenia and icterus have been reported. In addition, water retention, hyponatraemia and alcohol intolerance have been observed, mainly with chlorpropamide (Jackson and Bressler, 1981).

Prolonged hypoglycaemia

As sulphonylureas lower blood glucose by increasing insulin release, hypoglycaemic reactions should be expected to occur. Normally, hypoglycaemia promotes release of blood glucose elevating hormones such as adrenaline and glucagon, whereby hypoglycaemia is counteracted through an increased hepatic glucose output. Moreover, the desensitizing effect of continuous exposure should minimize the risk of hypoglycaemia. However, in elderly patients hypoglycaemia may occasionally become prolonged and this condition may lead to permanent neurological damage and even death (Seltzer, 1979; Asplund et al, 1983; Berger et al, 1986). It should be noted that prolonged hypoglycaemia may be misdiagnosed as a cerebrovascular insult.

Prolonged hypoglycaemia can occur only if there is a sustained suppression of hepatic glucose output. This is most likely to occur with long-lasting sulphonylureas, such as chlorpropamide (Seltzer, 1979) and glibenclamide (Asplund et al, 1983; Berger et al, 1986; Melander et al, 1988) in combination with some complicating factor (see below). At similar plasma concentrations, glibenclamide causes a 50% greater suppression of hepatic glucose output than glipizide (Groop et al, 1987) and this helps to explain why glibenclamide may be more liable to provoke prolonged hypoglycaemia than is glipizide.

Almost all severe prolonged hypoglycaemic cases have involved patients over the age of 75 years. In addition, some complicating factor has almost invariably been implicated, e.g. a drug interaction or acute energy deprivation (Asplund et al, 1983). This warrants particular caution in using sulphonylureas, especially long-lasting ones, in elderly NIDDM patients. Unless subjective symptomatic hyperglycaemia necessitates use of sulphonylureas, these drugs should perhaps be entirely avoided in people over the age of 75 years.

DRUG INTERACTIONS

Several drugs may interact with sulphonylureas (Seltzer, 1979; Jackson and Bressler, 1981; Asplund et al, 1983; Berger et al, 1986; Melander et al, 1988). Alcohol, aspirin, sulphonamides and trimethoprim have been involved in serious cases of sulphonylurea-related hypoglycaemia. The risk of interactions with aspirin and similar drugs should be particularly emphasized, as the use of analgesic drugs is common among elderly patients.

While (non-selective) beta-blockers may inhibit the counter-regulatory effect of adrenaline in hypoglycaemia, there are also data to support the assumption that beta-blockers may reduce the efficacy of sulphonylureas (Zaman et al, 1982). Thiazides may also reduce the long-term blood glucose lowering effects of sulphonylureas (Murphy et al, 1982).

SELECTION AND DOSAGE OF SULPHONYLUREAS

There are few appropriate prospective controlled long-term comparisons between different sulphonylureas. Such studies are also difficult to design and carry out due to the heterogeneity of the disease, the variation in dietary compliance, the possibility that the dose-response curve is bell-shaped, and the fact that the steady state levels of several, if not all, sulphonylureas show a large interindividual variation following standard doses (Ferner & Chaplin, 1987; Melander et al, 1988). Moreover, the absorption rate and the time of appearance of sulphonylurea in blood relative to the meal intake may be more important than the dose size (Sartor et al, 1980; Hartling et al, 1987; Melander et al, 1988).

The limited comparative data indicate that there is little or no difference in clinical efficacy between sulphonylureas in the short term. This, together with the fact that short-acting sulphonylureas may be safer than the long-acting ones, would favour selection of the former e.g. tolbutamide or glipizide. This is also the opinion of the European NIDDM Policy Group of the European Association for the Study of Diabetes. An additional argument in this direction is derived from the concept that the long-term efficacy of sulphonylureas may be best maintained by discontinuous sulphonylurea exposure, i.e. by a rapid- and short-acting agent given in a low- and/or once-daily maintenance dose (Table 2).

Time of administration

To obtain the most appropriate effect on insulin release relative to meals, (rapid-acting) sulphonylureas should be administered some time before the meal(s). The effects of glipizide, glibenclamide and tolbutamide are increased when given 30 minutes before meals (Melander et al, 1988) (Table 2).

Table 2. Suggested steps in the treatment of NIDDM

1. Early detection of NIDDM by simple screening, e.g. random non-fasting blood glucose >7 mmol/l.
2. Strict dietary regulation, hypocaloric in overweight subjects.
3. Addition of rapid- and short-acting sulphonylurea (e.g. glipizide) after 3 months of dietary regulation.
    N.B. persistence in dietary regulation!
4. Slow dosage increase from 2.5 mg (glipizide) once daily ½ h before breakfast, increase by 2.5 mg at a time up to 20 mg once daily ½ h before breakfast.
5. When euglycaemia or near-normal glucose has been reached, try dose reduction.

EFFICACY OF TREATMENT

As pointed out initially, there is reason to assume that sulphonylureas should be introduced early in the management of NIDDM, as a complement to (hypocaloric) dietary regulation. Even treatment of IGT subjects may be considered. On the other hand less than 50% of IGT subjects develop manifest NIDDM, and screening for IGT can hardly be carried out as a routine measure. Hence it would seem most rational to screen for early NIDDM, which can be simply done by a random non-fasting blood glucose in out-patient care (Bitzén and Scherstén, 1986).

The efficacy of dietary regulation and sulphonylurea (glipizide) has been evaluated in NIDDM patients found by such screening. A small number could maintain normal fasting blood glucose levels for more than 5 years by hypocaloric dietary regulation alone. The combination of hypocaloric dietary regulation and glipizide achieved normal fasting blood glucose in about 50% of the cases, and they also had an improved insulin action. Blood glucose control was kept close to normal for about 4 years, without increasing basal insulin secretion, without chronic hyperinsulinaemia, and without weight increase (Bitzén et al, 1988c). In about 25% of the cases there was little or no reduction of fasting blood glucose even after maximum drug therapy. The main reason for this failure was a low compliance with dietary regulation rather than a lack of response to sulphonylurea. Of those who responded to the drug, only those who had discontinuous exposure ($\leqslant 10$ mg once daily) maintained long-term improvement of acute insulin release, and they also had the most pronounced improvement of postprandial glucose control (Bitzén et al, 1988c).

PRIMARY AND SECONDARY FAILURES OF SULPHONYLUREAS

Several NIDDM patients never show any therapeutic response to sulphonylureas (primary failures), and among those who do respond initially there is often a subsequent (secondary) failure. In many cases the drug failure can be blamed on insufficient compliance with dietary regulation (Liu et al, 1985; Bitzén et al, 1988c), and it is also possible that some secondary failures could be due to chronic, continuous sulphonylurea exposure at high dosage. A common cause of both primary and secondary failures is that sulphonylureas have not been introduced until the disease is advanced, i.e. that the vicious circle of hyperglycaemia has been established and attenuated B cell function.

As appropriate use of (rapid- and short-acting) sulphonylureas does not seem to accelerate but rather counteract the deterioration of B cell function, the rate of sulphonylurea failure might be minimized by early introduction of the drug. However, it is re-emphasized that sulphonylurea therapy is bound to fail unless combined with (hypocaloric) dietary regulation.

CONCLUSION

Sulphonylureas are usually needed as a complement to dietary regulation in order to attain euglycaemia. If introduced in screening-detected NIDDM and combined with hypocaloric dietary regulation, (rapid- and short-acting) sulphonylureas are able to attain and maintain (near) normal blood glucose levels for several years. If introduced in a pre-NIDDM phase, sulphonylureas may postpone the NIDDM development and reduce the increase in cardiovascular morbidity and mortality. It is crucial that weight reducing dietary regulation is maintained, otherwise sulphonylurea therapy will fail. Maintenance sulphonylurea therapy should be carried out at low and/or once-daily dosage so as to promote discontinuous exposure. Long-acting sulphonylureas may be more liable than others to provoke prolonged and hence dangerous hypoglycaemia in elderly subjects. Sulphonylureas should not be combined with alcohol, beta-adrenergic blockers, thiazides, sulpho namides, aspirin or aspirin-like drugs.

REFERENCES

Andersson A & Borg LAH (1980) Effects of glipizide on the insulin production by isolated mouse pancreatic islets. *Acta Endocrinologica* **239 supplement:** 37–41.

Asplund K, Wiholm B-E & Lithner F (1983) Glibenclamide-associated hypoglycaemia: A report on 57 cases. *Diabetologia* **24:** 412–417.

Berger W, Cardiff, F, Pasquel M & Rump A (1986) Die relative Häufigkeit der schweren Sulfonylharnstoff-Hypoglykämie in den letzten 25 Jahren in der Schweiz. *Schweizerische Medizinische Wochenschrift* **116:** 145–151.

Bitzén P-O & Scherstén B (1986) Assessment of laboratory methods for detection of unsuspected diabetes in primary health care. *Scandinavian Journal of Primary Health Care* **4:** 85–95.

Bitzén P-O, Melander A, Scherstén B & Svensson M (1988a) Efficacy of dietary regulation in primary health care patients with screening-detected hyperglycaemia. *Diabetic Medicine* (in press).

Bitzén P-O, Melander A, Scherstén B & Wåhlin-Boll E (1988b) The influence of glipizide on early insulin release and glucose disposal before and after dietary regulation in diabetic patients with different degrees of hyperglycaemia. *European Journal of Clinical Pharmacology* **35:** 31–37.

Bitzén P-O, Melander A, Scherstén B & Svensson M & Wåhlin-Boll E (1988c) Long-term normalisation of blood glucose by dietary regulation and glipizide treatment in patients with screening-detected NIDDM. (submitted for publication).

Cerasi E, Efendic S & Luft R (1973) Dose response relation between insulin and blood glucose levels during oral glucose loads in prediabetic and diabetic subjects. *Lancet* **i:** 794–797.

DeFronzo RA, Ferrannini E & Koivisto V (1983) New concepts in the pathogenesis and treatment of non-insulin-dependent diabetes mellitus. *American Journal of Medicine* **74: (supplement 1A)** 52–81.

Donahue RP, Abbott RD, Reed DM & Katsuhiko Y (1987) Postchallenge glucose concentration and coronary heart disease in men of Japanese ancestry. Honolulu Heart Program. *Diabetes* **36:** 689–692.

Ferner RE & Chaplin S (1987) The relationship between the pharmacokinetics and pharmacodynamic effects of oral hypoglycaemic drugs. *Clinical Pharmacokinetics* **12:** 379–401.

Ferner R, Stephenson P & Alberti KGMM (1987) Improved B-cell response correlates with reduced fasting blood glucose in non-insulin-dependent diabetes. *Diabetic Medicine* (in press).

Fuller JH, Shipley MJ, Rose G, Jarrett RJ & Keen H (1980) Coronary-heart-disease risk and impaired glucose tolerance. *Lancet* **i:** 1373–1376.

Greenfield MS, Doberne L, Rosenthal M et al (1982) Effect of sulfonylurea treatment on in vivo insulin secretion and action in patients with non-insulin-dependent diabetes mellitus. *Diabetes* **31:** 307–312.

Groop L, Luzi L, Melander A et al (1987) Different effects of glyburide and glipizide on insulin secretion and hepatic glucose production in normal and NIDDM subjects. *Diabetes* **36:** 1320–1328.

Hadden DR, Blair ALT, Wilson EA et al (1986) Natural history of diabetes presenting age 40–69 years: a prospective study of the influence of intensive dietary therapy. *Quarterly Journal of Medicine, New Series 59,* **230:** 579–598.

Hartling SG, Faber OK, Wegmann M-L, Wåhlin-Boll E & Melander A (1987) Interaction of ethanol and glipizide in humans. *Diabetes Care* **10:** 683–686.

Hellman B, Sehlin J & Taljedal I-B (1984) Glibenclamide is exceptional among hypoglycaemic agents in accumulating progressively in B-cell rich pancreatic islets. *Acta Endocrinologica* **105:** 385–390.

Jackson EJ & Bressler R (1981) Clinical pharmacology of sulphonylurea hypoglycaemic agents. *Drugs* **22:** 211–245 and 295–320.

Janbon M, Chaptal J, Vedel A & Schaap J (1942) Accidents hypoglycemiques graves par un sulfamidothiodiazol. *Montpellier Medicale* **21/22:** 441–444.

Jarrett RJ, McCartney P & Keen H (1982) The Bedford Survey: Ten year mortality rates in newly diagnosed diabetics, borderline diabetics and normoglycaemic controls and risk indices for coronary heart in borderline diabetics. *Diabetologia* **22:** 79–84.

Karam JH, Sanz N, Salamon E & Nolte MS (1986) Selective unresponsiveness of pancreatic B-cells to acute sulfonylurea stimulation during sulfonylurea therapy in NIDDM. *Diabetes* **35:** 1314–1320.

Knowler WC, Sartor G & Scherstén B (1987) Effects of glucose tolerance and treatment of abnormal tolerance on mortality in Malmöhus County, Sweden. *Diabetologia* **30:** 541A.

Lebovitz HE, Feinglos MN, Bucholtz HK & Lebovitz FL (1977) Potentiation of insulin action:

a probable mechanism for the anti-diabetic action of sulfonylurea drugs. *Journal of Clinical Endocrinology and Metabolism* **45:** 601–604.

Liu GC, Coulston AM, Lardinois CK et al (1985) Moderate weight loss and sulfonylurea treatment of non-insulin-dependent diabetes mellitus. *Archives of Internal Medicine* **145:** 665–669.

Melander A, Bitzén P-O, Faber O & Groop L (1988) Sulphonylurea antidiabetic drugs: An update on their clinical pharmacology and rational therapeutic use. *Drugs 1988* (in press).

Murphy MB, Lewis PJ, Kohner E, Schumer B & Dollery CT (1982) Glucose intolerance in hypertensive patients treated with diuretics; a fourteen-year follow up. *Lancet* **ii:** 1293–1295.

O'Rahilly SP, Rudenski AS, Burnett MA et al (1986) Beta-cell dysfunction, rather than insulin insensitivity, is the primary defect in familial type 2 diabetes. *Lancet* **ii:** 360–363.

Persson G (1977) Cardiovascular complications in diabetics and subjects with reduced glucose tolerance. *Acta Medica Scandinavica* **supplement** 605.

Reaven GM & G Hoffman BB (1987) A role for insulin in the aetiology and course of hypertension. *Lancet* **2:** 435–436.

Sartor G, Scherstén B, Carlström S et al (1980) Ten-year follow-up of subjects with impaired glucose tolerance. Prevention of diabetes by tolbutamide and diet regulation. *Diabetes* **29:** 41–49.

Seltzer HS (1979) Severe drug-induced hypoglycemia. A review. *Comprehensive Therapy* **5:** (4) 21–29.

Siconolfi-Baez L & Lebovitz HE (1985) Charactersitics of a specific plasma membrane sulfonylurea receptor. *Diabetes* **34 (supplement 1):** 228–232.

Simonson DC, Ferrannini E, Bevilacqua S et al (1984) Mechanism of improvement in glucose metabolism after chronic glyburide therapy. *Diabetes* **33:** 838–845.

Turtle JR (1970) Glucose and insulin secretory response patterns following diet and tolazamide therapy in diabetics. *British Medical Journal* **3:** 606–610.

UK prospective study of therapies of maturity-onset diabetes (1983) 1. Effect of diet, sulfonylurea, insulin or biguanide therapy on fasting plasma glucose and body weight over one year. *Diabetologia* **24:** 404–411.

Unger RH & Grundy S (1985) Hyperglycemia as an inducer as well as a consequence of impaired islet cell function and insulin resistance: implications for the management of diabetes. *Diabetologia* **28:** 119–121.

Wåhlin-Boll E, Sartor G, Melander A & Scherstén B (1982) Imparied effect of sulfonylurea following increased dosage. *European Journal of Clinical Pharmacology* **22:** 21–25.

Zaman R, Kendall MJ & Biggs PI (1982) The effect of acebutolol and propranolol on the hypoglycaemic action of glibenclamide. *British Journal of Clinical Pharmacology* **13:** 507–512.

11

Treatment—metformin

C. J. BAILEY
M. NATTRASS

Following the introduction of the first sulphonylurea (1954), the main biguanide drugs metformin and phenformin (1957) emerged as an additional class of orally active glucose-lowering agents. Their history lies in the use of *Galega officinalis* (Goat's rue or French lilac) as a traditional treatment for diabetes in Europe. The active substance, guanidine, and many of its derivatives, including biguanides, were evaluated in the 1920s. Some proved too toxic for clinical use and all were quickly superceded by insulin (Sterne, 1969; Beckmann, 1971). The rediscovery of biguanides in the 1950s led to the widespread use of phenformin and metformin for the treatment of non-insulin-dependent diabetes mellitus (NIDDM). Phenformin was regarded as the more potent drug and received greater use, but it was withdrawn in most countries at the end of the 1970s due to an association with lactic acidosis (Nattrass and Alberti, 1978). Metformin shows many qualitative and quantitative differences from phenformin and continues to receive extensive use (Schafer, 1983; Bailey, 1983). This review considers current information on the actions of metformin and examines the present place of metformin in the treatment of NIDDM.

PHARMACOKINETICS OF METFORMIN

The chemistry, pharmacokinetics and toxicology of metformin have been thoroughly reviewed elsewhere (Sterne, 1969; Beckmann, 1971; Hermann, 1979; Schafer, 1983). Briefly, metformin (Figure 1) is absorbed mainly from the small intestine with an estimated absorption half-time of 0.9–2.6 h and a bioavailability of 50–60% (Noel, 1979; Pentikainen et al, 1979; Vidon et al,

$$CH_3 \diagdown \underset{CH_3 \diagup}{N} - \overset{\overset{NH}{\|}}{C} - NH - \overset{\overset{NH}{\|}}{C} - NH_2 . HCl$$

Figure 1. Metformin hydrochloride (dimethylbiguanide hydrochloride).

1988). Plasma concentrations up to about 1–2 μg/ml (approximately 10^{-5} mol/l) are achieved some two hours after oral doses (500 mg or 1 g) of the proprietary brand Glucophage® (Sirtori et al, 1978; Pentikainen et al, 1979; Tucker et al, 1981). Metformin does not bind to plasma proteins and it is rapidly eliminated (average plasma $t_{1/2}$ estimated at 1.7–4.5 h). Virtually all of the drug is excreted unchanged in the urine with 90% being cleared in 12 h. Thus metformin appears to be stable and non-metabolized or almost non-metabolized (Pentikainen et al, 1979; Tucker et al, 1981). Since renal clearance is greater than the glomerular filtration rate it has been suggested that the drug is secreted by the proximal convoluted tubules (Tucker et al, 1981).

ANTIHYPERGLYCAEMIC EFFECT

The glucose-lowering effect of metformin is distinctly different from that of sulphonylureas (Bailey, 1988; Bailey et al, 1988). Metformin does not normally reduce glucose concentrations below euglycaemia (Hermann, 1979), even if the drug is consumed in marked excess with suicidal intent (Sterne and Junien, 1981; McLelland, 1985). Moreover, the glucose-lowering effect of metformin is difficult to demonstrate in non-diabetic subjects unless glucose concentrations are artificially raised (Hermann, 1979). Since metformin does not induce clinical hypoglycaemia (Bailey et al, 1988), this drug should be regarded as an 'antihyperglycaemic' agent rather than a hypoglycaemic agent (Bailey, 1985).

The antihyperglycaemic efficacy of metformin in NIDDM has been evaluated during monotherapy and in combination with a sulphonylurea. Early studies have been thoroughly reviewed by Hermann (1979). Some of these studies are difficult to interpret due to variable criteria for patient inclusion and poor discrimination between drug effects and the influence of dietary adjustments and weight control. However, the concensus of these studies indicates that metformin monotherapy of 1.5–3 g/day to obese or non-obese NIDDM patients typically reduced basal glucose concentrations by 20% or more (usually 2 mmol/l). Where reported, at least 80–90% of patients showed an improvement in glycaemic control. Long-term studies showed that the effectiveness of metformin was normally maintained over several years.

Recent studies designed to investigate the mode of action of metformin have confirmed the efficacy of the drug (Table 1). These studies recruited diet-failed patients who were maintained on a constant diet and exercise regimen during the study and showed a constant body weight. Although the studies usually comprised only small groups of patients and short periods of investigation, they affirm that there is no obvious predictor of the extent to which a patient will respond. There was no apparent association between the extent of the glucose-lowering effect and the degree of pre-treatment hyperglycaemia, the duration of diabetes, age, obesity or the prevailing basal insulin concentration. In addition to demonstrating reductions in basal glucose concentrations of 16–37% (1.4–4.6 mmol/l) and reductions in the

Table 1. Effect of metformin monotherapy on glycaemic control in NIDDM*

Authors	Date	Obese – O Nonobese – NO (n)	Dose of metformin (g/day)	Duration†	Design‡	Basal plasma glucose (mmol/l)			Basal plasma insulin
						Start	End	%↓	
Lord et al	1983a	O (8)	1.5	4 w	Open	11.5	9.1	20	NC
Prager & Schernthaner	1983	O (10)	1.7	2 w	DBCX	9.8	6.1	37	NC
Trischitta et al	1983	O (6)	2.5	4 d	Open	11.5	8.0	30	NC
UK Prospective	1985	O (6)	2.5	1 y	Open	8.6	7.2	16	—
Fantus & Brosseau	1986	O (11) NO (7)	2.0	1 w	Open	11.6	8.7	25	NC
Prager et al	1986	O & NO (12)	1.7	4 w	Open	13.5	8.8	34	NC
Rizkalla et al	1986	O (6)	1.7	2 w	DBCX	12.8	10.6	17	NC
Campbell et al	1987	O (14)	1–3	6 m	Open	11.5	7.7	33	NC
Nosadini et al	1987	O (7)	2.5	4 w	Open	8.6	6.2	27	NC

* All patients were diet-failed or sulphonylurea-failed obese or nonobese NIDDM. Patients were requested to maintain diet and exercise throughout the period of study.

† d = days, w = weeks, m = months, y = year, (n) = number.

‡ Open studies used each patient as his/her own pretreatment control. DBCX = double blind cross-over.

%↓ = percentage decrease.

NC = no significant change.

percentage of glycated haemoglobin, improvements of oral glucose tolerance have been consistently noted (Lord et al, 1983b; Prager and Schernthaner, 1983; Fantus and Brosseau, 1986). This may be compared with the Edinburgh studies (Clarke and Duncan, 1968; Clarke and Campbell, 1977) which noted larger reductions in random plasma glucose concentrations (mean reductions of 43–50%). Several studies have suggested that the antihyperglycaemic effect of metformin is more effective against postprandial excursions of glucose, as evidenced by measurments of daily glucose profiles (Rigas et al, 1968; Leatherdale and Bailey, 1986).

Extending earlier reports reviewed by Hermann (1979), Table 2 shows four studies in which addition of metformin in combination with a sulphonylurea, reduced basal glucose concentrations (18–40%) similarly to metformin monotherapy. Patients included in these studies were stable but failed to achieve adequate glycaemic control with diet plus sulphonylurea therapy. The small number of patients involved showed no apparent differences in the effect of metformin that could be attributed to the type of sulphonylurea, obesity or the level of hyperglycaemia. The studies were only of short duration and the long-term benefits of combined sulphonylurea and metformin therapy remain to be conclusively established, although several centres have commented anecdotally that they see merit in the long-term use of combined therapy.

Mechanism of antihyperglycaemic effect

The antihyperglycaemic action of metformin is not due to increased insulin concentrations. Basal insulin concentrations and insulin concentrations during glucose tolerance tests are unchanged or slightly reduced by metformin treatment despite lower blood glucose concentrations (Hermann, 1979; Lord et al, 1983b; Prager and Schernthaner, 1983; Trischitta et al, 1983; Fantus and Brosseau, 1986; Jackson et al, 1987). Also, metformin is not effective in the total absence of insulin (Sterne, 1969). These findings point strongly to the possibility that the drug might improve insulin action. An impaired hypoglycaemic action of insulin (insulin resistance) is a major factor contributing to the hyperglycaemia of NIDDM. Insulin resistance affects the liver—resulting in excess hepatic glucose production—and peripheral insulin target tissues such as muscle and fat, thereby reducing glucose uptake and metabolism (DeFronzo et al, 1983). At the cellular level insulin resistance is attributable partly to a decreased number of insulin receptors, but, more importantly, to one or more defects at postreceptor sites of insulin action (Olefsky et al, 1985).

Hepatic glucose output

Accompanying a reduction in the basal blood glucose concentration of 27% (mean value of 8.6 reduced to 6.2 mmol/l), Nosadini et al (1987) noted a small reduction (9%) of basal hepatic glucose output (mean value of 2.2 reduced to 2.0 mg kg^{-1} min^{-1}) in a group of seven obese NIDDM patients treated with metformin (2.5 g/day for 4 weeks). Since the effect was

Table 2. Effect of metformin in addition to a sulphonylurea on glycaemic control in NIDDM*

Authors	Date	Obese – O Nonobese – NO (n)	Sulphonylurea treatment (mg/day)	Dose of metformin (g/day)	Duration†	Design‡	Basal plasma glucose mmol/l		
							Start	end	% ↓
Higginbotham & Martin	1979	O & NO (17)	Glibenclamide (10–20 mg)	1.0	2 m	DBCX	12.4	9.9	20
Capretti et al	1982	O (15)	Glibenclamide (7.5 mg)	1.5	5 d	CX	10.5∅	6.9∅	34
Holman et al	1987	O & NO (17)	Tolbutamide/ Chlorpropamide/ Glibenclamide	1.5–2.5	2 m	CX	8.9	7.3	18
Jackson et al	1987	NO (10)	Glibenclamide	2.0–2.5	3 m	Open	9.5	5.7	40

* All patients were stable but inadequately controlled by diet plus a sulphonylurea. Patients were requested to maintain diet and exercise throughout the period of study.
† d = days, m = months, (n) = number.
‡ Open study used each patient as his/her own pretreatment control. DBCX = double blind cross-over. CX = single blind cross-over.
% ↓ = percentage decrease.
∅ Values estimated from an illustration.

achieved at lower insulin concentrations (mean value of 9 versus 15 mU/l), the authors suggested that metformin increased the sensitivity of the liver to insulin. A greater decrease (17%) in basal hepatic glucose output (mean value of 2.67 decreased to 2.20 mg kg^{-1} min^{-1}) was observed in 10 non-obese NIDDM men receiving metformin (1–1.5 g/day) for at least three months (Jackson et al, 1987). This was associated with a 40% decrease in basal glucose concentrations (mean value of 9.5 decreased to 5.7 mmol/l) and no change in basal insulin. The reduction in hepatic glucose output was maintained during an oral glucose tolerance test.

Alterations in hepatic glycogen mobilization appear unlikely to account for the suppression of basal hepatic glucose output by metformin, since this effect of metformin has been observed after an overnight fast when hepatic glycogen is largely depleted (Arky, 1979). Therapeutic concentrations of metformin have little effect or increase liver glycogen in diabetic patients and animals. However the drug decreases liver glycogen in non-diabetic animals irrespective of any effect on blood glucose (Laastuen and Todd, 1969; Sterne, 1969) and decreases glycogenesis in cultured rat hepatocytes (Alengrin et al, 1987).

Animal studies have provided evidence that the metformin-induced decrease in hepatic glucose output is due to a decrease in gluconeogenesis. Metformin reduced gluconeogenesis in normal guinea-pigs (Meyer et al, 1967) and high concentrations (10^{-3} mol/l and above) of the drug reduced basal and glucagon-stimulated gluconeogenesis by isolated animal liver and kidney tissue in the absence of insulin (Meyer et al, 1967; Cooke et al, 1973; Alengrin et al, 1987). However, therapeutic concentrations (e.g. 10^{-5} mol/l) of metformin acted synergistically with physiological concentrations of insulin to suppress gluconeogenesis by isolated rat hepatocytes (Wollen and Bailey, 1988a). Indeed metformin and insulin in combination, reduced gluconeogenesis with very low concentrations of each agent which were not effective alone. The additional antigluconeogenic effect of therapeutic concentrations of metformin in the presence of insulin was in the order of 10–16% for a range of a gluconeogenic substrates (lactate, pyruvate, gluta-mine, alanine and glycerol), and the effect was not attributable to any changes in the energy status or redox state of the cells (Wollen and Bailey, 1988b).

Suppression of hepatic gluconeogenesis by metformin appears to be proportionally smaller (9–17% in NIDDM patients) than the decrease in basal glucose concentrations (27–40% in the same patients) (Jackson et al, 1987; Nosadini et al, 1987). Moreover the antigluconeogenic effect would not account for the apparently greater reduction in postprandial glycaemia during metformin treatment, indicating the involvement of other actions.

Peripheral glucose uptake

Improved glucose tolerance without increased insulin concentrations in NIDDM patients suggests that metformin may improve insulin-mediated glucose disposal (Hermann, 1979; Bailey, 1988). This has been substan-tiated using hyperinsulinaemic glucose clamp procedures in which hepatic glucose output is almost completely suppressed. Prager et al (1986) noted that metformin (1.7 g/day for four weeks) improved glucose disposal by 23% (from a mean value of 4.4 to 5.4 mg kg^{-1} min^{-1}) in 12 obese and non-obese NIDDM patients studied with a hyperglycaemic (approximately 8.3 mmol/l) hyperinsulinaemic (140 mU/l) clamp. Using a euglycaemic (approximately 5.0 mmol/l) hyperinsulinaemic clamp Nosadini et al (1987) studied seven obese NIDDM patients before and after four weeks on metformin (2.5 g/day). At lower insulin concentrations (approximately 90 mU/l) glucose disposal was increased by 43% (from 3.44 to 4.94 mg kg^{-1} min^{-1}) during metformin treatment, and at higher insulin concentrations (approximately 1860 mU/l) glucose disposal was increased by 22% (from 7.34 to 8.99 mg kg^{-1} min^{-1}). These data suggest that metformin can increase both insulin sensitivity and insulin responsiveness as indicated by increased glucose disposal at submaximally- and maximally-stimulating insulin concentrations (Bailey et al, 1984).

Further evidence that metformin can improve insulin action is derived from reports that metformin reduced insulin requirements, glycosuria and blood glucose concentrations, in overweight insulin-treated NIDDM patients (Leblanc et al, 1987) and in some patients with insulin-dependent diabetes mellitus (IDDM) (Ferguson et al, 1961; Schatz et al, 1975; Hermann, 1979; Coscelli et al, 1984). In a double blind trial with IDDM patients, addition of metformin (1.7 g/day for two days) to the insulin regimen reduced by 26% the postprandial insulin requirement assessed using an artifical pancreas after a mixed meal. This was also associated with lower mean blood glucose concentrations (Gin et al, 1982). A group of IDDM patients receiving metformin (2.5 g/day) for four to six weeks showed an overall 25.8% reduction in insulin requirement assessed with an artificial pancreas during a 24 h profile (Pagano et al, 1983). This was also associated with lower glucose concentrations, and there was a greater reduction (about 50%) in insulin requirement postprandially. Using a euglycaemic (4.3 mmol/l) hyperinsulinaemic (approximately 90 mU/l) clamp, Gin et al (1985) noted that IDDM patients receiving a metformin supplement (1.7 g/day for seven days) showed an 18% improvement in glucose uptake.

GLUCOSE METABOLISM BY MUSCLE

Metformin increases insulin-mediated glucose uptake and metabolism by skeletal muscle of diabetic animals. Soleus muscles isolated from streptozotocin diabetic mice treated with metformin (250 mg kg^{-1} day^{-1} for three weeks) showed an increase of about 20% in insulin-mediated glucose uptake and oxidation at physiological and supraphysiological insulin concentrations (Bailey and Puah, 1986). Glycogenesis was similarly increased by high concentrations of insulin in the isolated muscles after metformin treatment, but the amount of glycogen stored in the muscle in the hypoinsulinaemic environment in vivo was not affected (Bailey and Puah, 1986). In vitro studies have shown that metformin acts directly on skeletal muscle to promote glucose uptake and oxidation (Bailey et al, unpublished data). A study with isolated hemidiaphragms of alloxan diabetic rats noted a 27% increase in insulin-mediated glucose uptake in the presence of a therapeutic concentration of metformin (Frayn and Adnitt, 1972). Consistent with the lack of effect of metformin on glycaemia in the euglycaemic non-diabetic state (Sterne, 1969; Hermann, 1979; Bailey and Broadbent, 1981) there is little effect of the drug on glucose metabolism of normal muscle (Frayn and Adnitt, 1972; Bailey and Puah, 1986). Metformin does exert a small stimulatory effect on glycogenesis in isolated normal soleus muscles exposed to high insulin concentrations (Bailey and Puah, 1986), whereas a small decrease in muscle glycogen has been noted during in vivo metformin treatment of normal animals (Sterne, 1969).

Glucose metabolism by adipose tissue. The effect of metformin on adipose tissue is less clear. The drug increased by 19% insulin-mediated glucose uptake by normal rat adipocytes, and a smaller increase in basal glucose uptake was recorded (Jacobs et al, 1986). Metformin increased (about 30%) insulin-stimulated glucose incorporation into triglyceride of fat tissue taken from normal human subjects (Cigolini et al, 1984). The effect of metformin on the metabolism of fat tissue from diabetic humans or animals has not been reported. However, consistent clinical observations that the drug does not increase adiposity and may facilitate weight loss in NIDDM patients (Hermann, 1979; Bailey, 1988) mitigates against a net increase in glucose conversion to stored triglyceride in these patients. Increased lipolysis and substrate cycling in adipose tissue might then be suspected, but there is no evidence of such an effect. Metformin did not affect lipolysis in adipose tissue of normal subjects (Cigolini et al, 1984) and consistent changes in plasma glycerol and free fatty acid concentrations have not been reported during metformin treatment in NIDDM patients (Schonborn et al, 1975; Hermann, 1979; Nattrass et al, 1979; Campbell et al, 1987; Jackson et al 1987). Recent studies have noted that metformin increased (25%) insulin-mediated glucose oxidation by normal human fat and increased (58%) basal glucose oxidation by normal rat adipocytes (Cigolini et al, 1984; Fantus and Brosseau, 1986). This raises the possibility that the drug can promote energy expenditure in adipose tissue. Preliminary observations in obese rats have indicated that metformin may increase glucose utilization by brown fat (Ferre et al, 1988) and it has been reported that metformin (1.5 g/day for 2 weeks) enhanced the thermogenic response to noradrenaline in IDDM patients (Leslie et al, 1986).

Insulin receptor and postreceptor effects

Increased insulin receptor binding has been considered as one mechanism through which metformin might potentiate insulin action. Metformin can increase insulin receptor binding in a range of cell types including erythrocytes, monocytes, hepatocytes, adipocytes and muscle cells (Holle et al, 1981; Lord et al, 1983a, b; Pagano et al, 1983; Trischitta et al, 1983; Bailey and Puah, 1986; Fantus and Brosseau, 1986; Rizkalla et al 1986; Cigolini et al, 1987). This is due almost entirely to an increased number of low affinity binding sites. The effect is direct, dose-related and reversible, and does not require *de novo* protein biosynthesis (Holle et al, 1981; Pezzino et al, 1982; Lord et al, 1983a; Fantus and Brosseau, 1986; Rizkalla et al, 1986). However there is only a poor correlation between the effects of metformin on insulin receptor binding and glucose metabolism (Bailey, 1988). For example, metformin can improve glucose homeostasis in diabetic humans and animals under circumstances in which insulin binding is unaltered (Lord et al, 1983a, 1985; Prager and Schernthaner, 1983; Fantus and Brosseau, 1986; Prager et al, 1986; Nosadini et al, 1987) and metformin can increase insulin receptor binding in the non-diabetic state without a measurable change of glucose metabolism (Holle et al, 1981; Lord et al, 1983a; Cigolini et al, 1984; Fantus and Brosseau, 1986; Jacobs et al, 1986). Thus, in part, metformin may help to improve insulin sensitivity in diabetic states through increased insulin receptor binding in individuals with a reduced number of insulin receptors (Fantus and Brosseau, 1986; Cigolini et al, 1987). The drug acts to potentiate the action of insulin on glucose metabolism predominantly at a site distal to the insulin receptor and its kinase activation (Jacobs et al, 1986). This interpretation is consistent with insulin dose-response studies which have shown increased glucose disposal in NIDDM patients (Nosadini et al, 1987) and glucose uptake by soleus muscles of streptozotocin diabetic mice (Bailey and Puah, 1986) at maximally effective insulin concentrations. Moreover, metformin restored the ability of insulin to inhibit adenylate cyclase activity of liver plasma membranes from streptozotocin diabetic rats. This was a postreceptor effect which was independent of the guanine nucleotide regulatory protein G_i (Gawler et al, 1988).

Insulin independent effects

Although metformin does not exert a significant antihyperglycaemic effect in the absence of insulin (Sterne, 1969), this does not preclude an effect of the drug on non-insulin mediated glucose uptake: for example, on the mass effect of glucose. Tissues may require a chronic influence of insulin to produce appropriate amounts of glucoregulatory enzymes (for example glucokinase) without depending upon insulin for the acute facilitation of glucose uptake and metabolism (or example the liver) (Pilkis, 1975; Davidson, 1981; Spence et al, 1986). Initial observations suggest that metformin can increase non-insulin mediated glucose uptake by IM-9 human lymphocytes (Purrello et al, 1987).

A proposed mechanism of action concerns the propensity of biguanides to bind with biological membranes, especially organelles such as mitochondria (Schafer, 1980). In this way biguanides alter surface charges and modify transmembrane ion fluxes. Through an effect on mitochondrial membranes, phenformin has been shown to impair oxidative phosphorylation, thereby reducing adenosine triphosphate (ATP) concentrations (Schafer, 1980). This might account in part for the increased anaerobic glycolysis and increased lactate production induced by phenformin. Moreover, a reduction of ATP concentrations increases glucose transport into some tissues, providing a rationale for increased glucose disposal. Differences in the pharmacokinetic properties and metabolic effects of metformin and phenformin (Sterne, 1969; Beckmann, 1971; Schafer, 1983; Bailey, 1988) suggest differences in their cellular mechanism of action. The membrane binding affinity of biguanides is dependent on the hydrocarbon side chains, and the dimethyl side chains of metformin enable only 2% of the binding affinity of phenformin for mitochondrial membranes (Schafer, 1980). Unlike phenformin, metformin does not appear to alter redox state or impair energy status at therapeutic concentrations (Meyer, 1960; Wollen and Bailey, 1988b). Indeed, metformin increased glucose oxidation in adipocytes and soleus muscles (Cigolini et al, 1984; Bailey and Puah, 1986; Fantus and Brosseau, 1986). Also, metformin did not increase lactate production by skeletal muscle (Bailey and Puah, 1986), consistent with the much lower risk of lactic acidosis with this biguanide (Berger, 1985; Campbell, 1985).

Intestinal glucose absorption

Although metformin lowers fasting glucose concentrations and improves intravenous glucose tolerance in NIDDM patients (Frayn et al, 1971), the postprandial antihyperglycaemic effect might involve a reduction in the rate of intestinal glucose absorption. Metformin is concentrated by the intestinal mucosa (Sterne, 1969), and high concentrations of metformin (10^{-3} mol/l) have been reported to suppress glucose transport by rat and hamster intestine in vitro (Lorch, 1971; Caspary and Creutzfeld, 1971), although this might partly reflect increased intestinal glucose utilization (Ferre et al, 1988; Bailey, unpublished observations). A reduction of the hepatic portal glucose concentration has been noted after metformin administration to normal subjects given an intraduodenal glucose challenge (Berger and Kunzli, 1970) but evidence that therapeutic concentrations of metformin reduce glucose absorption in NIDDM patients is lacking. Despite reports of abdominal discomfort and diarrhoea during initial treatment with metformin, gastric emptying in non-diabetic subjects and NIDDM patients was not significantly altered by metformin (Leatherdale and Bailey, 1986; Vidon et al, 1988).

Body weight control and appetite

Unlike sulphonylureas or insulin, metformin does not cause weight gain in NIDDM patients and often promotes weight loss—especially in patients who observe an energy-restricted diet (Hermann, 1979; Wales, 1980; UK prospective diabetes study, 1985). In groups of obese and non-obese NIDDM patients, one year of metformin therapy was associated with an average weight loss of 1.2 kg and 1.5 kg respectively, compared with average increments in body weight of 5.2 kg and 4.6 kg respectively on chlorpropamide therapy (Clarke and Duncan, 1968; Clarke and Campbell, 1977).

Weight loss in NIDDM patients during long term metformin therapy appears to level out at an average of 1–3% below pretreatment weight. However in a group of predominately obese non-diabetic diet restricted women, metformin increased weight loss by 20% (Pedersen, 1965). There is no obvious association between the amount of weight loss and the reduction in glucose concentrations in NIDDM patients (Hermann, 1979) and the mechanism responsible for weight loss (or lack of weight gain) is unknown. Increased thermogenesis is one possibility (Leslie et al, 1986). Another suggestion has been an anorectic effect, but evidence here is anecodotal, based on reports of reduced appetite during inital therapy when patients may experience transient abdominal discomfort. Small changes of energy balance are difficult to record accurately in long term clinical studies, and no data are available for metformin. In animal studies a large bolus of metformin (250 mg/kg) produced a transient anorectic effect, but chronic administration of the drug (up to $250 \, \text{mg} \, \text{kg}^{-1} \, \text{day}^{-1}$) did not alter normal daily food consumption (Bailey et al, 1986).

EFFECT UPON LIPID METABOLISM

Whereas certain chronic complications of NIDDM, particularly those involving microvascular disease, appear to be associated to some extent with the duration and severity of hyperglycaemia (Kilo, 1985), other complications such as macrovascular disease do not show an association (Panzram, 1987). Abnormalities of lipid and lipoprotein metabolism in NIDDM may contribute to the premature development of arterial vascular disease (Taskinen et al, 1984; Pyorala et al, 1987).

Metformin reduces total circulating triglyceride, especially in patients with hypertriglyceridaemia (Gustafson et al, 1971; Fedele et al, 1976; Sirtori et al, 1977, 1984; Janka, 1985). In hypertriglyceridaemic NIDDM patients and non-diabetic subjects metformin (2.5 g/day for 6 months) reduced total triglyceride on average by greater than 50% (Montaguti et al, 1979), although reductions of 10–20% are more likely in non-hypertriglyceridaemic subjects. The hypertriglyceridaemic effect of metformin is largely due to a decrease in very low-density lipoprotein (VLDL) triglyceride, and studies in metformin treated fructose fed rats have shown a decrease in the VLDL production rate (Zavoroni et al, 1984).

Total cholesterol concentrations were slightly but significantly lowered (about 4%) by metformin in NIDDM and non-diabetic subjects (Fedele et al, 1976; Montaguti et al, 1979), and a more prominent effect was observed in hypertriglyceridaemic animals (Sirtori et al 1977, 1979). However, no significant change in total cholesterol was observed in other studies involving non-hypertriglyceridaemic diabetic and non-diabetic animals and human subjects (Gustafson et al, 1971; Billingham et al, 1980, 1981; Janka, 1985; Campbell et al, 1987). High density lipoprotein (HDL) cholesterol was not significantly altered by metformin in normal and diabetic animals (Billingham et al 1980, 1981), but a small increase (about 8%) was observed in metformin treated NIDDM patients (Janka, 1985) and non-diabetic subjects (Sirtori et al, 1984).

METFORMIN IN CLINICAL PRACTICE

Indications

Metformin is used in the treatment of non-insulin-dependent diabetic patients either as monotherapy or in combination with a sulphonylurea. In general terms monotherapy may be useful in the obese patient who cannot, or will not follow a weight-reducing diet. Combination therapy may be useful in obese or non-obese patients as a way of delaying or avoiding insulin therapy. Behind these simple statements lie very difficult clinical decisions capable of prompting fervent argument between dedicated protagonists and antagonists of metformin use.

Monotherapy. The obese diabetic patient poorly controlled by a weight reducing diet presents the commonest, and perhaps the most difficult, therapeutic decision. It can be argued whether this stems from unrealistic, inappropriate or inadequate dietary advice or social pressure, minimal willpower, or general cussedness on the part of the patient. On the assumption that diet has been advised and reiterated sufficiently for the conclusion to be drawn that it will not be adequate to obtain control, the options of metformin, sulphonylurea or insulin remain. Probably the major consideration in a decision is the propensity for sulphonylureas (Clarke and Duncan, 1968; Clarke and Campbell, 1977) and insulin (Peacock and Tattersall, 1984; UK prospective diabetes study, 1985) to promote weight gain. Thus to choose either of those options entails weighing the evidence of 'greatest risk'. Which poses the greater long-term risk factor for morbidity and mortality—hyperglycaemia or obesity? Given that many would concede the difficulties of finding a clear answer to this question the metformin option emerges with a certain appeal. Metformin has the major advantage of, at least, not prompting weight gain or, at best, of promoting weight loss (Hermann, 1979; Wales, 1980; UK prospective diabetes study, 1985; Bailey, 1988). In addition, while the potential for lower blood glucose concentrations without increased body weight is attractive in this situation there is a further consideration. The antihyperglycaemic effect of metformin is achieved with lower or relatively lower circulating insulin concentrations. In turn this may relate to the lack of weight gain, but there may be other potential benefits in this approach. Peripheral hyperinsulinaemia has been proposed as a risk factor for arterial vascular disease (Stout 1979). Together with the reported antiatherogenic effect of metformin in animals (Sirtori et al, 1977; Marquie, 1978, 1983), plus reports of decreased sensitivity to platelet aggregating agents (Feruglio et al, 1979; Tremoli et al, 1982) and increased fibrinolytic activity (Chakrabarti et al, 1965; DeSilva et al, 1979; Vague et al, 1987), a possible vasoprotective effect of metformin warrants consideration and further investigation.

Combination therapy. The introduction of a second class of oral hypogly-caemic agents to a patient poorly controlled on either a sulphonylurea or metformin monotherapy presents a further therapeutic dilemma. Here the choice is combination therapy or insulin. Insulin has been traditionally regarded by the physician as the last refuge in the therapeutic armamen-tarium, and by the patient as a necessary evil when all-else fails. These views have been challenged (Peacock and Tattersall, 1984) but it is of note that only in retrospect do patients moderate their views.

Combination therapy allows delay or avoidance of insulin therapy. The physician will obviously consider the suitability of the patient for this treatment in the light of known side-effects and contra-indications. More than this, reassurance will be needed that the patient is not at risk of developing contra-indications to the drug or, at least, they will promptly be detected and treated should they develop. Also, it will not be advantageous to delay a difficult decision simply to buy time. As patients get older it becomes more difficult to learn new techniques such as insulin injection; other diseases may occur; renal function may deteriorate; and they may become dependent upon others for meals. A prerequisite therefore is to ensure adequate supervision and regular assessment, not only of blood glucose control but also of social circumstances and medical condition. A patient approaching 80 years of age taking metformin (1.5 g/day) and a sulphonylurea cannot have the metformin withdrawn without admitting that to do so is tantamount to a positive decision to use insulin. Tablets or insulin in this situation continues as a subject of considerable debate (Peacock and Tattersall, 1984; Nattrass, 1986).

Extent of use

Metformin accounts for approximately 25% of prescriptions for oral hypo-glycaemic drugs in Great Britain (information courtesy of DHSS Statistics and Research Division) about one-third being given as monotherapy and two-thirds in combination with a sulphonylurea.

Efficacy

The occurrence of primary failures has been reported at 5–20%, but this is not necesarily a primary failure of the drug to improve glycaemic control. More often the figure has included patients who discontinued the drug due to initial gastrointestinal reactions, although these are usually only tran-sient. In reality about 3% of patients are unable to tolerate the drug, and more than 90% of treated patients show an improvement in glycaemic control, that is, a primary failure rate of less than 10%. Secondary failures, in patients who fail to maintain an improvement of glycaemic control, are reported to be 5–10% per annum (Hermann, 1979). Thus primary and secondary failure rates for metformin are similar or slightly less than those reported for sulphonylureas (Lebovitz and Feinglos, 1983). This has been

confirmed in studies that have directly compared metformin with a sulphonylurea (Clarke and Duncan, 1968; Clarke and Campbell, 1977).

It is clear, however, that assessments of primary and secondary failure are
entirely dependent upon definition. This can be an improvement in glycaemic control, improvement of greater than $x\%$ (arbitrary) in blood glucose
concentration or ability to achieve a pre-set goal e.g. a given fasting blood
glucose. With this is mind it should be acknowledged that recently proposed
guidelines for good control—fasting blood glucose concentration less than
6.7 mmol/l (Alberti and Gries, 1987)—may not be achieved. Indeed many
studies have noted that a proportion of patients failed to meet the European
consensus requirements for moderate control of a fasting blood glucose
concentration of less than 7.8 mmol/l. Information on how successful insulin
or sulphonylureas are in this respect must await rigorous study.

Side-effects

Acute side-effects of metformin therapy have been reported in 5–20% of
patients (Hermann, 1979). These are mainly gastrointestinal disturbances
such as anorexia, abdominal discomfort, nausea or diarrhoea. With the
exception of diarrhoea they are usually transient and do not normally
require discontinuation of the drug. Diarrhoea during metformin treatment
is often needlessly investigated and abates following withdrawal of the drug.
Gastrointestinal side-effects are greatly minimized if the drug is taken with
meals and if the dose is increased slowly.

After several years of therapy intestinal absorption of vitamin B_{12} is
impaired in 30% of patients (Tomkin, 1973). Similarly folate absorption
may be decreased (Bergman et al, 1978). These findings are of no clinical
significance and there is only one report of anaemia attributable to metformin (Callaghan et al, 1980). Of other adverse reactions a single case of
vasculitis and pneumonitis is documented (Klapholz et al, 1986).

Lactic acidosis occupies a special place in the history of biguanide usage.
Phenformin was withdrawn from use in many countries because of an
unacceptably high incidence of lactic acidosis during treatment with the
drug. Similar fears have dogged metformin use since that time. Because of
its importance it is considered in more detail below.

Caution in prescribing

Contra-indications to prescribing metformin for a patient are difficult to
define quantitatively. With the exception of pregnancy where it is considered unsuitable, all depend upon the presence of other medical problems.
While it is relatively easy to draw up a list of associated conditions which cast
doubt upon metformin use it is considerably more difficult to say how much
associated disease must be present or to give particular weight to a specific
disease. The fear of lactic acidosis is central to reservations about, and
contra-indications to, metformin use. Some of the caution is justified, but a
proportion derives from extrapolation of phenformin use and phenformin-
associated lactic acidosis. This extrapolation is unjustified.

Lactate metabolism during metformin treatment

The increase in blood lactate which accompanies metformin is usually small (less than 2 mmol/l), exceeding the typical range for NIDDM patients only during postprandial excursions (Alexander and Hayes, 1979; Nattrass et al, 1979; Campbell et al, 1987; Jackson et al, 1987). The source of the excess lactate is uncertain. Potentially it could arise from increased peripheral production, increased intestinal or hepatic production or decreased hepatic clearance. It does not appear to originate from skeletal muscle (Bailey and Puah, 1986) and probably results from over production in the splanchnic bed (Jackson et al, 1987).

These abnormalities of blood lactate which are seen with metformin use either alone or in combination with a sulphonylurea are accompanied by small but significant elevations of circulating concentrations of the other gluconeogenic precursors pyruvate and alanine. (Nattrass et al, 1977, 1979; Jackson et al, 1987).

Co-existing medical conditions which are a contra-indication to metformin use

These considerations lead logically to the avoidance of metformin when diabetes coexists with certain other diseases. An associated disease which allows accumulation of metformin may enhance the hyperlactataemic effect and serves therefore as a contra-indication. Similarly any disease with the potential to increase peripheral lactate production or decrease hepatic clearance may exacerbate hyperlactataemia from metformin. Top of the list of contra-indications is impairment of renal function which has a profound effect upon metformin excretion.

This is followed by hepatic disease which impairs lactate clearance, and circulatory and respiratory diseases which, through peripheral hypoxia, enhance peripheral lactate production. Hepatic disease in non-diabetic subjects is associated with similar elevations in blood lactate to those produced by metformin in NIDDM patients (Stewart et al, 1983). Peripheral hypoxia from circulatory impairment is a major cause of lactic acidosis independent of diabetes (Alberti and Nattrass, 1977), while in patients with peripheral vascular disease there is a marked increase in lactate with exercise—reflecting hypoxia (Pernow et al, 1975). Small, but significant elevations of lactate are also reported in non-diabetic patients with chronic lung disease (Stubbs and Alberti, 1980). Further contra-indications are a previous history of lactic acidosis, suicidal intent and alcoholism.

In clinical practice the problems come, not in deciding on the introduction of metformin therapy when patients can be adequately assessed for the presence of contra-indications, but when patients on the drug move towards unsuitability. There are no clear solutions to the problems posed by deteriorating renal function with age, development of retinopathy and presumably nephropathy, or development of angina or claudication in a patient taking metformin.

Even a rational approach to the use of metformin can be confounded by acute illness. Myocardial infarction and septicaemia cannot be predicted and both demand immediate cessation of therapy.

Lactic acidosis

Metformin-associated lactic acidosis has been reported in 0–0.08 cases/1000 patient years, with a mortality risk of 0–0.024 cases/1000 patient years (Table 3). The incidence and mortality risk are much lower than for phenformin, and the incidence is lower than sulphonylurea-induced hypoglycaemia although the mortality risk is similar (Lucis, 1983; Berger, 1985; Campbell, 1984, 1985). As reviewed by Hermann (1979), in almost all patients who developed metformin-associated lactic acidosis described in the literature there were contra-indications to the drug or the patients attempted suicide. Renal insufficiency was the most commonly overlooked contra-indication, indicating that lactic acidosis usually occurs only if there is an accumulation of the drug. Recent accounts of metformin-associated lactic acidosis emphasize the importance of observing contra-indications (Ryder, 1984; Hutchinson and Catterall, 1987). As shown by the Canadian experience (1972–1982), strict adherence to the prescribing recommendations avoided any cases of metformin-associated lactic acidosis (Lucis, 1983).

SUMMARY

The hyperglycaemia of NIDDM is associated with insulin resistance due, in part, to reduced insulin receptor binding and more especially postreceptor defects. Metformin is an antihyperglycaemic agent which can be used to ameliorate insulin resistance. It appears to act directly on insulin target cells to enhance insulin action. Although metformin may increase insulin-receptor binding, its main effect appears to be directed at the postreceptor level of insulin action. Accordingly the drug potentiates insulin-suppression of hepatic gluconeogenesis and increases insulin-mediated peripheral glucose uptake and metabolism. It does not stimulate insulin release, does not cause weight gain and does not cause clinical hypoglycaemia. The risk of lactate accumulation should be appreciated in patients with renal insufficiency, liver dysfunction and following acute illness with hypoxia, when therapy should be stopped. Although metformin is often bracketed with phenformin in the context of lactic acidosis, different pharmacodynamics and adherence to prescribing guidelines render such a comparison unwarranted.

REFERENCES

Alberti KGMM & Gries FA (1987) Proposal for a consensus on the management of NIDDM. Proceedings of EASD Symposium: *The management of NIDDM: a European consensus*, pp 1–10. Berlin.
Alberti KGMM & Nattrass M (1977) Lactic acidosis. *Lancet* **ii**: 25–29.

Table 3 Incidence and mortality risk of metformin-associated lactic acidosis compared with phenformin-associated lactic acidosis and sulphonylurea-induced hypoglycaemic coma.*

	Patient years of treatment	Total cases (non-fatal/fatal)	Incidence (Total cases/1000 patient years)	Mortality rate (fatal cases/1000 patient years)
Metformin-associated lactic acidosis				
UK 1976–86	~400,000	11 (4/7)	0.027	0.017
Switzerland 1972–77	~29,800	2 (2/0)	0.067	—
Canada 1972–82	~56,000	0	—	—
Sweden 1972–81	~83,500	7 (5/2)	0.084	0.024
Phenformin-associated lactic acidosis				
Switzerland 1972–77[a]	~6,200	4 (1/3)	0.64	0.48
Sweden 1975–77	~20,000	13 (7/6)	0.64	0.30
Sulphonylurea-induced hypoglycaemic coma				
Switzerland 1960–69[b]	~350,000	88 (83/5)	0.251	0.014
Sweden 1972–81[c]	~300,000	57 (47/10)	0.190	0.033

* Based on survey data reported by Cohen 1979; Lucis 1983; Berger 1985; Campbell 1984, 1985.
[a] Excluding Basel
[b] Various sulphonylureas
[c] Glibenclamide

Alengrin F, Gossi G, Canivet B & Dolais-Kitagi J (1987) Inhibitory effects of metformin on insulin and glucagon action in rat hepatocytes involve post-receptor alterations. *Diabete et Metabolisme* **13**: 591–597.

Alexander WD & Hayes TM (1979) Metformin and sulphonylureas; a comparison of their effect on lactate levels in diabetics with and without complications. *Research and Clinical Forums* **1**: 65–68.

Arky RA (1979) Hypoglycemia. In Degroot LJ, Cahill GF, Odell WD et al (eds) *Endocrinology* **2**, pp 1099–1123. New York: Grune and Stratton.

Bailey CJ (1985) The antihyperglycaemic action of metformin. *Royal Society of Medicine International Congress and Symposium Series* **79**: 17–26.

Bailey CJ (1988) Metformin revisited: its actions and indications for use. *Diabetic Medicine* **5**: 315–320.

Bailey CJ & Broadbent ME (1981) Chronic effects of glibenclamide, chlorpropamide and metformin on plasma glucose and insulin in non-diabetic rats. *General Pharmacology* **12**: 323–326.

Bailey CJ & Puah JA (1986) Effect of metformin on glucose metabolism in mouse soleus muscle. *Diabete et Metabolisme* **12**: 212–218.

Bailey CJ, Lord JM & Atkins TW (1984) The insulin receptor and diabetes. In Nattrass M & Santiago J (eds) *Recent Avances in Diabetes* 1, pp 27–44. Edinburgh: Livingstone.

Bailey CJ, Flatt PR & Ewan C (1986) Anorectic effect of metformin in lean and genetically obese hyperglycaemic (ob/ob) mice. *Archives Internationales de Pharmacodynamie et de Therapie* **282**: 233–239.

Bailey CJ, Flatt PR & Marks V (1988) Drugs inducing hypoglycaemia. *Journal of Pharmacology and Experimental Therapeutics* (in press).

Beckmann R (1971) Biguanide. In Maske H (ed) *Handbook of Experimental Pharmacology*, **29**: pp 439–596. Berlin: Springer-Verlag.

Berger W (1985) Indicence of severe side effects during therapy with sulphonylureas and biguanides. *Hormone and Metabolic Research* **15 (supplement)**: 111–115.

Berger W & Kunzli H (1970) Effect of dimethylbiguanide on insulin, glucose and lactic acid contents observed in portal vein blood and peripheral venous blood in the course of intraduodenal glucose tolerance tests. *Diabetologia* **6**: 37.

Bergman U, Boman G & Wiholm BE (1978) Epidemiology of adverse drug reactions to phenformin and metformin. *British Medical Journal* **2**: 464–466.

Billingham MS, Hall RA, Simpson S & Bailey CJ (1980) Lack of effect of glibenclamide, chlorpropamide and metformin on plasma cholesterol and HDL-cholesterol in non-diabetic rats. *Hormone and Metabolic Research* **12**: 340–341.

Billingham MS, Hall RA, Simpson S & Bailey CJ (1981) Plasma high density liproprotein cholersterol in streptozotocin diabetic and non-diabetic mice after prolonged administration of glibenclamide, chlorpropamide and metformin. *Diabete et Metabolisme* **7**: 271–274.

Callagham TS, Hadden DR & Tomkin GH (1980) Megaloblastic anaemia due to vitamin B12 malabsorption associated with long-term metformin treatment. *British Medical Journal* **280**: 1214–1215.

Campbell IW (1984) Metformin and glibenclamide: comparative risks. *British Medical Journal* **289**: 289.

Campbell IW (1985) Metformin and the sulphonylureas: the comparative risk. *Hormone and Metabolic Research* **15 (supplement)**: 105–111.

Campbell IW, Duncan CD, Patton NW et al (1987) The effect of metformin on glycaemic control, intermediary metabolism and blood pressure in non-insulin-dependent diabetes mellitus. *Diabetic Medicine* **4**: 337–341.

Capretti L, Bonora E, Coscelli C & Butturini U (1982) Combined sulphonylurea-biguanide therapy for non-insulin dependent diabetics. Metabolic effects of glibenclamide and metformin or phenformin in newly diagnosed obese patients. *Current Medical Research and Opinion* **7**: 677–683.

Caspary WF & Creutzfeld W (1971) Analysis of the inhibitory effect of bigunides on glucose absoption: inhibition of sugar transport. *Diabetologia* **7**: 379–385.

Chakrabarti R, Hocking ED & Fearnley GR (1965). Fibrinolytic effect of metformin in coronary artery disease. *Lancet* **ii**: 256–259.

Cigolini M, Bosello O, Zancanaro C et al (1984) Influence of metformin on metablic effect of insulin in human adipose tissue in vitro. *Diabete et Metabolisme* **10**: 311–315.

Cigolini M, Zancanaro C, Benati D et al (1987) Metformin enhances insulin binding to in vitro down regulated human fat cells. *Diabete et Metabolisme* **13**: 20–22.

Clarke BF & Duncan LJP (1968) Comparison of chlorpropamide and metformin treatment on weight and blood glucose response of uncontrolled obese diabetics. *Lancet* **i**: 123–126.

Clarke BF & Campbell IW (1977) Comparison of metformin and chlorpropramide in non-obese maturity-onset diabetics uncontrolled by diet. *British Medical Journal* **275**: 1576–1578.

Cohen RD (1979) The relative risks of different biguandides in the causation of lactic acidosis. *Research and Clinical Forums* **1**: 125–134.

Cooke DE, Blair JB, Gilfillan C & Lardy HA (1973) Mode of action of hypoglycaemic agents. IV. Control of the hypoglycaemic activity of phenethylbiguanide in rats and guinea pigs. *Biochemical Pharmacology* **22**: 2121–2128.

Coscelli C, Palmari V, Saccardi F, Alpi O & Bonora E (1984) Evidence that metformin addition to insulin induces an amelioration of glycaemic profiles in type 1 (insulin-dependent) diabetes mellitus. *Current Therapy Research* **35**: 1058–1069.

Davidson MB (1981) Autoregulation by glucose of hepatic glucose balance: permissive effects of insulin. *Metabolism* **30**: 279–284.

DeFronzo R, Ferrannini E & Koivisto V (1983) New concepts in the pathogenesis and treatment of non-insulin dependent diabetes mellitus. *American Journal of Medicine* **74 (supplement)**: 52–81.

DeSilva SR, Shawe JE, Patel H & Cudworth AG (1979) Plasma fibrinogen in diabetes mellitus. *Diabete et Metabolisme* **5**: 201–206.

Fantus IG & Brosseau R (1986) Mechanism of action of metformin: insulin receptor and postreceptor effects in vitro and in vivo. *Journal of Clinical Endocrinology and Metabolism* **63**: 898–905.

Fedele D, Tiengo A, Nosadini R et al (1976) Hypolipidaemic effects of metformin in hyper-prebetalipoproteinaemia. *Diabete et Metabolisme* **2**: 127–134.

Ferguson AW, De La Harpe PL & Farquhar JW (1961) Dimethybiguanide in the treatment of diabetic children. *Lancet* **i**: 1367–1369.

Ferre P, Hitier Y, Penicaud L & Girard J (1988) Effects of the biguanide metformin on glucose metabolism in the obese Zucker rat. In Shafrir E & Renold AE (eds) *Lessons from animal diabetes II* abstract 326. London: Libbey.

Feruglio FS, Calabrese S, Giansante C & Cattin L (1979) Metformin and platelet aggregation. *Research and Clinical Forums* **1**: 105–112.

Frayn KN & Adnitt PI (1972) Effects of metformin on glucose uptake by isolated diaphragm from normal and diabetic rats. *Biochemical Pharmacology* **21**: 3153–3162.

Frayn KN, Adnitt PI & Turner P (1971) The hypoglycaemic action of insulin. *Postgraduate Medical Journal* **47**: 777–780.

Gawler D, Milligan G & Houslay MD (1978) Treatment of streptozotocin-diabetic rats with metformin restores the ability of insulin to inhibit adenylate cyclase activity and demonstrates that insulin does not exert this action through the inhibitory guanine nucleotide regulatory protein G_i. *Biochemical Journal* **249**: 537–542.

Gin H, Slama G, Weissbrodt P et al (1982) Metformin reduces postprandial insulin needs in type 1 (insulin dependent) diabetic patients: assessment by the artificial pancreas. *Diabetologia* **53**: 24–36.

Gin H, Messerchmitt C, Brottier E & Aubertin J (1985) Metformin improved insulin resistance in type 1 insulin-dependent, diabetic patients. *Metabolism* **34**: 923–925.

Gustafson A, Bjorntorp P & Fahlen M (1971) Metformin administration in hyperlipidaemic states. *Acta Medica Scandinavica* **190**: 491–494.

Hermann LS (1979) Metformin. A review of its pharmacological properties and therapeutic use. *Diabete et Metabolisme* **5**: 233–245.

Higginbotham L & Martin FIR (1979) Double-blind trial of metformin in the therapy of non-ketotic diabetes. *Medical Journal of Australia* **2**: 154–156.

Holle A, Mangels W, Dreyer M, Kuhnau J & Rudiger HW (1981) Biguanide treatment increases the number of insulin-receptor sites on human erythrocytes. *New England Journal of Medicine* **305**: 563–566.

Holman RR, Steemson J & Turner RC (1987) Sulphonylurea failure in type 2 diabetes: treatment with a basal insulin supplement. *Diabetic Medicine* **4**: 457–462.

Hutchinson SMW & Catterall JR (1987) Metformin and lactic acidosis – a reminder. *British*

Journal of Clinical Practice **41:** 673–674.

Jackson RA, Hawa MI, Jaspan JV et al (1987) Mechanism of metformin action in non-insulin-dependent diabetes. *Diabetes* **36:** 632–640.

Jacobs DB, Hayes GR, Truglia JA & Lockwood DH (1986) Effects of metformin on insulin receptor tyrosine kinase activity in rat adipocytes. *Diabetologia* **29:** 798–801.

Janka HU (1985) Platelet and endothelial function tests during metformin treatment in diabetes mellitus. *Hormone and Metabolic Research* **15 (supplement 1):** 120–122.

Kilo C (1985) Value of glucose control in preventing complications of diabetes. *American Journal of Medicine* **79 (supplement 2B):** 33–37.

Klapholz L, Leitersdorf E & Weinrauch L (1986) Leucocytoclastic vasculitis and pneumonitis induced by metformin. *British Medical Journal* **293:** 483.

Laastuen L & Todd WR (1969) Rat liver glycogen-lowering activity of fed creatine – a retraction. *Journal of Nutrition* **99:** 446–448.

Leatherdale BA & Bailey CJ (1986) Acute antihyperglycaemic effect of metformin without alteration of gastric emptying. *IRCS Medical Science* **14:** 1085–1086.

Leblanc H, Marre M, Billault B & Passa Ph (1987) Combined continuous subcutaneous insulin infusion in 10 overweight insulin requiring diabetic patients. *Diabete et Metabolisme* **13:** 613–617.

Lebovitz HE & Feinglos MN (1983) The oral hypoglycemic agents. In Ellenberg M & Rifkin H (eds) *Diabetes mellitus: theory and practice, 3rd edn,* pp 591–610. New York: Medical Examination Publishing Co.

Leslie P, Jung RT, Isles TE et al (1986) Effect of optimal glyceamic control with continuous subcutaneous insulin infusion on energy expediture in type I diabetes mellitus. *British Medical Journal* **293:** 1121–1126.

Lorch E (1971) Inhibition of intestinal absorption and improvement of oral glucose tolerance by biguanides in the normal and in the streptozotocin diabetic rat. *Diabetologia* **7:** 195–203.

Lord JM, Atkins TW & Bailey CJ (1983a) Effect of metformin on hepatocyte insulin receptor binding in normal streptozotocin diabetic and genetically obese diabetic (ob/ob) mice. *Diabetologia* **25:** 108–113.

Lord JM, White SI, Bailey CJ et al (1983b) Effect of metformin on insulin receptor binding and glycaemic control in type II diabetes. *British Medical Journal* **286:** 830–831.

Lord JM, Puah JA, Atkins TW & Bailey CJ (1985) Postreceptor effect of metformin on insulin action in mice. *Journal of Pharmacy and Pharmacology* **37:** 821–823.

Lucis OJ (1983) The statusi of metformin in Canada. *Canadian Medical Association Journal* **128:** 24–26.

McLelland J (1985) Recovery from metformin overdose. *Diabetic Medicine* **2:** 410–411.

Marquie G (1978) Effect of metformin on lipid metabolism in the rabbit aortic wall. *Atherosclerosis* **30:** 165–170.

Marquie G (1983) Mettormin action on lipid metabolism in lesions of experimental aortic atherosclerosis of rabbits. *Atherosclerosis* **47:** 7–17.

Meyer F (1960) Etude sur le mode d'action des biguanides hypoglycemiants. *Compte Rendu* **251:** 1928–1930.

Meyer F, Ipaktchi M & Clauser H (1967) Specific inhibition of gluconeogenesis by biguandides. *Nature* **213:** 203–204.

Montaguti U, Celin D, Ceredi C & Descovich GC (1979) Efficacy of the long-term administration of metformin in hyperlipidaemic patients. *Research and Clinical Forums* **1:** 95–103.

Nattrass M (1986) Treatment of type II diabetes. *British Medical Journal* **292:** 1033–1034.

Nattrass M & Alberti KGMM (1978) Biguanides. *Diabetologia* **14:** 71–74.

Nattrass M, Todd PG, Hinks L, Lloyd B & Alberti KGMM (1977) Comparative effects of phenformin, metformin and glibenclamide in metabolic rhythms in maturity-onset diabetics. *Diabetologia* **13:** 145–152.

Nattrass M, Hinks L, Smythe P, Todd PG & Alberti KGMM (1979) Metabolic effects of combined sulphonylurea and metformin therapy in maturity-onset diabetics. *Hormone and Metabolic Research* **11:** 332–337.

Noel M (1979) Kinetic study of normal and sustained release dosage forms of metformin in normal subjects. *Research and Clinical Forums* **1:** 35–50.

Nosadini R, Avogaro A, Trevisan R et al (1987) Effect of metformin on insulin-stimulated glucose turnover and insulin binding to receptors in type II diabetes. *Diabetes Care* **10:** 62–67.

Olefsky JM, Revers RR, Prince M et al (1985) Insulin resistance in non-insulin dependent (type II) and insulin dependent (type I) diabetes mellitus. *Advances in Experimental and Medical Biology* **189:** 176–205.

Pagano G, Tagliaferro V, Carta Q et al (1983) Metformin reduces insulin requirement in type 1 (insulin dependent) diabetes. *Diabetologia* **24:** 351–354.

Panzram G (1987) Mortaity and survival in type 2 (non-insulin-dependent) diabetes mellitus. *Diabetologia* **30:** 123–131.

Peacock J & Tattersall RB, (1984) The difficult choice of treatment for poorly controlled maturity onset diabetes: tablets or insulin? *British Medical Journal* **288:** 1956–1959.

Pedersen J (1965) The effect of metformin on weight loss in obesity. *Acta Endocrinologica* **49:** 479–486.

Pentikainen PJ, Neuivonen PJ & Penttila A (1979) Pharmacokinetics of metformin after intravenous and oral administration to man. *European Journal of Clinical Pharmacology* **16:** 195–202.

Pernow B, Saltin B, Wahren J, Cronenstrand R & Ekestrom S (1975) Leg blood flow and muscle metabolism in occlusive arterial disease of the leg before and after reconstructive surgery. *Clinical Science and Molecular Medicine* **49:** 265–275.

Pezzino V, Trischitta V, Purrello F & Vigneri R (1982) Effect of metformin on insulin binding to receptors in cultured human lymphocytes and cancer cells. *Diabetologia* **23:** 131–135.

Pilkis SJ (1975) Glucokinase of rat liver. *Methods in Enzymology* **42:** 31–33.

Prager R & Schernthaner G (1983) Insulin receptor binding to monocytes, insulin secretion and glucose tolerance following metformin treatment. *Diabetes* **32:** 1083–1086.

Prager R, Schernthaner G & Graf H (1986) Effect of metformin on peripheral insulin sensitivity in non insulin dependent diabetes mellitus. *Diabete et Metabolisme* **12:** 346–350.

Purrello F, Gullo D, Brunetti A et al (1987) Direct effect of biguanides on glucose utilization in vitro. *Metabolism* **36:** 774–776.

Pyorala K, Laakso M & Uusitupa M (1987) Diabetes and atherosclerosis: an epidemiologic view. *Diabetes Metabolism Reviewes* **3:** 491–494.

Rigas AN, Bittles AH, Hadden DR & Montgomery DAD (1968) Circadian variation of glucose, insulin and free fatty acids during long-term use of oral hypoglycaemic agents in diabetes mellitus. *British Medical Journal* **4:** 25–28.

Rizkalla SW, Elgrably F, Tchobroutsky G & Slama G (1986) Effects of metformin treatment on erythrocyte insulin binding in normal weight subjects, in obese non diabetic subjects and type 1 and type 2 diabetic patients. *Diabete et Metabolisme* **12:** 219–224.

Ryder REJ (1984) Lactic acidotic coma with multiple medication including metformin in a patient with normal renal function. *British Journal of Clinical Practice* **38:** 229–230.

Schafer G (1980) Guanidines and biguanides. *Pharmacology and Therapeutics* **8:** 275–295.

Schafer G (1983) Biguanides. A review of history, pharmacodynamics and therapy. *Diabete et Metabolisme* **9:** 148–163.

Schatz H, Winkler G, Jonatha EM & Pfeiffer EF (1975) Studies on juvenile-type diabetes in children. *Diabete et Metabolisme* **1:** 211–220.

Schonborn J, Heim K, Rabast U & Kasper H (1975) Oxidation rate of plasma free fatty acids in maturity onset diabetics. Effect of metformin. *Diabetologia* **11:** 375.

Sirtori CR, Tremoli E, Sirtori M, Conti F & Paoletti R (1977) Treatment of hypertriglyceridemia with metformin. *Atherosclerosis* **26:** 853–862.

Sirtori CR, Franceschini G, Galli-Kienle M et al (1978) Disposition of metformin (N, N-dimethylbiguanide) in man. *Clinical Pharmacology and Therapeutics* **24:** 683–693.

Sirtori CR, Weber G, Losi M et al (1979) Metformin and lipid metabolism. *Research and Clinial Forums* **1:** 117–121.

Sirtori CR, Franceschini G, Gianfranschi G et al (1984) Metformin improves peripheral vascular flow in nonhyperlipidemic patients with arterial disease. *Journal of Cardiovascular Pharmacology* **6:** 914–923.

Somogyi A, Stockley C, Keal J, Rolan P & Bochner F (1987) Reduction of metformin renal tubular secretion by cimetidine in man. *British Journal of Clinical Pharmacology* **23:** 44–50.

Spence JT, Merrill MJ & Pitot HC (1981) Role of insulin, glucose and cyclic GMP in the regulation of glucokinase in cultured hepatocytes. *Journal of Biological Chemistry* **265:** 1598–1603.

Sterne J (1969) Pharmacology and mode of action of hypoglycaemic guanidine derivatives. In

Campbell GD (ed) *Oral hypoglycaemic agents*, pp 193–245. London: Academic Press.

Sterne J & Junien JL (1981) Metformin: Pharmacological mechanisms of the antidiabetic and antilipidic effects and clinical consequences. *Royal Society of Medicine International Congress and Symposium* **48:** 3–16.

Stewart A, Johnston DG, Alberti KGMM, Nattrass M & Wright R (1983) Hormone and metabolic profiles in alcoholic liver disease. *European Journal of Clinical Investigation* **13:** 397–403.

Stout RW (1979) Diabetes and atherosclerosis. The role of insulin. *Diabetologia* **16:** 141–150.

Stubbs WA & Alberti KGMM (1980) The lung, whole body metabolism and disease. In Porter R & Whelan J (eds) *Metabolic activities of the lung, Ciba Foundation Symposium* **78:** pp 351–372. Amsterdam: Exerpta Medica.

Taskinen M-R, Harno K & Nikkila EA (1984) Serum lipids and lipoproteins in type 2 diabetes. *Acta Endocrinologica* **105 (supplement 263):** 95–99.

Tomkin G (1973) Malabsorption of vitamins B_{12} in diabetic patients treated with phenformin: a comparison with metformin. *British Medical Journal* **3:** 673–675.

Tremoli E, Ghiselli G, Maderna P, Collis S & Sirtori CR (1982) Metformin reduces platelet hypersensitivity in hypercholesterolemic rabbits. *Atherosclerosis* **41:** 53–60.

Trischitta V, Gullo D, Pezzino V & Vigneri R (1983) Metformin normalizes insulin binding to monocytes from obese nondiabetic subjects and obese type II diabetic patients. *Journal of Clinical Endocrinology and Metabolism* **57:** 713–718.

Tucker GT, Casey C, Phillips PJ, Connor H, Ward JD & Woods HF (1981) Metformin kinetics in healthy subjects and in patients with diabetes mellitus. *British Journal of Clinical Pharmacology* **12:** 235–246.

UK prospective diabetes study. II (1985) Reduction in HbA1c with basal insulin supplement, sulfonylurea or biguanide therapy in maturity-onset diabetes. *Diabetes* **34:** 793–798.

Wales JK (1980) Treatment of the obese diabetic patient. In Bjorntorp P, Cairelli M & Howard AN (eds) *Recent advances in obesity research*, 3 pp 184–189. London: Libbey.

Wollen N & Bailey CJ (1988a) Metformin potentiates the antihyperglycaemic action of insulin. *Diabete et Metabolisme* **14:** 88–91.

Wollen N & Bailey CJ (1988b) Inhibition of hepatic glucoeogenesis by metformin: synergism with insulin. *Biochemical Pharmacology* (in press).

Vague Ph, Juhan-Vague I, Alessi MC, Badier C & Valadier J (1987) Metformin decreases the high plasminogen activator inhibition capacity, plasma insulin and triglyceride levels in non-diabetic obese subjects. *Thrombosis Haemostasis* **57:** 326–328.

Vidon N, Chaussade S, Noel M, Franchisseur C, Hachet B & Bernier JJ (1988) Metformin in the digestive tract. *Diabetes Research and Clinical Practice* **4:** 223–229.

Zavaroni I, Dall Aglio E, Bruschi F, Alpi C, Coscelli C & Butturini U (1984) Inhibition of carbohydrate-induced hypertriglyceridemia by metformin. *Hormone and Metabolic Research* **16:** 85–87.

12

Insulin treatment of non-insulin-dependent diabetes mellitus

ROBERT J. HEINE

Non-insulin-dependent diabetes represents one of the major chronic ill-nesses in the elderly population. Despite this large and growing number of patients (Neil et al, 1987) no consensus of opinion exists on who to treat this important cause of morbidity and mortality (Panzram, 1987). One reason is that until recently most of the clinical research interest has gone into the field of insulin-dependent diabetes mellitus, where much effort is spent in finding the best way to achieve normoglycaemia. Since the role of good metabolic control in the prevention of long term complications has been recognized, the strict treatment targets in these patients have been accepted (Cahill et al, 1976). A completely different view still seems to exist where non-insulin-dependent diabetic patients are concerned (Tattersall, 1984; Tattersall and Scott, 1987). Diabetes in elderly patients is often referred to as being mild when it is treated with diet or oral hypoglycaemic agents but when looking at the morbidity and mortality statistics another opinion might be more appropriate (Tattersall, 1984; Morley et al, 1987).

Age- and sex-related overall mortality rates are approximately twice as high as in non-diabetic individuals. Cohort studies in NIDDM patients have demonstrated a very poor prognosis: 44% of patients dying within ten years of diagnosis (Panzram and Zabel-Langhennig, 1981). Numerous investigations provide unequivocal evidence for cardiovascular and cerebrovascular disease as the leading cause of death in NIDDM patients (Panzram, 1987). Only in those patients in whom the diagnosis was made past the age of 75 was there no significant increase in mortality due to diabetes. Another important consequence of diabetes is its impingement on the quality of life, as reflected by the high frequency of amputations, blindness, fatigue, infections and neuropathy due to diabetes. From this it seems evident that the treatment targets in NIDDM patients should be defined very carefully and, in general, follow the same principles as those already accepted in younger patients.

AIMS OF TREATMENT

The defined objectives of therapy (Table 1) will determine the intensity of treatment. These objectives will usually be either relief of hyperglycaemic

Table 1. Objectives of treatment.

Improvement of quality of life.
Prevention of metabolic catastrophies.
Prevention of long-term micro- and macrovascular complications.
Relief of hyperglycaemic symptoms.
Avoidance of frequent episodes of hypoglycaemia.

symptoms or, in order to prevent acute and chronic complications, (near) normoglycaemia. In elderly patients with severe complications there is no sense in trying to achieve normoglycaemia as no evidence exists that established complications will reverse with better control. In these patients the improvement of general well-being will be the prime aim. Only a few studies have documented the effect of insulin treatment on impaired physical performance of NIDDM patients. Selz et al (1980), studied the well-being before and after one year of therapy in 11 NIDDM patients over 55 years of age. A moderate improvement of metabolic control was accompanied by a better well-being. Other results were obtained in a prospective study in 58 patients who no longer responded to maximum doses of oral hypoglycaemic agents. They were given once daily lente insulin at a dose which was limited to 48 U/day (Peacock and Tattersall, 1984). In only 18 patients was a significant improvement of the glycaemic control obtained and only 22 patients reported an improvement of their well-being. In this study the outcome probably was influenced to a great extent by the limitation of the insulin dosage to 48 U daily. Since most patients with NIDDM are insulin resistant a higher dose is, at least initially, often required (Unger and Grundy, 1985; Garvey et al, 1985). More studies are required urgently to establish the beneficial effect of insulin treatment on physical and neuro-psychological performance, and general well-being in patients failing to respond sufficiently to oral hypoglycaemic agents.

In younger patients with NIDDM without advanced macrovascular complications the same targets should be set as in IDDM, i.e. to achieve glucose levels as close to the normal range as possible. This recommendation is supported by the existing evidence that near physiological control of glycaemia is advantageous to the diabetic patient (Cahill et al, 1976; Tchobroutsky, 1978; Unger, 1982). Obviously the treatment objectives have to be set according to individual needs and available resources. Table 1 lists the various objectives of treatment which determine the glycaemic control to be obtained.

INDICATIONS FOR INSULIN THERAPY

In general, treatment of NIDDM comprises a prescription of oral hypo-glycaemic agents and/or a diet aiming for weight reduction. An adequate weight loss is, despite tremendous efforts from health care providers and patients, not accomplished in the majority of patients (Wing et al, 1987a;

Table 2. Indications for insulin treatment in non-insulin-dependent diabetes.

Hyperglycaemic symptoms accompanied by fasting blood glucose levels of above 15 mmol/l.

Primary drug failure.

Secondary drug failure.

Temporary insulin treatment in patients on oral drugs or diet alone undergoing surgery or in periods of poor control due to other diseases.

1987b). Oral hypoglycaemic agents have, in most patients, only a temporary effect. Approximately 10% of NIDDM patients no longer have satisfactory control after one year and 90% after five years' therapy with a sulphonylurea (Lebovitz and Feingloss, 1978; Schoffling, 1980). When diet and oral hypoglycaemic agents fail to induce the metabolic control which was aimed for, insulin therapy is indicated (Table 2). The decision tree in Figure 1 gives a strategy guideline for the therapy of NIDDM.

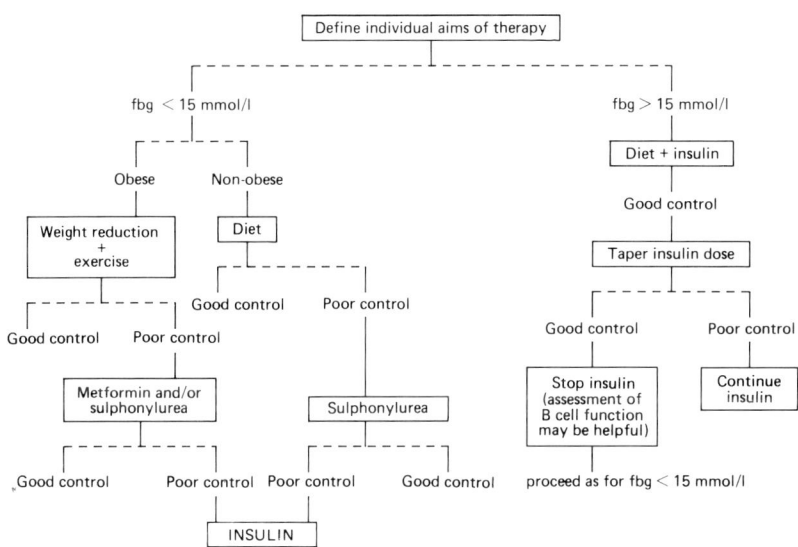

Figure 1. Decision tree for the therapy of NIDDM patients. fbg = fasting blood glucose level.

Primary insulin treatment

The decision tree indicates a possibility of primary treatment of the NIDDM patient with insulin. The patients in whom insulin treatment is prudent from the onset are indicated by being clinically ill or having severe hyperglycaemic symptoms, a short history, marked weight loss, first degree family history of IDDM and ketonuria (Wilson et al, 1985; Tattersall and Scott, 1987). A considerable number of these patients are likely to have insulin-dependent diabetes diagnosed after the age of 30. Their prevalence is generally underestimated. In a group of 154 patients in the age range 35 to 75 years with non-ketotic diabetes, 14% were found to be islet cell antibody positive (Groop et al, 1986). These patients, frequently women, are further characterized by often having other auto-immune endocrine diseases. As these patients rapidly develop insulin deficiency it is obvious that insulin treatment is indicated.

Also patients who are not classified as type 1b or late onset IDDM, but present with severe symptoms and high fasting blood glucose levels, above 15 mmol/l, are preferably treated with insulin. At these fasting blood glucose levels the insulin secretory capacity is invariably diminished and insulin sensitivity severely decreased (Faber and Damsgaard, 1984; Ward et al, 1984). When fasting blood glucose levels are 15 mmol/l or higher, oral hypoglycaemic agents are not likely to induce normoglycaemia in NIDDM patients. In a recent study by Hollenbeck and Reaven (1987) in 10 moderately obese NIDDM patients with a mean fasting blood glucose level of approximately 16 mmol/l, glipizide administration did not succeed in lowering the glucose levels below 10 mmol/l. Some of these patients will be found later to have absolute insulin deficiency, requiring insulin treatment in order to achieve acceptable metabolic control. Early insulin treatment reduces the risk of the development of hyperosmolar or ketoacidotic coma due to insulin deficiency. This risk should not be underestimated. A UK study revealed that approximately 30% of hyperosmolar or ketoacidotic episodes occurred in patients over 50 years of age (Gale et al, 1981). The mortality in this group was 56%. This high mortality could, in most instances, be attributed to late diagnosis and inadequate treatment. When initial treatment consists of insulin, a rapid correction of the hyperglycaemia can be achieved avoiding the risk of metabolic catastrophies. At a later stage the insulin dose may be gradually discontinued and oral hypoglycaemic agents and/or diet alone may be substituted. Obviously this should occur under vigilant metabolic control monitoring.

Most often, clinical criteria and metabolic assessment will be sufficient to determine whether patients are likely to respond favourably to oral hypo-glycaemic agents. When considerable uncertainty exists, B cell secretory capacity assessment after stimulation with either glucagon or an oral glucose load can be of help in deciding whether withdrawal of insulin is likely to be successful (Rendall, 1983; Grant et al, 1984).

The same approach is applicable to the obese NIDDM patient presenting with fasting hyperglycaemia, regardless of the fact that energy restriction is supposed to be the cornerstone of therapy. Clinically the most important question is whether it is more important to achieve normal weight or good metabolic control in the obese NIDDM patients. Several studies in which considerable effort has been put into a weight reduction programme, including diet, exercise and behavioural therapy, have shown a poor prognosis for both sustained weight loss and achieved glycaemic control (Wing et al, 1987a, 1987b; Korhonen et al, 1987). A recent study assessed the efficacy of a behavioural weight control programme in 114 obese patients with NIDDM (Wing et al, 1987a). The mean sustained weight loss after one year was 4.5 kg. It was shown that only 26 patients, who lost more than 6.9 kg, experienced significant improvement in glycaemic control. The authors concluded that with present weight loss techniques only modest long term results can be expected. If we accept that no more than a minority can achieve a significant weight reduction despite extensive efforts it seems more appropriate to initiate insulin treatment when objectives of therapy are not otherwise accomplished.

It is also of considerable interest to note that in this study no evidence was found that diabetes treatment affected weight loss. Patients receiving insulin demonstrated similar reduction in weight and improvements in HbA1 percentages compared with those on diet alone or taking oral hypoglycaemic agents.

Another indication for primary insulin treatment in NIDDM is the existence of contraindications to the use of sulphonylurea or metformin. These are dealt with elsewhere in this volume.

Secondary failure

Since the University Group Diabetes Programme (UGDP) reported their results from the large scale multicentre study which started in 1961, much controversy has arisen on the use of oral hypoglycaemic agents. It was suggested that the use of oral hypoglycaemic agents, i.e. tolbutamide and phenformin, more likely resulted in death due to cardiovascular disease than no treatment and that insulin treatment was of no value in preventing this (University Group Diabetes Programme, 1976). However, most aspects of this study have been criticized severely and the results refuted (Kilo et al, 1980).

The use of oral hypoglycaemic agents has since gained in interest, mainly due to the claimed advantages of having a beneficial effect on insulin sensitivity and of inducing a more physiological insulin response to carbohydrate loading as opposed to exogenous insulin administration (Mandarino and Gerich, 1984). A recent study has compared the influence of insulin therapy and tolazamide administration on hepatic and peripheral insulin sensitivity in NIDDM patients. Both treatments induced similar metabolic control and insulin action improved to a comparable degree (Firth et al, 1986a). From this study it can be concluded that as far as insulin action is concerned no specific advantages can be claimed for either form of therapy, provided good glycaemic control is achieved. Of equal importance is to know what the long-term effects are of primary treatment of NIDDM patients with diet alone, oral hypoglycaemic agents and insulin on the progression of diabetic complications and achieved metabolic control.

A new multicentre study has started in the UK to answer these essential questions. This UK Prospective Study of Therapies of Maturity Onset Diabetes (1983) was initiated in 1980 and will enroll 4000 patients by 1988. We have to wait for the results of this study in 1992 before firm conclusions can be drawn as to the advantages and disadvantages of either forms of therapy.

Temporary treatment with insulin

Temporary insulin treatment is advocated in patients with NIDDM on oral hypoglycaemic agents and/or diet treatment who are undergoing major surgery and during other periods with severe stress (Alberti et al, 1983; Clark et al, 1985). In these circumstances it is preferable to use highly purified porcine or human insulin and to refrain from bovine insulin which is the most immunogenic. Acute allergic reactions can be a considerable problem in patients previously sensitized to bovine insulin preparations (Reeves, 1986).

As indicated in the decision tree (Figure 1) it is advisable to treat patients presenting severe symptoms and/or fasting blood glucose levels of above 15 mmol/l with insulin.

After having accomplished good control with insulin, some patients may respond well to either oral hypoglycaemic agents and/or diet. Since good glycaemic control will improve insulin sensitivity and insulin secretion, a favourable response to oral hypoglycaemic agents is more likely to occur in patients already controlled adequately with insulin than in hyperglycaemic patients.

PRESUMED DISADVANTAGES OF INSULIN THERAPY

Risk factor for cardiovascular disease

When discussing insulin therapy in non-insulin-dependent diabetes mellitus it is of importance to know what the effects of insulin administration are on the known risk factors for macrovascular disease (Table 3). These risk factors in the general population, i.e. hyperlipidaemia, obesity, hypertension and smoking, are also operative in the diabetic population (Pyörälä et al, 1987). Of special interest is the link which seems to exist between

Table 3. Insulin therapy in non-insulin-dependent diabetes.

Concern	Recommendation
Promotion of macrovascular disease	Achievement of good metabolic control lowers the known risk factors for cardiovascular disease.
Weight gain	Dietary counselling will prevent excessive weight gain. Small weight gain is due mainly to water repletion.
Frequent hypoglycaemic episodes	Home blood glucose monitoring and patient education will reduce the risk for hypoglycaemia.
Compliance and convenience in elderly patients	Involvement of the district nurse or family in the care for patients who are unable to inject themselves. Pen-like insulin delivery systems will enhance convenience and acceptance.

insulin resistance and the risk factors for cardiovascular disease: low HDL2-cholesterol levels, hypertriglyceridaemia, hyperinsulinaemia and hypertension (Ginsberg, 1987; Ferrannini et al, 1987; Pyörälä et al, 1987). It is tempting to speculate that insulin resistance in itself plays a key role in the twofold enhancement of cardiovascular disease in patients with diabetes (Modan et al, 1985, 1987; Taskinen, 1987). Insulin therapy has been implicated in enhancing the risk for macrovascular disease by causing hyperinsulinaemia (Stout, 1979) and by promoting weight gain (Lipson, 1986). Clinically, it is important to assess the potential benefits and disadvantages of insulin therapy for each individual patient by considering insulin sensitivity, insulinaemia, serum lipid levels and body weight.

Hyperinsulinaemia/insulin resistance

High insulin levels have been found to favour the development of atherosclerosis (Stout, 1979). This has caused reluctance to start insulin treatment in patients with NIDDM and fear of high insulin dosages. The association between high insulin levels and cardiovascular disease has been found in several epidemiological studies. The involvement of insulin in atherogenesis is further suggested by the fact that insulin is known to cause smooth muscle cell proliferation and lipid accumulation in arterial wall in vitro (Stout, 1985). At present, however, a causative relationship between insulin and atherogenesis is largely speculative.

As outlined earlier it can be argued that not hyperinsulinaemia in itself but insulin resistance accompanied by hyperinsulinaemia is the link to the excess large vessel disease in NIDDM (Chen et al, 1987; Modan et al, 1985).

So far it is not possible to distinguish between hyperinsulinaemia per se and the metabolic consequences of poorly controlled diabetes in the development of large vessel disease. It is of interest to know that treatment of diabetes, regardless of diet, oral hypoglycaemic agents or insulin, causes an enhancement of insulin sensitivity. It has been shown convincingly that insulin treatment in non-insulin-dependent diabetic patients restores insulin sensitivity and also results in an improvement of B cell function (Scarlett et al, 1982; Garvey et al, 1985; Razenberg et al, 1985; Hollenbeck and Reaven, 1987). Garvey et al (1985) treated 14 NIDDM patients for three weeks with continuous subcutaneous insulin infusion. In these patients, normalization of basal and postprandial blood glucose levels were achieved at the expense of high insulin dosages of approximately 140 U/day during the initial week of treatment. Despite the induction of hyperinsulinaemia the in vivo insulin sensitivity, which was assessed after three week CSII therapy, improved remarkably. The insulin stimulated glucose disposal rate which was measured at several insulin levels during euglycaemic clamping was significantly greater following insulin treatment.

The shift of the insulin dose response curve was consistent with a partial reversal of the postbinding defect in insulin action. The improved insulin sensitivity was reflected clinically by a decrease of 23% in the insulin requirement during the second week which stabilized throughout the final (third) week of treatment with maintenance of normoglycaemia. The basal hepatic glucose output decreased by approximately 40% to a rate which was not significantly different from normal. Endogenous insulin secretion, which was assessed both after meals and after an i.v. glucose challenge, improved considerably despite the lower glycaemia after three weeks intensive insulin treatment. From this short-term intensive insulin treatment study it may be concluded that reversal of various metabolic defects results in improvement of the sensitivity to insulin and enhances the B-cell secretory capacity.

Recently we completed a study in 15 NIDDM patients who were no longer responding satisfactorily to sulphonylureas (secondary failures). This trial was undertaken to evaluate the effects of longer term insulin therapy in an outpatient setting on B cell function and in vivo insulin sensitivity. Patients were treated for six months with twice daily combinations of short acting and neutral protamine Hagedorn (NPH) insulin. A sustained improvement of metabolic control, albeit not normoglycaemia, was achieved in all patients. The mean HbA1 percentage dropped from 12.3 to 9.3% (upper normal: 7.5%) after six months. Endogenous insulin secretory capacity and insulin sensitivity in vivo were assessed after two and six months insulin treatment. A significant incremental increase of the C-peptide responses to a mixed meal was demonstrated after six months insulin treatment. Insulin-stimulated glucose disposal rates were significantly enhanced following two and six months insulin treatment. These results support the findings of the shorter term studies and are in accordance with the hypothesis that long-lasting hyperglycaemia is detrimental to the B cell and impairs insulin action beyond the insulin binding site (Unger and Grundy, 1985). This hypothesis is further supported by recent animal and in vitro studies which suggested that hyperinsulinaemia with maintenance of normal glucose levels enhances the sensitivity of tissues to insulin (Wardzala et al, 1985; Watanabe et al, 1986). Therefore, it seems justified to conclude that impaired insulin sensi-tivity can be restored by sustained stringent metabolic control. Insulin requirements may initially be very high, reflecting the insulin resistant state, but will diminish as soon as good metabolic control is accomplished.

Serum lipid levels

Hypertriglyceridaemia in association with low HDL2 cholesterol levels, is the most common lipid abnormality encountered in NIDDM (Uusitupa et al, 1986). From an epidemiological point of view, this lipoprotein pattern is considered to be atherogenic (Laakso et al, 1985; Pyörälä et al, 1987). High triglyceride levels are a consequence of both enhanced production and impaired clearance of very low-density lipoprotein (VLDL), which prob-ably is a result of a subnormal lipoprotein lipase (LPL) activity (Taskinen, 1987). These defects are a common finding in NIDDM and in obesity, especially when insulin resistance is present (Chen et al, 1987). Correction of hyperglycaemia *per se* has been shown to reduce triglyceride levels by enhancing the catabolic rate and by decreasing the production of VLDL. It should be noted that this can be established regardless of the application of diet, oral hypoglycaemic agents or insulin, indicating that the correction of the metabolic disorder is the primary factor and not the way by which it is established (Taskinen, 1987). Overproduction of triglyceride rich particles has been attributed to hyperinsulinaemia (Reaven and Greenfield, 1981). The fact that insulin treatment reverses high triglyceride levels does not contradict this association, but supports the concept that by decreasing triglyceride-precursors, i.e. free fatty acids and glycerol levels, and by improving insulin sensitivity, triglyceride metabolism can be ameliorated (Taylor et al, 1979; Taskinen, 1987). Moreover, insulin therapy has also been shown to enhance HDL2-cholesterol levels in NIDDM patients not responding to sulphonylurea drugs (Razenberg et al, 1985). This may be explained by the inverse relationship between HDL-cholesterol and VLDL triglyceride levels which is mediated mainly by adipose tissue LPL. Correction of hyperglycaemia by insulin enhances LPL activity and thereby lowers VLDL triglyceride levels and concomitantly increases HDL2 cholesterol concentration. These beneficial effects of insulin therapy on the lipoprotein profile result in a lower atherogenic risk. Prospective studies in NIDDM patients are necessary to establish the value of lowering these atherogenic risk factors.

Body weight

Weight gain has been considered to be one of the major drawbacks of insulin therapy, while weight loss is the recommended form of therapy for obese patients with NIDDM. This potential disadvantage has been a reason to limit the maximum allowed daily insulin dosage (Peacock and Tattersall, 1984). This approach, governed by the fear of weight gain, does not allow assessment of the efficacy of insulin treatment in these patients. It is now well known that in many cases high insulin dosages have to be given initially in order to achieve appropriate control (Lipson, 1986; Garvey et al, 1985), after which insulin dosages can be reduced as a result of a lesser degree of insulin resistance and improved B cell function. The mean weight gain in our study in 15 NIDDM patients was 3.5 kg (77.5 to 81 kg), which occurred mainly in the initial two months of insulin treatment. Part of this weight gain probably can be attributed to repletion of fluid and reduction of glycosuria. Similar weight gain has been observed in patients with sulphonylurea drugs. In the UK prospective study both sulphonylurea and insulin treatment for one year resulted in similar weight gain, which was approximately 2 kg more than in those patients treated with diet alone or metformin (UK Prospective Study, 1983).

There is no doubt that obesity plays a role in the development of the risk factors for cardiovascular disease in NIDDM. These particularly concern hyperlipidaemia, insulin resistance, hyperglycaemia and hypertension. However, the evidence for an independent relationship between obesity and cardiovascular risk is at least conflicting (Pyörälä et al, 1987). Furthermore, recent reports suggest that body composition, i.e. body fat mass, and not body weight, is associated with increase of cardiovascular disease risk factors. Excess adiposity was found to be related to high diastolic blood pressure, elevated LDL-cholesterol and low HDL-cholesterol levels and elevated insulin levels in the fasting state and after glucose challenge (Segal et al, 1987). Since most atherogenic risk factors associated with diabetes become attenuated with better glycaemic control, it is evident that normoglycaemia should be aimed for, even at the expense of a (small) weight gain.

Insulin therapy and hypoglycaemia

The occurrence of hypoglycaemia is always a risk when insulin therapy is initiated. When hypoglycaemic episodes occur repeatedly it may demoralize patients. It is therefore of great importance to educate the patients thoroughly and to teach them home blood glucose monitoring. The patients should be aware of the possibility that insulin requirements may decline with the improvement of metabolic control. The occurrence of hypoglycaemia is by no means exclusively confined to insulin treated patients. With sulphonylureas the risk of hypoglycaemic episodes is not small (Asplund et al, 1983). It should also be realized that in elderly patients altered drug disposition due to decreased hepatic, renal or cardiac function may lead to severe hypoglycaemia of long duration (Lebovitz and Feingloss, 1978).

Insulin therapy and convenience

Many physicians and patients are afraid of starting insulin therapy. It is widely believed that elderly patients cannot cope with insulin therapy because of arthritis, memory loss or poor eye sight. Patients consider insulin therapy as a last resort and as evidence of the severity of their diabetes. It is crucial to reassure patients that insulin therapy does not represent an undue hardship but, on the contrary, may reduce their hyperglycaemic complaints and improve their quality of life. Problems with insulin therapy resulting from poor eye sight or other physical inability should be overcome by asking relatives or a district nurse to prepare injections. A major advantage over conventional syringes are the pen-like devices, which may enable most patients to take insulin injections in an easy and convenient way.

INSULIN THERAPY REGIMENS

The insulin therapy regimens which have been advocated are derived mostly from practical experience in IDDM patients. The pathophysiology of NIDDM however, is different from that of IDDM and another approach might therefore be more appropriate (Olefsky and Kolterman, 1981; DeFronzo et al, 1983). Hyperglycaemia in NIDDM is a consequence of insufficient inhibition of basal hepatic glucose output and of enlarged postprandial glucose excursions. It seems reasonable to aim for a normalization of the hepatic glucose output by providing an adequate insulin availability during the night (DeFronzo et al, 1985; Firth et al, 1986b). In most patients it is not possible to achieve this by injecting an intermediate or long acting insulin in the morning, due to the limited duration of action of the available insulin preparations (Heine, 1988). A normal fasting blood glucose level can more easily be obtained by injecting an intermediate or long acting insulin at bedtime, as suggested by Riddle (1985).

Preliminary reports on studies comparing bedtime and morning NPH insulin administration suggest that this approach is effective. Bedtime NPH insulin in 11 NIDDM patients resulted in better glycaemic control than with injections of NPH insulin in the morning (Seigler et al, 1987). Normalization of the fasting blood glucose levels will influence beneficially the endogenous insulin response to carbohydrate ingestion and thereby lower daytime glycaemia (Turner and Holman, 1978; Garvey et al, 1985; Rosetti et al, 1987). After having achieved normoglycaemia in the basal state some patients still may require additional treatment dependent on the ability of the endogenous insulin secretory capacity to control postprandial blood glucose excursions. Then the second step will be to administer an additional injection of insulin before breakfast, either intermediate acting insulin or a mixture of short acting and NPH insulin. More studies comparing this more physiological approach with the conventional insulin regimens used in IDDM patients would be of interest.

Insulin + sulphonylurea

The hypoglycaemic effect of sulphonylurea drugs is considered not only to be a result of improving insulin secretion, but also to be mediated by an enhancement of insulin stimulated glucose utilization (Gerich, 1985). The addition of sulphonylurea to basal insulin treatment in patients with secondary sulphonylurea failure seems therefore appealing when aiming for control of postprandial glycaemic excursions. Several studies in NIDDM patients have suggested that combination therapy may provide better metabolic control, compared with insulin therapy alone or comparable control at a lower insulin dose (Groop et al, 1984; Simonson et al, 1987). A recent study has shown that the addition of glibenclamide to insulin therapy in 20 NIDDM patients who failed to respond adequately to sulphonylurea, lowered the insulin requirements from 62.5 to 34.6 U/day. Furthermore the B cell response to mixed meals was enhanced as reflected by higher meal-stimulated C-peptide levels. The achieved metabolic control and in vivo insulin sensitivity were not clearly different (Gutniak et al, 1987). In another study the efficacy of a combination of sulphonylurea with ultralente insulin was compared with that of ultralente alone in NIDDM patients with fasting hyperglycaemia while on maximal sulphonylurea therapy. The addition of sulphonylurea to ultralente insulin reduced the insulin requirement, but mean HbA1 levels were similar (Holman et al, 1987). From these studies it seems most likely that the sulphonylureas exert their action mainly by stimulating the B cells rather than by facilitating insulin action. Before adapting a combination of two drugs with separate, known side effects and risks in clinical practice it seems prudent to await further evidence of clear advantages of the combined drug regimen in long-term studies.

Intermittent insulin therapy?

As insulin therapy in NIDDM patients restores, at least partly, insulin sensitivity and B cell function, a short course of insulin therapy may be sufficient to induce lasting physiological improvements. This hypothesis was recently studied in 10 NIDDM patients who were treated for four weeks with insulin. As demonstrated earlier both insulin secretion and insulin action improved. However, within a few weeks of withdrawing insulin treatment, glucose tolerance and C-peptide response to oral glucose had nearly returned to pre-treatment values (Gormley et al, 1986). These preliminary observations make it very unlikely that intermittent insulin therapy will be of any benefit when compared with sustained insulin administration.

Insulin versus proinsulin

Biosynthetic human proinsulin has now been introduced for clinical studies as an alternative to intermediate acting insulin. The hypoglycaemic activity has been found to be approximately 8% of that of insulin. Several studies have suggested that proinsulin exerts a preferential inhibitory effect on hepatic glucose production compared to its effect on peripheral glucose uptake (Revers et al, 1984; Glauber et al, 1987). This implies that when glucose output is suppressed by proinsulin at a rate identical to that achieved with insulin, peripheral glucose uptake will be less stimulated by proinsulin.

The reduced clearance and the longer half life of proinsulin compared to that of insulin, and its absorption characteristics from the subcutaneous tissue, results in a time action course which resembles that of an intermediate acting insulin (Revers et al, 1984; Heine et al, 1987). In a recent study the efficacy of a bedtime injection of proinsulin was compared with NPH insulin in obese NIDDM patients with fasting hyperglycaemia. In these patients proinsulin lowered fasting glycaemia primarily by reducing the hepatic glucose output. When NPH insulin was injected in the same dose (0.2 U/kg) fasting glycaemia was hardly improved in these patients. From this acute metabolic study it was concluded that NPH insulin had, on a unit-for-unit basis, a lesser glucose-lowering potency than proinsulin (Glauber et al, 1987). However, larger doses of NPH insulin would probably have produced effects similar to those of proinsulin. Since the hypoglycaemic effect of proinsulin was achieved mainly by suppressing hepatic glucose production rather than stimulating peripheral glucose uptake, the risk for hypoglycaemic episodes may be less than with NPH insulin. Before therapeutic recommendations can be made, results from long-term studies including large groups of patients are necessary. Currently it would seem unlikely that these studies will be performed since all clinical trials with proinsulin have been suspended.

SUMMARY

The standard treatment of NIDDM consists of diet, oral hypoglycaemic agents and, mostly as a last resort, insulin. Indications for insulin therapy cannot be generalized for the whole population of NIDDM patients. The defined objectives of therapy for the individual patient will determine the choice and intensity of therapy. These will usually be either a relief of hyperglycaemic symptoms in the elderly patient or normoglycaemia, as in the insulin-dependent diabetic patients, in order to prevent acute and chronic complications. Primary insulin treatment is advisable in patients with hyperglycaemic symptoms and fasting blood glucose levels above 15 mmol/l, as in these patients the major defect will be insulin deficiency rather than insulin resistance.

The correction of long lasting hyperglycaemia partly restores insulin sensitivity and B cell function, thereby allowing sequential reduction of insulin dosage. When metabolic control can be sustained with low insulin dosages some of these patients may later respond well to oral hypoglycaemic agents or to diet alone. In the management of non-insulin-dependent diabetic patients it is of great importance to recognize in time when treatment with oral hypoglycaemic agents fails. Insulin therapy should not be withheld on the presumption that it will cause weight gain and will promote development of macrovascular disease. Weight gain can be reduced by adequate dietary counselling and the level of macrovascular risk factors reduces with improved metabolic control. In this context also it should be realized that the correction of hypertension, hyperlipidaemia and the cessation of cigarette smoking is probably of equal importance. Insulin therapy regimens which have been used in non-insulin-dependent diabetic patients have been the same as prescribed for insulin dependent patients. When considering the fact that hepatic overproduction of glucose is the major determinant of fasting blood glucose level and that postprandial glycaemic excursions are superimposed on this level it seems reasonable to aim for normalization of the basal hepatic glucose production. A bedtime injection of an intermediate or long acting insulin can be used for this aim. Other therapeutical approaches which have been studied recently are the use of combinations of insulin and oral hypoglycaemic agents and the use of proinsulin as an alternative for intermediate acting insulin. Before these forms of therapy can be advocated long-term clinical studies are necessary to define their therapeutic role.

REFERENCES

Alberti KGMM, Gill GV & Elliott MJ (1982) Insulin delivery during surgery in the diabetic patient. *Diabetes Care* **5 (supplement 1):** 65–77.

Asplund K, Wilholm BE & Lithner F (1983) Glibenclamide associated hypoglycaemia: a report on 57 cases. *Diabetologia* **24:** 412–417.

Cahill GF, Etzweiler DD & Freinkel N (1976) Control and diabetes. *New England Journal of Medicine* **294:** 1004–1005.

Chen YDI, Jeng C-Y & Reaven GM (1987) HDL metabolism in diabetes. *Diabetes/Metabolism Reviews* **3:** 653–688.

Clark RS, English M, McNeill GP & Newton RW (1985) Effects of intravenous infusion of insulin in diabetes with acute myocardial infarction. *British Medical Journal* **291:** 303–305.

DeFronzo RA, Ferrannini E & Koivisto V (1983) New concepts in the pathogenesis and treatment of non-insulin-dependent diabetes mellitus. *American Journal of Medicine* **74:** 52–81.

DeFronzo RA, Gunnarson R, Björkman O, Olsson M & Wahren J (1985) Effects of insulin on peripheral and splanchnic glucose metabolism in non-insulin-dependent (type II) diabetes mellitus. *Journal of Clinical Investigation* **76:** 149–155.

Faber OK & Damsgaard EM (1984) Insulin secretion in type II diabetes. *Acta Endocrinologica* **105 (supplement 262)**: 47–50.

Ferrannini E, Buzzigoli G, Bonadonna R et al (1987) Insulin resistance in essential hypertension. *New England Journal of Medicine* **317**: 350–357.

Firth RC, Bell PM & Rizza RA (1986a) Effects of tolazamide and exogenous insulin on insulin action in patients with non-insulin-dependent diabetes mellitus. *New England Journal of Medicine* **314**: 1280–1286.

Firth RG, Bell PM, Marsh HM, Hansen I & Rizza RA (1986b) Postprandial hyperglycaemia in patients with non-insulin-dependent diabetes mellitus. Role of hepatic and extrahepatic tissues. *Journal of Clinical Investigation* **77**: 1525–1532.

Gale EAM, Dornan TL & Tattersall RB (1981) Severely uncontrolled diabetes in the over fifties. *Diabetologia* **21**: 15–28.

Garvey WT, Olefsky JM, Griffin J, Hamman RF & Kolterman OG (1985) The effect of insulin treatment on insulin secretion and insulin action in type 2 diabetes mellitus. *Diabetes* **34**: 222–234.

Gerich JE (1985) Sulfonylureas in the treatment of diabetes mellitus—1985. *Mayo Clinics Proceedings* **60**: 439–443.

Ginsberg HN (1987) Very low density lipoprotein metabolism in diabetes mellitus. *Diabetes/Metabolism Reviews* **3**: 571–589.

Glauber HS, Henry RR, Wallace P et al (1987) The effect of biosynthetic human proinsulin on carbohydrate metabolism in non-insulin-dependent diabetes mellitus. *New England Journal of Medicine* **316**: 443–449.

Gormley MJJ, Hadden DR, Woods R, Sheridan B & Andrews WJ (1986) One month's insulin treatment of type II diabetes: the early- and medium-term effects following insulin withdrawal. *Metabolism* **35**: 1029–1036.

Grant PJ, Barlow E & Miles DW (1984) Plasma C-peptide levels identify insulin treated diabetic patients suitable for oral hypoglycaemic therapy. *Diabetic Medicine* **1**: 284–286.

Groop L, Harno K & Tolppanen EM (1984) The combination of insulin and sulphonylurea in the treatment of secondary drug failure in patients with type II diabetes. *Acta Endocrinologica* **106**: 97–101.

Groop LC, Botazzo GF & Doniach D (1986) Islet cell antibodies identify latent type 1 diabetes in patients aged 35–75 years at diagnosis. *Diabetes* **35**: 237–241.

Gutniak M, Karlander S-G & Efendic S (1987) Glyburide decreases insulin requirement, increases β cell response to mixed meal, and does not affect insulin sensitivity: effects of short- and long-term combined treatment in secondary failure to sulfonylurea. *Diabetes Care* **10**: 545–554.

Heine RJ (1988) The insulin dilemma: which one to use? In Krall L and Alberti KGMM (eds) World Book of Diabetes **3**. Amsterdam: Elsevier. In press.

Heine RJ, Oolbekkink M & van der Veen EA (1987) Absorption kinetics of human proinsulin and human NPH insulin from the deltoid, abdominal and femoral region. *Diabetologia* **30**: 529 (abstract).

Hollenbeck CB & Reaven GM (1987) Treatment of patients with non-insulin-dependent diabetes mellitus: diabetic control and insulin secretion and action after different treatment modalities. *Diabetic Medicine* **4**: 311–316.

Holman RR, Steemson J & Turner RC (1987) Sulphonylurea failure in type 2 diabetes: treatment with a basal insulin supplement *Diabetic Medicine* **4**: 457–462.

Kilo C, Miller JP & Williamson JR (1980) The crux of the UGDP: spurious results and biologically inappropriate data analysis. *Diabetologia* **18**: 179–185.

Korhonen T, Uusitupa M, Aro A et al (1987) Efficacy of dietary instructions in newly diagnosed non-insulin-dependent diabetic patients. *Acta Medica Scandinavica* **222**: 323–331.

Laakso M, Voutilainen E, Pyörälä K & Sarlund H (1985) Association of low HDL and HDL2 cholesterol with coronary heart disease in non-insulin-dependent diabetics. *Arteriosclerosis* **5**: 653–658.

Lebovitz ME & Feingloss MN (1978) Sulphonylurea drugs: mechanisms of antidiabetic action and therapeutic usefulness. *Diabetes Care* **1**: 189–198.

Lipson LG (1986) Diabetes in the elderly: diagnosis, pathogenesis and therapy. *American Journal of Medicine* **80**: 10–21.

Mandarino LJ & Gerich JE (1984) Prolonged sulfonylurea administration decreases insulin resistance and increases insulin secretion in non-insulin-dependent diabetes mellitus:

evidence for improved insulin action at a postreceptor site in hepatic as well as extrahepatic tissues. *Diabetes Care* **7 (supplement 1):** 89–99.

Modan M, Halkin H, Almog S et al (1985) Hyperinsulinaemia—a link between hypertension, obesity and glucose intolerance. *Journal of Clinical Investigation* **75:** 809–817.

Modan M, Halkin H, Karasik A & Lusky A (1987) Elevated serum uric acid—a facet of hyperinsulinaemia. *Diabetologia* **30:** 713–718.

Morley JE, Mooradian AD, Rosenthal MJ & Kaiser FE (1987) Diabetes mellitus in elderly patients. Is it different? *American Journal of Medicine* **83:** 533–544.

Neil HAW, Gatling W, Mather HM et al (1987) The Oxford community diabetes study: Evidence for an increase in the prevalence of known diabetes in Great Britain. *Diabetic Medicine* **4:** 539–543.

Olefsky JM & Kolterman OG (1981) Mechanisms of insulin resistance in obesity and non-insulin-dependent (type II) diabetes. *American Journal of Medicine* **70:** 151–167.

Panzram G (1987) Mortality and survival in type II (non-insulin-dependent) diabetes mellitus. *Diabetologia* **30:** 123–131.

Panzram G and Zabel-Langhennig R (1981) Prognosis of diabetes mellitus in a geographically defined population. *Diabetologia* **20:** 587–591.

Peacock I & Tattersall RB (1984) The difficult choice of treatment for poorly controlled maturity onset diabetes: tablets or insulin? *British Medical Journal* **288:** 1956–1959.

Pyörälä K, Laakso M & Uusitupa M (1987) Diabetes and atherosclerosis: an epidemiologic view. *Diabetes/Metabolism Reviews* **3:** 463–525.

Razenberg PPA, Venekamp WJRR, Sikkenk AC, Heine RJ & van der Veen EA (1985) Effects of insulin treatment in type II diabetes on insulin sensitivity and insulin responsiveness. *Diabetes Research and Clinical Practice* **(supplement 1):** 465 (abstract).

Reaven GR & Greenfield MS (1981) Diabetic hypertriglyceridemia. Evidence for three clinical syndromes. *Diabetes* **30 (supplement 2):** 66–75.

Reeves WG (1986) The immune response to insulin characterisation and clinical consequences. In Alberti KGMM & Krall LP (eds) *The Diabetes Annual/2*, pp 81–93. Amsterdam: Elsevier.

Rendell M (1983) C peptide levels as a criterion in treatment of maturity onset diabetes. *Journal of Clinical Endocrinology and Metabolism* **57:** 1198–1206.

Revers RR, Henry R, Schmeiser L et al (1984) The effects of biosynthetic human proinsulin on carbohydrate metabolism. *Diabetes* **33:** 762–770.

Riddle MC (1985) New tactics for type 2 diabetes: regimens based on intermediate-acting insulin taken at bedtime. *Lancet* **i:** 193–195.

Rosetti L, Schulman GI, Zawalich W & DeFronzo (1987) Effect of chronic hyperglycaemia on in vivo insulin secretion in partially pancreatectomized rats. *Journal of Clinical Investigation* **80:** 1037–1044.

Scarlett JA, Gray RS, Griffin J, Olefsky JM & Kolterman OG (1982) Insulin treatment reverses the insulin resistance of type 2 diabetes mellitus. *Diabetes Care* **5:** 353–363.

Schöffling K (1980) Orale diabetes therapie. *Endokrinologie* **1:** 3–18.

Segal KR, Dunaif A, Gutin B et al (1987) Body composition, not body weight, is related to cardiovascular disease risk factors and sex hormone levels in men. *Journal of Clinical Investigation* **80:** 1050–1055.

Seigler DE, Olsson M & Skyler JS (1987) Morning versus bedtime NPH insulin in type 2 (non-insulin-dependent) diabetes mellitus. *Diabetologia* **30:** 581 (abstract).

Selz B, Nyffenbegger U & Burgi H (1980) Wann sollen stabile altersdiabetiker auf insulin umgestellt werden? *Schweizerische Medizinische Wochenschrift* **110:** 1534–1537.

Simonson DC, Delprato S, Castellino P, Groop L & DeFronzo RA (1987) Effect of glyburide on glycemic control, insulin requirement, and glucose metabolism in insulin treated diabetic patients. *Diabetes* **36:** 136–146.

Stout RW (1979) Diabetes and atherosclerosis: the role of insulin. *Diabetologia* **16:** 141–150.

Stout RW (1985) Overview of the association between insulin and atherosclerosis. *Metabolism* **34:** 7–12.

Taskinen MR (1987) Lipoprotein lipase in diabetes. *Diabetes/Metabolism Reviews* **3:** 551–570.

Tattersall RB (1984) Diabetes in the elderly—a neglected area? *Diabetologia* **27:** 167–173.

Tattersall RB & Scott AR (1987) When to use insulin in the maturity onset diabetic. *Postgraduate Medical Journal* **63:** 859–864.

Taylor KG, Galton DJ & Holdsworth G (1979) Insulin-independent diabetes: a defect in the activity of lipoprotein lipase in adipose tissue. *Diabetologia* **16:** 313–317.

Tchobroutsky G (1978) Relation of diabetic control to development of microvascular complications. *Diabetologia* **15:** 143–152.

Turner RC & Holman RR (1978) Beta cell function during insulin or chlorpropamide treatment of maturity-onset diabetes mellitus. *Diabetes* **27 (supplement 1):** 241–246.

UK Prospective Study of Therapies of Maturity Onset Diabetes (1983) The effect of diet, sulphonylurea, insulin or biguanide therapy on fasting plasma glucose and body weight over 1 year. *Diabetologia* **24:** 404–411.

Unger RH (1982) Meticulous control of diabetes: benefits, risks and precautions. *Diabetes* **31:** 479–483.

Unger RH & Grundy S (1985) Hyperglycaemia as an inducer as well as a consequence of impaired islet cell function and insulin resistance: implications for the management of diabetes. *Diabetologia* **28:** 119–121.

University Group Diabetes Program (1976) A study of the effects of hypoglycaemic agents on vascular complications in patients with adult-onset diabetes. *Diabetes* **25:** 1129–1153.

Uusitupa M, Siitonen O, Voutilainen E et al (1986) Serum lipids and lipoproteins in newly diagnosed non-insulin-dependent (type II) diabetic patients, with special reference to factors influencing HDL-cholesterol and triglyceride levels. *Diabetes Care* **9:** 17–22.

Ward WK, Beard JC, Halter JB, Pfeifer MA & Porte D (1984) Pathophysiology of insulin secretion in non-insulin-dependent diabetes mellitus. *Diabetes Care* **7:** 491–502.

Wardzala LJ, Hirshman M, Pofcher E et al (1985) Regulation of glucose utilisation in adipose cells and muscle after long-term experimental hyperinsulinaemia in rats. *Journal of Clinical Investigation* **76:** 460–469.

Watanabe N, Kobayashi M, Maegawa H et al (1986) Long-term in vitro effects of insulin on insulin binding and glucose transport. *Diabetes Research and Clinical Practice* **2:** 1–8.

Wilson RM, Van der Minne P, Deverill I et al (1985) Insulin dependence: problems with the classification of 100 consecutive patients. *Diabetic Medicine* **2:** 167–172.

Wing RR, Koeske R, Epstein LH et al (1987a) Long-term effects of modest weight loss in type II diabetic patients. *Archives of Internal Medicine* **147:** 1749–1753.

Wing RR, Marcus MD, Epstein LH & Salate R (1987b) Type II diabetic subjects lose less weight than their overweight non-diabetic spouses. *Diabetes Care* **10:** 563–566.

13

Treatment—education

STEWART M. DUNN

'Education is a form of treatment for diabetes!'

The analogy to medication is quoted frequently in the literature and there are certainly significant parallels at one end of the scale. Medicine has never cured a case of diabetes—neither has education. Medicine has failed to develop an effective means of controlling the disease and preventing the development of complications—so too has education. It is well to remind ourselves of these limitations, at a time when diabetes education assumes the proportion of a growth industry and claims for its effectiveness approach the limits of credibility. Yet the potential contribution of education to promote healthy behaviour change in non-insulin-dependent diabetes (NIDDM) may well lie beyond those limits.

Education in diabetes pervades all levels of the health care system—from international planning and co-operation in the development of public health care and screening services, through professional education of medical and ancillary staff, to the individual patient confronted with the daily tasks of living with diabetes. This chapter reviews the specific case of patient education in the context of two basic questions. What is education and what is education supposed to achieve?

In an address to the Second European Symposium of the Diabetes Education Study Group, Grabauskas (1983), representing the World Health Organization, defined diabetes within the broad context of health education:

'Like general education, the goal of health education is a change in the knowledge, feelings and behaviour of people. . . . In order to be effective, the planning, methods and procedures must take into account the process by which people acquire knowledge and change their feelings and behaviour, as well as the factors that influence such changes.'

The questions addressed by diabetes education research in 1988 are increasingly more sophisticated and analytical. What sorts of educational intervention are effective with which sub-groups of patients? What aspects of an intervention affect which features of patient knowledge, attitudes, and behaviour? What is the relationship between these features and metabolic control? These questions reflect this broader definition of diabetes education.

Initial recognition for the integral role of education in comprehensive diabetes care came from the pioneering work of Joslin and Etzwiler in the USA and Assal in Europe. Recognition of the need for specificity in educational diagnosis was highlighted by Davis et al (1981) and has been formulated by the National Standards for Diabetes Education Programs (1984) in the form of a documented needs assessment for each patient.

The diabetes education literature is increasingly scientific, diverse and demanding, reflecting the variety of professional expertise required for comprehensive patient care and education. It is mandatory to have a basic understanding of the natural history of psychological reactions to diabetes and the impact of psychosocial events on metabolic control, since these form the substrate upon which any intervention must operate. The diabetes education team must be familiar with the principles of teaching and learning. Programme evaluation must be based on familiarity with the clinical course of diabetes and a realistic appreciation of the potential effects of programme-induced changes on behavioural and metabolic indices—many of which occur long after patient and practitioner have parted company.

In the last ten years we have accumulated a solid foundation of experimental data on the potential and limitations of diabetes education. Table 1 presents a representative selection from this database in respect of three major educational outcomes which are presumed to mediate improved diabetic control—knowledge, compliance and psychological adjustment. Essentially, we want to ask three questions of this database:

1. Can we measure these factors objectively and reliably?
2. Can we intervene so as to improve patient performance on these factors?
3. Will such improvement be associated with improved metabolic control?

KNOWLEDGE IS NOT POWER

Anderson (1986) has argued that the current practice of diabetes patient education is simply an extension of the information transfer approach found in most schools. According to this approach, lack of knowledge and skills accounts for the major portion of poor self-care behaviour. Anderson suggests that the emphasis on information transfer is probably partially attributable to the fact that it is easier to measure and evaluate. Research into the precise details of diabetes knowledge and its scientific measurement have seen possibly more rapid progress than any other area of diabetes education. It is certainly true that this reflects the relative ease of measuring *simple* knowledge among a plethora of psychosocial factors also implicated in metabolic control.

A variety of well-researched instruments—many developed from the pioneering work of Etzwiler (1962) and others—are available for the scientific assessment of diabetes knowledge (Windsor et al, 1981; Hess and Davis, 1983; Dunn et al, 1984b; Wise et al, 1986). Garrard et al (1987) recently added another from Etzwiler's group, reporting impressive evidence for content, concurrent, and discriminant validity of a 50–item Test of Patient

Table 1. Experimental and descriptive data on three potential outcomes of diabetes education.

	Knowledge	Compliance	Psychological adjustment
Can we measure it?	Yes	Yes	Yes
	Bloomgarden (1987)	Glasgow (1986)	Bradley (1984)
	Dunn (1984b)	Johnson (1986)	Delamater (1987)
	Falkenberg (1986)	Kaplan (1987)	Davis (1987)
	Garrard (1987)	Lockington (1987)	Dunn (1986b)
	Hess (1983)	Mazze (1984, 1985)	Harris (1985)
	Korhonen (1983)	Mazzuca (1986)	Peyrot (1985)
	Mazzuca (1986)	Schafer (1983)	Schafer (1983)
	Rettig (1986)	White (1986)	Tattersall (1985)
	Terrent (1985)	Wilson (1986)	
	Wise (1986)	Wing (1985)	
Can we improve it?	Yes	Yes	Yes
	Bloomgarden (1987)	Kaplan (1987)	Dunn (1986)
	Dunn (1984b)	Mazze (1985)	Tattersall (1985)
	Falkenberg (1986)	Mazzuca (1986)	
	Garrard (1987)		
	Rettig (1986)		
	Wise (1986)		
	No		
	Korhonen (1983)		
	Mazzuca (1986)		
Will it improve control?	Yes	Yes	Yes
	Mazzuca (1986)	Glasgow (1986)	Bradley (1984)
		Kaplan (1987)	Delamater (1987)
		Lockington (1987)	Dunn (1986)
		Mazzuca (1986)	Harris (1985)
	No	Schafer (1983)	Peyrot (1985)
	Bloomgarden (1987)	White (1986)	Tattersall (1985)
	Dunn (1984b)	Wilson (1986)	Wise (1986)
	Falkenberg (1986)		
	Korhonen (1983)	No	
	Rettig (1986)	Mazze (1984, 1985)	

Knowledge, as well as internal consistency, readability and sensitivity to instructional gains. There can be little excuse now for studies to use poorly-standardized knowledge tests.

The traditional thesis of diabetes education is that improvements in knowledge, attitudes and skills lead to improved compliance with treatment advice—and subsequently to better metabolic control. To date no evidence has been forthcoming to support the association between knowledge gain and metabolic improvement (Wise et al, 1986; Meadows et al, 1987) although many of the conflicting results stemmed directly from the poor standardization and reliability of the instruments used to assess knowledge in the early studies.

Bloomgarden et al (1987) reported a randomized study of 749 insulin-treated patients assigned to education and control groups. The nine education sessions were offered over a period of 1.6 years and 82 of the 145 patients in the education group attended the required number of sessions to graduate. Knowledge scores increased by slightly more than 6% in the education group (10% in graduates) but there was no change in the control group. Programme graduates also recorded a significant increase in scores on a behaviour assessment. Glycosylated haemoglobin (HbA_{1c}) fell in both groups but the difference was not significant. Various other outcome measures, which did not discriminate between the groups, included fasting blood glucose, body mass index, lipids, use of medical care, and associated illnesses. The authors argued that patient education is functionally meaningless unless predicated on the assumption that improvements in knowledge will lead to improved metabolic control.

The intervention provided patients with an overview of various aspects of diabetes, with particular emphasis on nutritional teaching. The authors deliberately did not design their programme as a therapeutic intervention aimed at improving metabolic control *per se*. They concluded that 'education is a weak intervention as a mode of treatment for diabetes', extending the medication analogy first proposed by Pichert (1983). Not surprisingly, the article led to vigorous debate principally on the grounds of: (a) inappropriate generalization from a highly specific and unrepresentative intervention which was isolated from other aspects of diabetes care; (b) defining patient education as a goal rather than as a tool; and (c) the unwarranted proposition that education alone will cause changes in metabolic status.

Additionally, the implicit assumption that education might be applied as the treatment of choice in all cases is clearly inappropriate. Some patients need education; some do not. The substantial issue for research is to determine the 'treatment specificity' of diabetes education.

As Table 1 indicates, a number of well-designed, randomized studies of diabetes education (Korhonen et al, 1983; Terrent et al, 1985; Mazzuca et al, 1986; Rettig et al, 1986) provide consistent evidence of significant improvements in diabetes knowledge without significant improvement in glycaemic control. This is an important limitation of diabetes education *per se*—in isolation from other aspects of integrated diabetes management. However, unsatisfactory diabetic control resulting from information lack may be a specific problem for some patients which is effectively and efficiently remedied by education programmes.

Innovative intervention represents one solution to the problems of treatment specificity in patients who lack specific information or skills. Falkenberg et al (1986) compared conventional classroom teaching with a 'problem oriented participatory education' programme, a method based on learner activity in group meetings. Their treatment group of 55–73 year-old NIDDM patients showed significant improvement in knowledge, but only transient improvement in HbA_{1c} and the authors concluded that group meetings would need to be continued beyond three months if metabolic improvement was to be maintained.

Wise et al (1986) randomized 174 IDDM and NIDDM patients to control groups, or to one of two interactive computer-based education systems: a teaching programme with text and animated graphics, and a multiple-choice programme with optional presciptive feedback. Patients in both pro-grammes showed similar significant knowledge gains at the 4–6 months follow-up, together with mean falls in HbA_{1c} of approximately 1%. There were no changes in the respective control groups. In the absence of any correlation between HbA_{1c} and knowledge status the authors suggested that enhanced motivation by the use of a novel teaching technique may be a more realistic explanation of the demonstrated improvement in diabetic control.

COMPLIANCE, ADHERENCE AND OTHER EUPHEMISMS

Compliance is frequently considered to be a pejorative term, yet a reason-able definition is 'the extent to which a person's behaviour coincides with medical advice'. As such, it involves a two-way process of communication between physician and patient, with rights and responsibilities on each side. In other contexts, the compliant patient—one who carried out any instruc-tion from someone in authority, no matter how onerous or unpleasant—is labelled dependent, or an 'authoritarian personality'. It is a fact that non-compliance is normal, healthy and perhaps even adaptive in some circum-stances (Dunn, 1986).

Recent studies of compliance have had two important implications for diabetes education. First is the important progress represented by the empirical approach to the measurement of compliant behaviour, which has been chronically relegated to the 'too hard' basket for many years. Second, the complexity which these studies identify in such behaviour emphasizes the naivety of many of our objectives in diabetes education, particularly the assumption that education automatically presumes knowledge which automatically presumes compliance.

The perceptions of health professionals are likely to be a significant determinant of the attitudes of patients. A survey of 30 NIDDM patients and 30 residents in internal medicine assessed their perceptions of the difficulties of complying with three aspects of diabetes treatment: medi-cation, diet, and urine testing (Pendleton et al, 1987). Resident staff rated each compliance component as significantly more difficult than did the patients. Whether these results represented over-estimation by the residents or under-estimation by the patients remains to be seen.

Lockington et al (1987) examined compliance, assessed by patients' carriage of sugar and diabetes identification, in 130 IDDM outpatients. The 58% of the sample who carried both sugar and ID had a mean HbA_{1c} of 8.4% compared with 10.3%–10.7% in those who carried only one or neither item. These patients also scored higher on a measure of 'general attitude to diabetes', and there were specific correlations, but no overall relationship, with HbA_{1c}. The authors concluded that absence of sugar or ID may represent a useful indicator of poor diabetic control and may assist in the definition of relevant attitudinal differences.

Johnson et al (1986) constructed 13 different measures of adherence behaviours based on three independent interviews with 168 young IDDM patients and their parents. Agreement between patient and parent was good on most behaviours with highest agreement in the 10–15 years age group. Overall teenagers were found to be less adherent than younger patients. The authors concluded from factor analysis of their data that adherence in childhood diabetes is a complex construct consisting of at least five different unrelated components.

Another area for behavioural intervention which continues to attract research interest is self-monitoring of blood glucose. Mazze et al (1984, 1985), in their research with glucose monitoring equipment containing a memory chip, have demonstrated the unreliability of patient-generated data using self-monitoring of blood glucose and shown that this performance may be improved by appropriately-designed intervention.

Wilson, Glasgow and their co-workers, have published several articles on aspects of compliance in diabetes (Glasgow et al, 1986; Wilson et al, 1986). They assessed four different self-care behaviours in 184 NIDDM patients: medication taking, glucose testing, diet, and exercise. Multiple measurements were collected of psychosocial variables including knowledge, stress, depression, anxiety, diabetes-specific health beliefs, and social support; metabolic control was measured by HbA_{1c}. They concluded that approximately 25% of the variance in self-care behaviours can be explained by psychosocial and demographic variables, but psychosocial variables were not significant predictors of diabetic control. The diabetes-specific measures were the most consistent and strongest predictors of self-care behaviour across all areas studied.

Davis et al (1987), in continued research with the Diabetes Educational Profile, report further evidence for the importance of discriminating among patients with different disease types and treatment modes. Other authors concur with the need for different norms for psychological adjustment, educational response, and diabetic control (Jenny, 1986).

Earlier evaluation studies were criticized for failing adequately to represent the poorly-motivated, lower socio-economic status patient (Dunn, 1986; Kaplan and Davis, 1986). In part, the studies published since 1985 have redressed this imbalance and several authors described randomized studies of creative programmes aimed at the poorly-educated, or illiterate patient. The Bloomgarden et al (1987) study reported the failure of a knowledge-based teaching programme to promote improved metabolic control, but several other authors have reported success in patients with low literacy using a variety of more flexible formats (Falkenberg et al, 1986; White et al, 1986; Mulrow et al, 1987; Vinicor et al, 1987; Wilson and Pratt, 1987).

Mazzuca et al (1986) studied 532 patients, predominantly elderly, black women with NIDDM of long duration, using random assignment to experimental and control groups. The experimental intervention included didactic instruction, skill exercises and behavioural modification techniques, and 275 patients (52%) were followed for up to four years. Differences in knowledge between experimental and control subjects 11–14 months after instruction were minimal, but self-care skills and compliance were significantly higher in the experimental group. Experimental group patients also experienced greater reductions in fasting blood glucose and HbA_{1c}, and in body weight, blood pressure and serum creatinine. In a more recent report, Vinicor et al (1987) described the random assignment of this group of patients, and their internal medicine residents, to one of four conditions: routine care, patient education, physician education, or both patient plus physician education. The combination of patient and physician education resulted in the greatest improvements in fasting and postprandial plasma glucose, HbA_{1c}, body weight, and diastolic blood pressure. However, obesity and hyperglycaemia still persisted in a large number of patients.

White et al (1986) compared the effects of conventional advice-education with a group management programme in 41 obese, NIDDM patients. Thirty-two completed the six month study. The patients were seen regularly for one hour sessions, and instructed in a number of self-management activities specifically aimed at improving metabolic control. Both groups showed a mean reduction in HbA_{1c}, but the group management programme recorded lower blood glucose than the advice/education programme. There were no differences between interventions in HbA_{1c} or obesity.

Kaplan et al (1987) randomized 76 adult NIDDM patients to one of four programmes: diet, exercise, diet plus exercise, or education (control). Each programme met weekly for ten weeks and 92% completed the follow-up study. The biggest reduction in HbA_{1c} was shown by the diet plus exercise group, who also showed significant improvements on a general quality of life measure. The authors concluded that the combination diet plus exercise programme benefits NIDDM patients and that the benefits may be independent of substantial weight loss.

In spite of the sophisticated nature of research into the efficacy of different approaches to motivating, inspiring, and cajoling NIDDM patients into recommended lifestyle changes, it remains a matter for concern that little of this information filters through to the bulk of health professionals. Hauenstein et al (1987) surveyed 500 dietitians, through the ADA Diabetes Care and Education Practice Group, to determine their use of motivational, counselling and teaching techniques aimed at behaviour change in NIDDM patients. They concluded that dietitians rarely use many techniques considered effective in obtaining dietary adherence.

PSYCHOLOGICAL ADJUSTMENT—IS FEELING BETTER DOING BETTER?

If the aim of diabetes education is to intervene to change patient's beliefs, attitudes or skills, it is of paramount importance that we have a thorough understanding of the psychology of diabetes. It is obviously not good enough to persist with any untested intervention on the basis that instinct says it ought to work. Several authors have begun to focus on the specific educational needs of the elderly diabetic patient (Waclawski et al, 1985; Knight and Kesson, 1986) and, as discussed above, many such interventions appear to offer more promising results than traditional classroom teaching approaches. Studies in neuropsychology and physiological psychology also expand our knowledge of the important link between physiology and behaviour in ways which are directly relevant to the design of educational intervention (Robertson-Tchabo et al, 1986).

The ability of individuals to adapt to the many stresses imposed by diabetes is determined, among other factors, by the coping strategies available to them. The majority of the research into this area has concentrated on coping strategies in the young IDDM patient. Perhaps the paucity of coping research in NIDDM reflects the ingrained belief that intervention based on such research results must be ineffective—on the grounds that 'you can't teach an old dog new tricks'.

Marteau and Johnson (1986) have shown that a family history of diabetes is an important determinant of psychological reactions in childhood diabetes. Parents of diabetic children rated the disease as significantly less serious if they had a diabetic relative in good health, compared with those having a relative in poor health or no family history. There is every reason to suppose that NIDDM patients and their families are subject to similar concerns.

The literature on coping strategies and psychological adjustment is complex and also concentrated on the young person with diabetes. Jacobson et al (1986), in a series of studies affirm that IDDM does not necessarily lead to psychological disruption and that early adjustment is embedded in a context of overall personality development. On the other hand, there is some evidence of profound effects on some children from IDDM diagnosed very early in life (Rovet et al, 1987a; 1987b). Delamater et al (1987) found that adolescents with IDDM in poor control were more inclined to use wishful thinking and avoidance/help-seeking coping strategies than were patients in good control.

Kovacs et al (1986) reported quite different findings. They suggested that coping and adjustment may well be independent of one another, at least in the beginning of IDDM, and that only with prolonged illness does such a relationship become evident. They also suggested that inability to cope and general maladjustment become evident only when a patient's psychologic status is relatively deviant. However, Kovac's research has used markers derived from the general psychiatric literature. There is now convincing evidence that measures of beliefs and emotional adjustment, developed specifically for diabetic populations, are more sensitive to relevant aspects of coping behaviour, adjustment and compliance (Dunn and Turtle, 1981; Dunn et al, 1986b; Delamater et al, 1987).

Consistent with other researchers, Kovacs et al (1986) observed that high use of positive behavioural coping strategies was somewhat related to pre-existing social adaptation, particularly the level of socially pertinent activities. In addition, they observed that behavioural strategy use shortly after diagnosis correlated highly with the same coping approach the following year, and suggested that some coping strategies may be trait-related rather than state-related.

The observation of long-term stability in several aspects of emotional adjustment in diabetes was reported by Dunn et al (1985; 1986) in a sample of older patients. Diabetes adjustment was assessed on the ATT39 Scale (Dunn et al, 1986b). Multivariate analyses of variance and covariance were used to assess the effects of treatment, and duration of diabetes, on adjustment as a function of age at diagnosis. Diabetes-related guilt was a major problem during the early years of diabetes for all patients and it reappeared many years later with the onset of diabetic complications. In the early-onset patient, the intervening years were characterized by stable adjustment. In older-onset patients, early adjustment was essentially normal, though largely dependent, and was replaced later by low frustration tolerance and guilt feelings. In patients diagnosed during mid-life, the adjustment profile remained unchanged with a pattern of constant stress and guilt, and feelings of personal inadequacy associated with diabetes. These results provide cross-sectional evidence that adjustment in diabetes involves unresolved and recurrent conflicts which are part of a normal ongoing reaction to an abnormal situation.

Such studies have important implications for the design of effective educational interventions which must be premised on a scientifically-based knowledge of the behavioural and metabolic outcomes associated with particular coping strategies. Having identified attitudes and adjustment strategies which are associated with improved compliance and/or control, it seems logical and feasible that we should be able to target educational interventions to encourage more 'metabolically effective' attitudes and strategies.

A pilot study with 273 insulin-treated patients (Dunn et al, 1986a) categorized emotional adjustment and examined its relationship to HbA_{1c} initially and at three months follow-up. Psychological adjustment was assessed on the ATT39 Scale and score profiles were determined by cluster analysis. ANOVA for between-cluster differences were highly significant on all six scales. Profiles dominated by profound disease conviction, or by denial strategies (stress and low frustration tolerance), were associated with poor initial metabolic control. In 'guilt-dominated' profiles control deteriorated over the three months, but it improved in patients who rated their own adjustment poorly, and in those who co-operated with medical providers whilst rejecting the chronic nature of their diabetes. Thus, discrete categories of psychological adjustment identified in this sample of IDDM patients had significant correlation with metabolic control.

In view of the enthusiasm for research on coping strategies and adjustment in childhood diabetes and IDDM, it is somewhat surprising that the major developments in specific educational interventions have been reserved for the NIDDM patient. In a review of the literature from 1986–1987 where some 20 publications reported specific intervention studies, only one involved childhood diabetes (Ryan, 1987). Significant studies were published in 1985 (Kaplan et al, 1985; Lucey and Wing, 1985); but, despite their reported success, no further studies have appeared and the bulk of the available data on interventions is derived from the evaluation of diabetes education programmes with predominantly NIDDM patients. We thus have the slightly absurd situation where the majority of psychosocial research has been conducted with the young IDDM patient, yet the majority of intervention research has concentrated on NIDDM where the psychosocial database for such intervention is less secure.

PUTTING THE PIECES TOGETHER

The experimental data presented in this chapter and categorized in Table 1 give the spurious impression that factors like knowledge, compliance and psychological adjustment act independently of each other and of diabetic control. The interactive nature of these responses to diabetes education requires multivariate analysis and longitudinal data collection, and these studies are now beginning to appear in the literature.

A preliminary report on a three year project involving comprehensive evaluation of 5 diabetes education programmes, compared with non-randomized outpatient controls has been presented (Dunn et al, 1986a). Knowledge of diabetes was assessed on the three parallel forms of the DKN Scales (Dunn et al, 1984b). Psychological adjustment was assessed on the ATT39 Scale (Dunn et al, 1986b). Metabolic control was measured by glycosylated haemoglobin. All measures were administered before and after the programmes and repeated at three month intervals for up to one year. Knowledge improvement was about 23% in all programmes and these improvements were maintained at follow-up in all programmes. DKN scores at three months were predicted (using stepwise multivariate regression) by higher initial DKN scores at entry to the programmes. Intelligence was also a predictor of knowledge at follow-up in shorter programmes, whereas personality factors were more important in the more extended interventions. Normalization of extreme scores for psychological adjustment was measured by regressing post-programme ATT39 scores on to pre-programme scores. Psychological adjustment was improved in all programmes, but this improvement was greatest in the extended programme. The small overall improvement in glycosylated haemoglobin was not statistically significant, and there were no between-programme differences. However, the three month patient turnover in the shortest programmes was almost twice that of the longest intervention. Thus future programme design must rationalize the demonstrated benefits of extended educational formats, with the size and needs of the local population, to provide the most cost-effective use of available resources.

The picture that now emerges from this research vindicates the belief that the primary task of any intervention is a clear statement of its goals and objectives. A well designed intervention which aims to teach factual knowledge to diabetic patients should achieve that objective. However, defining the objective as improved compliance or control, as a result of such knowledge improvement, is based on a premise which is probably false and, at best, unproven. Whether knowledge improvement is 'functionally meaningless', or constitutes a justifiable end-point for *some* diabetes education activities, is a matter for individual judgement. Equally clearly, it is possible to induce behaviour change in patients who have low literary skills by designing an intervention whose objective is direct behaviour change. However, even though this approach is generally effective, at this stage there seems little predictability in the pattern of changes among diabetic and metabolic parameters.

COMMUNICATION AND CO-ORDINATION

'In the case of patient/health-team-member communication, the effectiveness of the educational process will depend on the closeness between the teacher and the patient, and how successfully the teacher evaluates the motivation of the patient's behaviour and can adapt to its changes. Patient instruction alone does not guarantee improved control of the disease. Patients must be willing to use that increased knowledge in a cooperative programme of health care. Sustained behavioural changes require continuing communication and support.' Grabauskas (1983)

'Our concern is with the supposition that . . . understanding, motivation, and skills must be developed in an education program, rather than as integral parts of the interaction between health care providers and the patient, which is basic to the art and practice of medicine.' (Bloomgarden et al, 1987)

There are patent dangers in assigning a special role for patient education to one person or to one intervention. Too often this allows other professionals, who are *de facto* involved in the continuing education of the patient, to absolve themselves of this responsibility. Education is the one ongoing activity which involves every professional working with the diabetic patient and, thus, provides a unique opportunity for integration of individual management in the overall delivery of diabetes care (Beaven and Scott, 1987).

The powerful role of the physician as a patient educator is frequently underestimated and overlooked. Yet we have little insight into the processes by which some physicians are able to alter the adjustment and behaviour of some of their patients but not of others. In a study recently completed, we obtained measures of physician-patient rapport by comparing scores from 194 patients (mean age 63 years) on standardized measures of psychological adjustment (ATT39) and diabetes knowledge (DKN) with physician estimates of each patient's scores. Eighty-eight physician-patient pairs completed the same measures at a second visit. Patients' DKN scores and physician estimates of knowledge correlated 0.56 and mean scores did not differ significantly. Patients' ATT39 scores and physician estimates of adjustment correlated 0.23 (range −0.77 to +0.94). ANOVA revealed no significant differences among patients' scores across doctors but there were significant differences amongst physicians' estimates of ATT39 scores. Seventy-four percent of physicians consistently under-estimated patients' adjustment. There were no sex differences in patients' scores but both male and female physicians assessed female patients as more poorly adjusted than male patients. Highest rapport existed between physician and patient at the second visit, with patients' scores moving toward the physicians' initial estimate of their adjustment. Highest mean correlations at the second visit were found between same-sexed patient–physician pairs, reaching 0.78 for female–female pairs. The results suggest that attitude change in diabetic patients is influenced subtly by physicians' beliefs about their psychological adjustment.

SUMMARY

The educational model which proposed knowledge improvement as a necessary condition for behaviour change (or increased compliance!) is wrong. It ignores the reality that patients fail to comply for many reasons, the least of which is insufficient information. This is not to say that group programmes, or certain types of individual intervention, are not effective in producing change in variables other than factual knowledge, particularly psychosocial factors. There is increasing evidence that formal education programmes are associated with changes in attitude, which may be more a result of the interaction between participants than a response to educational content, and that it is these attitudinal changes which are the precursors to behavioural change.

The initial enthusiasm of the medical community for diabetes education as the solution to the major problem of non-compliance has now been replaced by a healthy skepticism. Diabetes education, by itself, has little to offer the patient whose metabolic control is inadequate. The effectiveness of formal education programmes in patients with compromised metabolic control is limted to the few cases where specific information, or a general understanding of diabetes in a newly-diagnosed patient, is lacking. Information deficit is a specific diagnosis with a specific remedy and in many cases the most efficient treatment may be formal education. For the vast majority of patients, however, the *information* gained from attending traditional diabetes education programmes has very limited implications for behaviour change.

REFERENCES

American Diabetes Association (1984) Quality recognition for diabetes patient education programs. Review criteria for national standards from the American Diabetes Association. *Diabetes Care* 9: xxxvi.

Anderson RM (1986) The personal meaning of having diabetes: implications for patient behaviour and education or kicking the bucket theory. *Diabetic Medicine* 3: 85–89.

Beaven DW & Scott RS (1987) Organising and evaluating diabetes care. In Alberti KGMM & Krall LP (eds) *The Diabetes Annual/3* pp 579–590. Amsterdam: Elsevier.

Bloomgarden ZT, Karmally W, Metzger MJ et al (1987) Randomized, controlled trial of diabetic patient education: improved knowledge without improved metabolic status. *Diabetes Care* 10: 263–272.

Bradley C, Brewin C, Gamsu DS & Moses JC (1984) Development of scales to measure perceived control of diabetes mellitus and diabetes-related health beliefs. *Diabetic Medicine* 1: 213–218.

Davis WK, Hull AL & Boutaugh ML (1981) Factors affecting the educational diagnosis of diabetic patients. *Diabetes Care* 4: 275–278.

Davis WK, Hess GE, Van Harrison R & Hiss RG (1987) Psychosocial adjustment to and control of diabetes mellitus: differences by disease type and treatment. *Health Psychology* 6: 1–14.

Delamater AM, Kurtz SM, Bubb J, White NH & Santiago JV (1987) Stress and coping in relation to metabolic control of adolescents with type I diabetes. *Journal of Developmental and Behavioural Pediatrics* 8: 136–140.

Dunn SM (1986) Reactions to educational techniques: coping strategies for diabetes and learning. *Diabetic Medicine* 3: 419–429.

Dunn SM & Turtle JR (1981) The myth of the diabetic personality. *Diabetes Care* 4: 640–646.

Dunn SM & Turtle JR (1984a) Coping strategies in diabetes. *Diabetes* 33 (**supplement**): 97 (abstract).

Dunn SM, Bryson JM, Hoskins P et al (1984b) Development of the Diabetes Knowledge (DKN) Scales: Forms DKNA, DKNB, and DKNC. *Diabetes Care* 7: 36–41.

Dunn SM, Beeney LJ & Turtle JR (1985) The (in)stability of adjustment in diabetes. *Proceedings of the Annual Scientific Meeting of the Australian Diabetes Society and Australian Diabetes Educators Association* 43 (abstract).

Dunn SM, Beeney LJ & Turtle JR (1986a) Evaluation of alternative approaches to diabetes education. *Proceedings of the Annual Scientific Meeting of the Australian Diabetes Society and Australian Diabetes Educators Association*, E4 (abstract).

Dunn SM, Smartt HH, Beeney LJ & Turtle JR (1986b) Measurement of emotional adjustment in diabetic patients: validity and reliability of the ATT39. *Diabetes Care* **9:** 480–489.

Etzwiler DD (1962) What the juvenile diabetic knows about his disease. *Pediatrics* **29:** 135–141.

Falkenberg MG, Elwing BE, Goransson AM, Hellstrand BE & Riis UM (1986) Problem oriented participatory education in the guidance of adults with non-insulin-treated type II diabetes mellitus. *Scandinavian Journal of Primary Health Care* **4:** 157–164.

Garrard J, Joynes JO, Mullen L et al (1987) Psychometric study of patient knowledge test. *Diabetes Care* **10:** 500–509.

Glasgow RE, McCaul KD & Schafer LC (1986) Barriers to regimen adherence in persons with insulin-dependent diabetes. *Journal of Behavioural Medicine* **9:** 65–77.

Grabauskas V (1983) Patient education—the viewpoint of the World Health Organization. In Assal JP, Berger M, Gay N & Canivet J (eds) *Diabetes Education: How to Improve Patient Education*, pp 8–11. Proceedings of the 2nd European Symposium of the Diabetes Education Study Group. Amsterdam: Excerpta Medica.

Harris R & Linn MW (1985) Health beliefs, compliance, and control of diabetes mellitus. *Southern Medical Journal* **78:** 162–166.

Hauenstein DJ, Schiller MR & Hurley RS (1987) Motivational techniques of dietitians counselling individuals with type II diabetes. *Journal of the American Dietetic Association* **87:** 37–42.

Hess GE & Davis WK (1983) The validation of a diabetes patient knowledge test. *Diabetes Care* **6:** 591–596.

Jacobson AM, Hauser ST, Wertlieb D, Wolfsdorf JI, Orleans J & Vieyra M (1986) Psychological adjustment of children with recently diagnosed diabetes mellitus. *Diabetes Care* **9:** 323–329.

Jenny JL (1986) Differences in adaptation to diabetes between insulin-dependent and non-insulin-dependent patients: Implications for patient education. *Patient Education and Counselling* **8:** 39–50.

Johnson SB, Silverstein J, Rosenbloom A, Carter R & Cunningham W (1986) Assessing daily management in childhood diabetes. *Health Psychology* **5:** 545–564.

Kaplan RM, Chadwick MW & Schimmel LE (1985) Social learning intervention to promote metabolic control in type I diabetes mellitus: pilot experiment results. *Diabetes Care* **8:** 152–155.

Kaplan RM & Davis WK (1986) Evaluating the costs and benefits of outpatient diabetes education and nutrition counselling. *Diabetes Care* **9:** 81–86.

Kaplan RM, Hartwell SL, Wilson DK & Wallace JP (1987) Effects of diet and exercise interventions on control and quality of life in non-insulin-dependent diabetes mellitus. *Journal of General Internal Medicine* **2:** 220–228.

Knight PV & Kesson CM (1986) Educating the elderly diabetic. *Diabetic Medicine* **3:** 170–173.

Korhonen T, Huttunen JA, Aro A et al (1983) A controlled trial on the effects of patient education in the treatment of insulin-dependent diabetes. *Diabetes Care* **6:** 256–261.

Kovacs M, Brent D, Steinberg TF, Paulauskas S & Reid J (1986) Children's self-reports of psychologic adjustment and coping strategies during first year of insulin-dependent diabetes mellitus. *Diabetes Care* **9:** 472–479.

Lockington TJ, Meadows KA & Wise PH (1987) Compliant behaviour: relationship to attitudes and control in diabetic patients. *Diabetic Medicine* **4:** 56–61.

Lucey D & Wing E (1985) A clinic based educational programme for children with diabetes. *Diabetic Medicine* **2:** 292–295.

Marteau TM & Johnston M (1986) Determinants of beliefs about illness: a study of parents of children with diabetes, asthma, epilepsy, and no chronic illness. *Journal of Psychosomatic Research* **30:** 673–683.

Mazze RS, Shamoon H, Pasmantier R et al (1984) Reliability of blood glucose monitoring by patients with diabetes mellitus *American Journal of Medicine* **77:** 211–217.

Mazze RS, Pasmantier R, Murphy JA & Shamoon H (1985) Self-monitoring of capillary blood glucose: changing the performance of individuals with diabetes. *Diabetes Care* **8:** 207–213.

Mazzuca SA, Moorman NH, Wheeler ML et al (1986) The Diabetes Education Study: A controlled trial of the effects of diabetes patient education. *Diabetes Care* **9:** 1–10.

Meadows KA, Lockington TJ & Wise PH (1987) Assessment of knowledge of diabetes by questionnaire. *Diabetic Medicine* **4:** 343 (letter).

Mulrow C, Bailey S, Sönksen PH & Slavin B (1987) Evaluation of an Audiovisual Diabetes Education Program: negative results of a randomized trial of patients with non-insulin-dependent diabetes mellitus. *Journal of General Internal Medicine* **2:** 215–219.

National Standards for Diabetes Education Programs (1984) National Diabetes Advisory Board. *Diabetes Care* **7:** xxxi–xxxv.

Pendleton L, House WC & Parker LE (1987) Physicians' and patients' views of problems of compliance with diabetes regimens. *Public Health Reports* **102:** 21–26.

Peyrot M (1985) Psychosocial factors in diabetes control: adjustment of insulin-treated adults. *Psychosomatic Medicine* **47:** 542–557.

Pichert JW (1983) Not all medicines (or patient education programs) are the same. *Diabetes Care* **6:** 618–619.

Rettig BA, Shrauger DG, Recker RR et al (1986) A randomized study of the effects of a home diabetes education program. *Diabetes Care* **9:** 173–178.

Robertson-Tchabo EA, Arenberg D, Tobin JD & Plotz JB (1986) A longitudinal study of cognitive performance in non-insulin dependent (Type II) diabetic men. *Experimental Gerontology* **21:** 459–467.

Rovet JF, Ehrlich RM & Hoppe M (1987a) Behaviour problems in children with diabetes as a function of sex and age at onset of disease. *Journal of Child Psycholosy and Psychiatry* **28:** 477–491.

Rovet JF, Ehrlich RM & Hoppe M (1987b) Intellectual deficits associated with early onset of insulin-dependent diabetes mellitus in children. *Diabetes Care* **10:** 510–515.

Ryan CM (1987) A team approach to the child with diabetes who is having academic difficulties. *Diabetes Educator* **13:** 58–60.

Schafer LC, Glasgow RE, McCaul KD & Dreher M (1983) Adherence to IDDM regimens: relationship to psychosocial variables and metabolic control. *Diabetes Care* **6:** 493–498.

Tattersall RB, McCulloch DK & Aveline MO (1985) Group therapy in the treatment of diabetes. *Diabetes Care* **8:** 180–188.

Terrent A, Hagfall O & Cederholm U (1985) The effect of education and self-monitoring of blood glucose on glycosylated hemoglobin in type 1 diabetes. A controlled 18-month trial in a representative population. *Acta Medica Scandinavica* **217:** 47–53.

Vinicor F, Cohen SJ, Mazzuca SA et al (1987) DIABEDS: a randomized trial of the effects of physician and/or patient education on diabetes patient outcomes. *Journal of Chronic Diseases* **40:** 345–356.

Waclawski ER, Fisher BM & Frier BM (1985) Is it a hypo? Knowledge of the symptoms of hypoglycaemia in elderly diabetic patients *Diabetic Medicine* **2:** 412 (letter).

White N, Carnahan J, Nugent CA, Iwaoka T & Dodson MA (1986) Management of obese patients with diabetes mellitus: comparison of advice education with group management. *Diabetes Care* **9:** 490–496.

Wilson W & Pratt C (1987) The impact of diabetes education and peer support upon weight and glycemic control of elderly persons with noninsulin dependent diabetes mellitus (NIDDM). *American Journal of Public Health* **77:** 634–635.

Wilson W, Ary DV, Biglan A, Glasgow RE, Toobert DJ & Campbell DR (1986) Psychosocial predictors of self-care behaviors (compliance) and glycemic control in non-insulin-dependent diabetes mellitus. *Diabetes Care* **9:** 614–622.

Windsor RA, Roseman J, Gartseff G & Kirk KA (1981) Qualitative issues in developing educational diagnostic instruments and assessment procedures for diabetic patients. *Diabetes Care* **4:** 468–475.

Wing RR, Epstein LH, Nowalk MP, Scott N & Koeske R (1985) Compliance to self-monitoring of blood glucose: a marked-item technique compared with self-report. *Diabetes Care* **8:** 456–460.

Wise PH, Dowlatshahi DC, Farrant S, Fromson S & Meadows KA (1986) Effect of computer-based learning on diabetes knowledge and control. *Diabetes Care* **9:** 504–508.

14

The long-term care of non-insulin-dependent diabetes

W. GATLING
R. D. HILL

Despite treatment with diet, oral hypoglycaemic agents or insulin, non-insulin-dependent diabetics have an increased mortality and morbidity when compared to non-diabetics (Shenfield et al, 1979). This is due to the development of long-term complications. Chronic hyperglycaemia appears to be associated with several pathophysiological processes. Damage to the small blood vessels at the capillary and arteriolar levels leads to micro-vascular complications e.g. retinopathy and nephropathy. Involvement of larger blood vessels produces early and advanced atherosclerotic changes leading to macrovascular complications e.g. coronary, cerebral and periph-eral vascular disease. In addition, disordered metabolism appears to be a factor leading to damage to the lens of the eye and the nerves. These pathological processes rarely occur in isolation and, for example in diabetic foot disease, combine to produce a complex mixture of ischaemia, neuro-pathy and infection.

In recent years, it has been recognized that there is a relationship between glycaemic control and the development of these complications. A large study of 4400 diabetics over 25 years showed an increasing prevalence of neuropathy, retinopathy and nephropathy with decreasing standards of glycaemic control (Pirart, 1978). Time is also an important factor. With increasing duration of diabetes, a larger proportion of patients will have demonstrable complications. However, the diagnosis of non-insulin-dependent diabetes is frequently made following a variable period of chronic hyperglycaemia. This means that the duration of known diabetes does not accurately reflect the total 'at risk' interval. It is not uncommon for non-insulin-dependent diabetics to have evidence of 'long-term compli-cations' at diagnosis. It is also known that impaired glucose tolerance is associated with an increased risk of macrovascular disease (Fuller et al, 1983).

Once the diagnosis of diabetes has been established and treatment initi-ated, it is essential to organize long-term follow up. The aims of this continuing care are listed in Table 1.

Table 1. The aims of follow-up of the diabetic patient.

1. To maintain patient morale.
2. To maintain patient's determination to continue self-care.
3. To continue education and revision.
4. To monitor glycaemic control.
5. To monitor weight.
6. To detect long term complications at an early stage.
7. To identify risk factors.
8. Advise on treatment.
9. To arrange an appointment and recall system.

THE AIMS OF LONG-TERM CARE OF THE DIABETIC PATIENT

Patient morale and education

All health workers involved in the care of patients with chronic medical conditions should recognize the importance of regular patient contact. This is especially important in diabetes where patients have such a central role in the management of their conditions. The aims of treatment need to be frequently stressed so that the patient understands the importance of good control and long-term health. The enthusiasm engendered at diagnosis may rapidly fade and renewed motivation for the years to come is essential. In addition, those patients who consistently fail to reach the goals set require support and understanding. It is clear that this role can be best achieved if the same medical staff see the patient at each visit.

Monitoring glycaemic control

All patients should be encouraged to monitor regularly their own diabetes and keep a chart or book for the results. This can then be reviewed at each visit.

Urine testing with a dipstick such as Diastix (Ames, UK) provides a simple method of measuring glycosuria and is suitable for the majority of diabetics treated by diet alone or diet with oral hypoglycaemic agents. The urine should be tested once each day at varying times. In this way, the patient can identify those times during the day when control is less than optimal. The aim should be to have the urine free of sugar at all times. Diabetics who achieve this must be praised but also encouraged to keep testing regularly so that deterioration in control can be quickly identified.

Home blood-glucose monitoring is not only useful in diabetics treated with insulin but also for those with either a low or high renal threshold even if treated with diet alone or diet plus tablets. Again, once daily testing is generally sufficient if the time of day (before meals, postprandial and before bed-time) is varied. Insulin-treated patients can be instructed to alter their dosage in response to the results to optimize control. The general aim of treatment should be for pre-meal glucose levels of 4–7 mmol/l (70–130 mg/100 ml) and postprandial levels of less than 10 mmol/l (180 mg/100 ml). However, the physician will need to set guidelines for each individual.

Laboratory testing of blood glucose and glycosylated haemoglobin (HbA_{1c}) are also essential components of monitoring glycaemic control. Maximal benefit will be gained if the results are available at the time of consultation. It is important to explain their significance to the patient and also relate this to their own monitoring. In one clinic, each diabetic was given a small co-operation book and at each visit, a note was made of the patient's weight, urine and blood results along with screening tests for complications (Hill, 1987). The booklet, kept by the patient, provided a valuable historical record of glycaemic control to which the patient can refer at any time.

Blood glucose levels in patients treated by diet alone or diet plus tablets do not fluctuate to the same extent during the day as do levels in patients treated with insulin. Thus, a fasting or timed postprandial blood glucose will be a good indicator of glycaemic control. However, a single blood glucose level in an insulin-treated diabetic is considerably less valuable and a HbA_{1c}, a longer term assessment of control, is essential.

With time, many non-insulin-dependent diabetics will require changes in their treatment. Diabetics initially well controlled on diet alone may need the addition of oral hypoglycaemic agents and some may require insulin. The deterioration in control is rarely rapid and it is useful to warn patients in advance of the likelihood of an impending change. This is particularly important for insulin therapy which many patients view with considerable fear.

Monitoring body weight

In conjunction with patients' home monitoring and laboratory results, changes in weight can provide valuable information. For example, weight gain in the face of poor glycaemic control suggests problems with dietary compliance. On the other hand, persistent weight loss in the non-obese patient with poor control suggests the need for insulin therapy.

The detection of complications

Non-insulin-dependent diabetes describes a heterogenous condition which is characterized by chronic hyperglycaemia. Diagnostic criteria have been carefully laid down (WHO, 1980), however, it is clear that whatever the aetiology, one consequence is the development of various complications. This is not inevitable, but at present it is impossible to identity those diabetics who will escape them. Thus, all diabetics need to be regularly reviewed to detect complications.

Diabetic eye disease

This represents a considerable problem. In the age group 30–64 years it is the single most common cause of blindness in the UK (Sorsby, 1972). It is also a substantial problem in the elderly (Table 2).

Table 2. The prevalence of sight-threatening retinopathy in a community based diabetic population in Poole. (W. Gatling, unpublished).

Prevalence of preproliferative or proliferative retinopathy	
Aged less than 65 years	6.0%
Aged 65 years and over	5.9%
Prevalence of maculopathy	
Aged less than 65 years	2.0%
Aged 65 years and over	6.8%

The manifestations of diabetic eye disease are as follows:

1. Transient refractory changes.
2. Cataract.
3. Diabetic retinopathy and its complications:
   a) maculopathy;
   b) vitreous haemorrhage/membrane formation;
   c) traction retinal detachment;
   d) rubeotic glaucoma.

Transient refractory changes. The osmolality of the blood and tissue fluids changes with the concentration of blood glucose. Chronic hyperglycaemia produces a change in the refractory media of the eye. Thus, blurred vision or deteriorating eyesight is not an uncommon presentation to the doctor or optician. The astute practitioner will be able to make a diagnosis of diabetes. The patient should be advised to have his eyes retested following treatment and stabilization of the blood glucose. These changes are usually transient and the patient may be reassured. However, it is essential that the fundi are carefully examined before this reassurance is given since serious retinopathy may be present at diagnosis.

Cataract. Accumulation of sorbitol in the lens is thought to account for the 'snowflake' cataract occasionally seen in the juvenile onset diabetic. However, the mechanism whereby non-insulin-dependent diabetics develop cataracts is not understood and probably represents an accelerated type of senile cataract.

Cataracts are commonly found in diabetics and can be surgically removed when visual acuity is severely impaired. Significant lens opacity can make screening for retinopathy with a direct ophthalmoscope very difficult. An ophthalmologist should be consulted as generally indirect ophthalmoscopy will give an adequate view. Cataract extraction should be considered if serious retinopathy is found so that future assessment and treatment can be carried out.

Diabetic retinopathy and its complications. The features of diabetic retinopathy are consequences of microvascular disease affecting the retina (Kohner et al, 1982). The earliest changes affect the capillaries; aneurysmal dilatation produces microaneurysms and later there is capillary closure. The blood–retinal barrier is breached at these damaged capillaries and plasma exudes into the extra-cellular space. This produces retinal oedema and lipid-rich deposits which appear as hard exudates on fundoscopy.

Thrombosis of microaneurysms and areas of capillary closure result in severe retinal ischaemia. Axoplasmic flow within the nerves is halted and axoplasm collects producing the whitish grey appearance of a 'cotton wool spot'. It is thought that chemical messengers coming from these ischaemic areas of the retina are the stimulus to new vessel production. Initially, these new vessels have no supporting connective tissue but gradually, as they extend away from the surface of the retina, fibrous proliferation occurs. Later, contraction of this tissue or the vitreous may lead to retinal detachment.

Damaged capillaries, microaneurysms and new vessels may bleed producing areas of haemorrhage. If they occur deep in the vascular layer or inner nuclear layer of the retina they have a round appearance and are called dot and blot haemorrhages. The former are indistinguishable from microaneurysms. Superficial haemorrhages have a flame shaped appearance as the blood tracks between the neurones. Pre-retinal vessels produce retrohyaloid haemorrhage with a fluid level and new vessels bleeding into the vitreous produce a diffuse vitreous haemorrhage with severe loss of vision.

The classification of diabetic retinopathy is valuable since it helps organize an approach to prognosis, follow-up and treatment. The prevalence of retinopathy in a community based diabetic population is shown in Table 3. Simple background retinopathy usually refers to the presence of dots and blots only. This does not cause any impairment of visual acuity. The prognosis is good and an annual review is generally sufficient. However, some patients will progress to more severe forms of retinopathy.

The presence of hard exudates with dots and blots is commonly classified as exudative retinopathy. If the lesions encroach upon the macula area, oedema is produced and there will be a gradual reduction in visual acuity. This is called maculopathy. Frequently, the patient is unaware of the early visual deterioration yet it has been clearly shown that treatment is more successful in preserving good vision if undertaken early (British Multicentre

Table 3. The prevalence of diabetic retinopathy in a community based population of non-insulin-dependent diabetics in the Poole area. (W. Gatling, unpublished).

	n	%
No retinopathy	472	73.8
Background retinopathy	114	17.8
Background retinopathy with maculopathy	17	2.7
Preproliferative retinopathy	15	2.3
Proliferative retinopathy	22	3.4
	640	100
Maculopathy	31	4.8

(6 had preproliferative retinopathy and 8 had proliferative retinopathy plus maculopathy).

Study Group, 1983). Patients with definite maculopathy or exudates likely to threaten the macula should be referred to a consultant ophthalmologist for assessment. Other patients with exudative retinopathy should be reviewed at 6–12 month intervals according to the extent of the retinopathy.

The presence of cotton wool spots indicates definite retinal ischaemia and signifies a pre-proliferative retinopathy. Many diabetics in this category will develop new vessels within two years. Other features suggesting a pre-proliferative phase are the presence of widespread capillary closure (the retina has an atrophic, featureless appearance but this is best seen on fluorescein angiography), deep dark round haemorrhages, intra-retinal microvascular abnormalities (IRMA) and venous abnormalities such as irregularity, tortuosity, beading and looping (Kohner et al, 1982). Patients in this category require close observation to detect progression to the proliferative phase and regular review by an ophthalmologist is desirable.

Diabetics who have evidence of new vessel formation whether at the optic disc or in the periphery are classified as having proliferative retinopathy and have a substantial risk of vitreous haemorrhage. In the past, approximately one-third of patients with either disc new vessels or those who had already suffered a vitreous haemorrhage were blind within three years (Caird et al, 1968). Timely photocoagulation will prevent blindness in 60% of such patients. Diabetics with proliferative retinopathy require urgent referral to an ophthalmologist.

Screening for diabetic eye disease. From the above description, it is clear that retinopathy represents a serious threat to the diabetic patient. It should also be apparent that the patient will generally be unaware of the changes occurring as visual acuity is only affected at a late stage. For this reason, it is essential to screen all diabetics at regular intervals to detect the early changes of retinopathy. Treatment can then prevent blindness.

Diabetics should have their eyes examined at diagnosis and thereafter at annual intervals. A full examination should include assessment of visual acuity (distant and near) with refractive errors corrected either by spectacles or a pinhole, and fundoscopy with a direct ophthalmoscope in a darkened room following pupillary dilatation. The latter is essential to obtain a good view of the retina and is especially important in the detection of lesions near the macula. Tropicamide 0.5–1% solution will dilate the pupils in approximately 10–15 minutes and the effect lasts for approximately three hours. Although near vision is often blurred, distant vision is not usually significantly affected by pupillary dilatation and reversal with pilocarpine is not necessary.

In the UK, there has been considerable debate about who should perform this screening (Waugh et al, 1986). The detection and assessment of retinopathy requires skill and yet the workload is considerable. The average health district in the UK with a catchment population of 250 000 has approximately 2525 diabetics (1894 with non-insulin-dependent diabetes) (Gatling et al, 1985). If detection and management of diabetic eye disease were the sole responsibility of one consultant ophthalmologist in the district, he would need to devote 4–5 sessions per week to screening alone. One session would be required for treatment and another for regular assessment of serious retinopathy. This would leave little time for general ophthalmology. At present, there is insufficient medical manpower to cover this.

Others believe that screening for retinopathy should be performed in the diabetic clinic. This represents a considerable workload. Also many clinics in the UK are staffed by junior doctors who have been shown to be poor at diagnosing retinopathy (Ryder et al, 1985). Screening facilities for retinopathy are also frequently inadequate (Royal College of Physicians and BDA, 1984). In addition, in some areas as many as 50% of diabetics do not attend the hospital diabetic clinic and yet these patients still require screening (Yudkin et al, 1980). Although general practitioners may supervise diabetic care, they are unlikely to provide an effective screening service. The average general practitioner will only encounter serious retinopathy occasionally. If the doctor has a list size of 2500 patients, there will be approximately 25 diabetics of whom two or three will have serious retinopathy and a new case would only be expected every three years (Hill, 1987).

Two other screening programmes have been suggested: the non-mydriatic retinal camera (Ryder et al, 1985); and the ophthalmic optician (optometrist) -based service (Hill, 1987). The new retinal cameras are capable of taking a single wide-angle (45°) picture of the retina and this is said to detect over 90% of lesions at the posterior pole. However, a skilled observer is required to review all the photogtraphs and this will amount to approximately 100 per week in an average district (50 patients per week). On the other hand, many diabetics, especially the elderly, already attend an optician to obtain spectacles. The annual eye examination can be conducted by the optometrist and usually includes screening for other eye disease e.g. glaucoma. These practitioners are skilled in fundoscopy and can diagnose retinopathy. Two successful schemes have so far been reported (Hill, 1981; Burns-Cox and Dean Hart, 1985).

Diabetics identified by the screening programme are best initially reviewed by a diabetologist with a good training in ophthalmology provided there is no unnecessary delay. At this time, not only can the findings be confirmed but also a full assessment of glycaemic control, risk factors and other long term complications be undertaken. Diabetics with serious retinopathy should be urgently referred to the ophthalmologist while others with a simple retinopathy can be kept under reveiw.

A joint clinic between consultant ophthalmologist and diabetologist is recommended for the care of diabetics with serious retinopathy (Spathis, 1986). This ensures that the patient receives supervision of his diabetes at the same time as the assessment of retinopathy thereby minimizing the number of hospital visits but also reinforcing the link between glycaemic control and complications. It is also very useful for the diabetologist to discuss regularly individual cases with his ophthalmologist colleague thus ensuring his skills in assessing retinopathy are maintained and maximizing co-operation between the two specialities.

Treatment of diabetic retinopathy. The effect of good glycaemic control on established retinopathy is variable. Some studies in insulin-dependent diabetics have shown a progression of retinopathy in the initial months of very strict diabetic control achieved by insulin infusion pumps. However, over longer periods of time the results have been more reassuring (Dahl-Jorgensen et al, 1986). The effect in non-insulin-dependent diabetes is unknown, however it would seem wise to optimize control gradually at least to try and prevent the development of other complications.

At present, no medical treatment has been successful in reversing established retinopathy. It is recognized that hypertension and cigarette smoking are significant risk factors in the development of retinopathy (WHO Multinational Study, 1985). Thus, uncontrolled hypertension should be treated and cigarette smoking strongly discouraged.

The only effective treatment for retinopathy is photocoagulation. This involves the direction of a high energy beam of photons on to the retina. The energy is absorbed, converted to heat and a burn is produced. Both the xenon arc and argon laser can be used for photocoagulation although the latter is preferable for use near the macula. Focal photocoagulation is used for the treatment of maculopathy and small areas of peripheral new vessels. Diabetics with disc new vessels or extensive peripheral new vessels are treated by pan photocoagulation. In this case, large areas of peripheral retina are photocoagulated in an attempt to destroy the ischaemic areas which are stimulating new vessel formation. Both forms of treatment have been shown in controlled randomized trials to be successful in preserving vision (British Multicentre Study Group, 1977, 1983).

Diabetic nephropathy

Diabetic nephropathy represents another microvascular complication of diabetes. The earliest change is a diffuse thickening of the glomerular capillary basement membrane. It is uncertain whether this is due to excessive production or a reduced breakdown of the basement membrane substance. Gradually, this material accumulates in the mesangium and leads to capillary damage. At the stage of nodular glomerulosclerosis large clumps of hyaline material collect and damage the glomerulus. These are the typical features of the 'Kimmelstiel-Wilson Kidney'. Destruction of large numbers of glomeruli eventually leads to renal failure (Ireland et al, 1982).

The glomerulus consists of a small knot of capillaries which act as a filtration barrier. Damage to the glomerular capillaries is manifest as proteinuria. The diagnostic hallmark of diabetic nephropathy is the presence of persistent proteinuria (greater than 500 mg protein/24 h). An earlier stage of diabetic renal disease is now detectable and this is identified by the presence of microalbuminuria.

Using immunological techniques, low concentrations of urinary albumin can be measured. The term microalbuminuria has been coined to describe urinary albumin excretion above normal (greater than 26 mg/24 h) but below that detectable by conventional methods (e.g. Albustix, less than 250 mg/24 h) (Viberti et al, 1984). Longitudinal studies in non-insulin-dependent diabetics have shown that a group of patients likely to develop nephropathy and also have a high mortality can be identified on the basis of micro-albuminuria (Mogensen, 1984; Jarrett et al, 1984).

Preliminary work has suggested that improved glycaemic control will reduce urinary albumin excretion (Mohamed et al, 1984). This implies that it may be possible to identify an earlier and potentially reversible stage of diabetic nephropathy.

Diabetics with nephropathy are usually asymptomatic until renal function becomes considerably impaired. Proteinuria is detectable using a dipstick method (e.g. Albustix), although in the initial stages these relatively crude tests may only be intermittently positive. Heavy proteinuria with hypo-proteinaemia and oedema, the features of nephrotic syndrome, is only occasionally seen in diabetics with nephropathy.

Hypertension is a frequent accompaniment and other complications are also usually found. Retinopathy is almost always present and its absence should lead the clinician to question the diagnosis of diabetic nephropathy. Macrovascular disease is a major problem in non-insulin-dependent diabetics with nephropathy and coronary artery disease is responsible for many deaths. Foot ulceration is also common since lowered resistance to infection, poor peripheral circulation and neuropathy are frequently found.

Screening for diabetic nephropathy. All diabetics should be screened for renal involvement at diagnosis and thereafter at annual intervals. The following tests are advisable:

1. Early morning urine specimen: dipstick for protein (Albustix): albumin/creatinine ratio.
2. Mid-stream urine specimen (MSU): culture and microscopy.
3. Serum creatinine.

These preliminary tests will identify diabetics with gross proteinuria (Albustix), microalbuminuria (albumin/creatinine ratio), urinary tract infection (MSU) and impaired renal function (serum creatinine).

The optimal urine sample to screen for nephropathy is debatable. Dipstick methods (e.g. Albustix) detect protein on the basis of a concentration. Thus, a very dilute or very concentrated urine sample might give a false negative or false positive result respectively. A urinary protein excretion rate would be preferable but timed urine collections are not feasible for screening purposes. The erect posture increases urinary protein excretion and so a daytime sample might be more sensitive for detecting proteinuria. However, the early morning urine sample has been shown to be useful in screening for microalbuminuria, a urinary albumin/creatinine ratio above 2 mg/mmol providing a sensitive cut off (Gatling et al, 1988a). If both an albumin/creatinine ratio and dipstick test are performed on the early morning urine sample, it is unlikely that patients with significant proteinuria will be missed.

Follow-up of diabetics with positive renal screen. Diabetics identified by the screening tests need further investigation. It should be noted that these tests do not specifically identify diabetic nephropathy. A thorough history and examination of the patient is essential and other causes of renal disease need to be excluded. This is particularly important in older patients since urinary tract infections, prostatic problems and renal calculi are common. If the diagnosis of diabetic nephropathy remains in doubt, a renal biopsy should be performed.

Diabetics found to have a positive screen for microalbuminuria (an albumin/creatinine ratio greater than 2 mg/mmol) should be instructed to collect a timed overnight urine sample for assessment of albumin excretion rate (AER). Those with an AER greater than 30 µg/min fall into the high risk group likely to develop diabetic nephropathy and have a high mortality (Mogensen, 1984; Jarrett et al, 1984). Those with an AER in the normal range (AER less than 7.1 µg/min in our laboratory) can be reassured and returned to an annual screen. Diabetics with an AER less than 30 but greater than 7.1 µg/min should be reassessed at 3–6 monthly intervals. At present, long term risks for diabetics in this 'grey area' remain unknown.

Management of diabetic nephropathy. In non-insulin-dependent diabetes, relatively little is known about the early stages of diabetic nephropathy identified on the basis of microalbuminuria. Work in insulin-dependent diabetics suggests there may be a phase of 'incipient nephropathy' and preliminary results indicate that this phase may be reversible or at least progression prevented by strict glycaemic control (Feldt-Rasmussen et al, 1986). Management of non-insulin-dependent diabetics with microalbuminuria should be aimed at optimising glycaemic control, treating hypertension and identifying other potential risk factors.

Improvements in glycaemic control have been shown to reduce urinary albumin excretion in non-insulin-dependent diabetics (Mohamed et al, 1984). This was brought about by dietary treatment alone. However, if dietary measures fail to control blood glucose levels adequately, oral hypoglycaemic agents or insulin therapy should be considered.

Blood pressure has been found to be an important determinant of urinary albumin excretion (Gatling et al, 1988b) and insulin-dependent diabetics with microalbuminuria have raised blood pressure (Mathiesen et al, 1984). Blood pressure requires careful monitoring and if found to be persistently raised then treatment should be commenced. It is important to consider the age of the patient in relation to the blood pressure and not use a single hypertension cut-off level. In insulin-dependent diabetics, the use of angiotensin converting enzyme inhibitors has been shown to reduce urinary albumin excretion and these agents deserve consideration (Hommel et al, 1986).

One longitudinal study of non-insulin-dependent diabetics with microalbuminuria identified a high mortality from cardiovascular disease (Jarrett et al, 1984). Assessment of macrovascular complications and risk factors, e.g. smoking, is recommended.

Diabetics with microalbuminuria should be reassessed at regular intervals and the following measured every 3–6 months:

1. Overnight AER.
2. Blood pressure.
3. Blood glucose.
4. HbA_{1c}.
5. Serum creatinine.
6. Glomerular filtration rate (chromium EDTA) (annual).

Serum creatinine should be normal but glomerular filtration rate may be elevated initially due to hyperfiltration.

Once a diabetic patient has developed persistent proteinuria (greater than 500 mg protein per 24 h), diabetic nephropathy has reached an irreversible stage. There follows a relentless deterioration in renal function. The rate of this decline, although highly variable between patients, appears to be steady for each individual (Jones et al, 1979). On average, it takes 5–7 years from the detection of persistent proteinuria to reach terminal renal failure. Management must be aimed at slowing this progression. Therapeutic manoeuvres include good glycaemic control, blood pressure control and dietary protein restriction.

There is some indirect evidence that good glycaemic control may reduce the rate of deterioration of renal function in insulin-dependent diabetics. It would seem sensible to optimize control in non-insulin-dependent diabetics. Dietary reappraisal is a good starting point. Certain oral hypoglycaemic agents are excreted by the kidneys (e.g. glibenclamide, metformin) and their use in diabetics with renal impairment is to be avoided. Glycaemic control often deteriorates with worsening renal function and insulin treatment may be necessary. It is important to try and maintain the HbA_{1c} in the normal range, whilst recognizing that this may give an over optimistic assessment of glycaemic control because of reduced red blood cell survival in renal failure.

Regular assessment of blood pressure and early treatment of mild hypertension is recommended. It is wise to monitor renal function closely since there can be a sharp fall in glomerular filtration rate with the start of antihypertensive treatment. However, in the long term there is a beneficial effect by reducing the rate of progressive decline in renal function (Mogensen, 1982).

Dietary protein restriction reduces the solute load on the kidney. Once the patient is in established renal failure, it will frequently lead to considerable symptomatic improvement. Research is in progress to investigate whether the earlier introduction of dietary protein restriction might significantly reduce the rate of deterioration in renal function.

The diabetic patient with nephropathy will need close supervision and monitoring. Other diabetic complications may develop and this may occur surprisingly rapidly. This is particularly true for retinopathy where proliferative changes may occur and lead to vitreous haemorrhage.

Once serum creatinine rises above 200 µmol/l it is wise to seek the advice of a nephrologist. The management of renal failure can be optimized and the long-term arrangements discussed with the patient. The majority of diabetics will now be accepted for renal replacement therapy and many diabetics are placed on the transplant list before commencing dialysis.

Macrovascular disease

Atherosclerosis appears to occur as a natural consequence of the ageing process in Western civilization. Diabetics have more extensive and diffuse disease at an earlier age when compared with matched controls. The manifestations of macrovascular disease depend upon the affected vessels but fall into three main groups: cerebrovascular disease producing transient ischaemic attacks and completed stroke; coronary artery disease causing angina and myocardial infarction; and peripheral vascular disease producing intermittent claudication and lower-limb ischaemia.

Patients with diabetes tolerate major vascular events such as stroke and myocardial infarction poorly. In diabetics, the mortality from myocardial infarction is twice that of non-diabetic patients (Clark et al, 1985).

Screening is based on a careful history and examination seeking evidence of macrovascular disease and potential risk factors (see Table 4). Cigarette smoking should be actively discouraged as it is a significant risk factor for macrovascular disease. Hyperlipidaemia should also be sought as this represents another potentially reversible risk factor. Further investigation of patients with positive features will be necessary. However, macrovascular disease usually affects more than one site. Consequently, it is wise to investigate all patients with any positive features for coronary artery disease especially if major surgery is planned. A resting and, if necessary, exercise electrocardiogram will identify a considerable number of diabetics with clinically unsuspected disease.

The medical treatment of macrovascular disease is important. During the acute event of a stroke or myocardial infarction, diabetes needs to be carefully controlled. Blood glucose levels may rise considerably during these stressful episodes and insulin treatment is often needed. Initially, a continuous insulin infusion with frequent blood glucose monitoring is necessary.

Table 4. Symptoms or signs suggestive of macrovascular disease.

History

1.	Cerebrovascular disease	– amaurosis fugax – transient motor/sensory/speech disturbance – transient vertigo – completed stroke
2.	Coronary artery disease	– angina/atypical chest pain myocardial infarction exertional dyspnoea/paroxysmal nocturnal dyspnoea
3.	Peripheral vascular disease	– intermittent claudication lower limb ulceration/slow healing rest pain
4.	General	– smoking history

Examination

1.	Cerebrovascular disease	– neurological signs carotid bruit
2.	Coronary artery disease	– left ventricular failure
3.	Peripheral vascular disease	– arterial bruits, decreased or absent peripheral pulses, dependent rubor, ischaemic changes in skin and its appendages, ankle/arm doppler pressure ratio less than 1
4.	General	– hypertension xanthelasma/xanthoma

With improvement in the patient's condition, this can be changed to preprandial subcutaneous insulin and, later, oral hypoglycaemic agents reintroduced.

After the acute event, medical treatment should be aimed at reducing symptoms and minimizing the risks of further episodes. Thus, in cerebro-vascular disease, anticoagulants or antiplatelet agents will be considered and hypertension, if present, adequately treated. Following a myocardial infarction, beta-blocker therapy may reduce the risk of sudden death. A cardioselective agent is preferable to reduce the risk of hypoglycaemic unawareness in the insulin-treated diabetic. However, these agents may be contraindicated if the patient also has significant peripheral vascular disease.

Hyperlipidaemia should be treated initially by dietary measures and weight reduction. Glycaemic control must also be optimized. If hyperlipidaemia persists despite these measures, lipid lowering agents can be introduced.

Diabetic neuropathy

Evidence of diabetic neuropathy is common when sought in diabetic patients. The pathophysiological processes involved in its evolution are complex and not clearly understood. Chronic hyperglycaemia leads to disturbances in metabolic pathways in the nerves. These undoubtedly produce alteration in function and are probably responsible for the symmetrical polyneuropathy seen in diabetes. It is likely that vascular factors also play a part. This is particularly important in the development of acute isolated lesions of mononeuritis. The clinical manifestations of diabetic neuropathy are listed in Table 5.

Symmetrical sensory polyneuropathy may be asymptomatic in some patients. Others will complain of numbness, paraesthesia and occasionally severe pain in their feet and legs. On examination, a symmetrical sensory impairment of pain, light touch and vibration sense is found with absent ankle reflexes. In rare cases, neuropathic arthropathy occurs (Charcot's joint) and there is a disruption of the joints of the foot.

Damage to the autonomic nervous system may be silent but can also produce a range of different symptoms according to the system involved (see Table 5). Cardiovascular involvement can be most serious causing sudden cardiorespiratory arrest (Ewing and Clarke, 1986). This may occur during the perioperative period when hypoxia or hypercapnia may be an important factor.

Table 5. The clinical manifestations of diabetic neuropathy.

1. Symmetrical sensory polyneuropathy
2. Autonomic neuropathy
    a) gastrointestinal tract—diabetic diarrhoea, gastroparesis/dilatation
    b) cardiovascular—postural hypotension, tachycardia, cardiorespiratory arrest
    c) sweating abnormality—gustatory sweating
    d) genitourinary tract—impotence, retrograde ejaculation, neurogenic bladder.
3. Mononeuritis and mononeuritis multiplex
4. Diabetic amyotrophy

Postural hypotension causes distressing dizziness and sometimes collapse when the patient attempts to stand up quickly. It is important to measure the blood pressure when lying and standing in all diabetic patients. A systolic fall on standing of more than 30 mm Hg is diagnostic of postural hypotension. These patients will often have systolic hypertension in the supine position. Antihypertensive treatment must be avoided since it will only exacerbate symptoms.

Mononeuritis is not uncommon among elderly diabetics. The third and fourth cranial nerves are frequently affected. The patient presents with pain and diplopia. Fortunately, these ocular palsies are usually transient and the patient can be reassured that full recovery will occur in 6–12 weeks.

Diabetic amyotrophy is a distressing condition. The patient frequently presents with severe pain and weakness. An asymmetric proximal muscle wasting with weakness and reduced reflexes will be found on examination. The muscles of the pelvic girdle and thighs are most commonly affected but the shoulders and arms can also be involved. In the early stages, it is not uncommon for the patient to complain of severe pain despite minimal physical signs.

Screening for diabetic neuropathy. A careful history and examination will identify most diabetics with significant neuropathy, although specific questioning may be necessary to detect those with impotence.

In asymptomatic patients, an objective test of peripheral and autonomic nerve function would be useful. These could be performed at intervals to detect any deterioration. Vibration threshold perception can be measured objectively using a biothesiometer (Bloom et al, 1984). Age standardized ranges have been produced. There is considerable inter-observer variation in this measurement and its repeated long term value has not been fully assessed. There are several tests of autonomic nerve function including beat to beat variation during forced ventilation and this can be readily performed during a resting electrocardiogram (Ewing and Clarke, 1986).

The management of diabetic neuropathy. The treatment of diabetic neuropathy is very difficult. Good glycaemic control is the best preventative measure. At present, there is no medical treatment which will reverse established neuropathy. Strict blood glucose control has been reported to produce symptomatic improvement in some cases of painful symmetrical neuropathy and amyotrophy (Boulton et al, 1982). It is wise to optimize control in all diabetics with symptomatic neuropathy and aim to achieve normoglycaemia. This will frequently require the use of insulin therapy but patients are usually well motivated because of the distressing symptoms.

Many patients receive multivitamin preparations in the belief that other metabolic factors may be contributing. There is no objective evidence that these are beneficial. Patients should be discouraged from smoking and heavy alcohol consumption.

Analgesia is a problem and a wide range of products need to be tried. These patients often require narcotic analgesia. Depression and weight loss are commonly associated symptoms. The prognosis for diabetics with amyotrophy is generally good, although recovery may take 6–24 months, however symmetrical polyneuropathy may be progressive.

The management of autonomic neuropathy is also unsatisfactory. Fludrocortisone has been used with some benefit in postural hypotension. Recently, domperidone has been found to be effective in some cases of gastroparesis, and poldine in neuropathic sweating (Ewing and Clarke, 1986).

It is important that anaesthetists are warned about diabetics known to have autonomic neuropathy prior to surgery. Special monitoring during the perioperative period can then be arranged.

Diabetic foot disease

Diabetic foot disease is not only common but also expensive. In the UK, more hospital beds are occupied by diabetics with foot problems than any other complication.

It is generally the result of a mixture of pathological processes: macrovascular disease reducing the blood supply; microvascular disease decreasing tissue perfusion at the capillary level; autonomic neuropathy producing arteriovenous shunting; and the loss of pain sensation depriving the patient of the normal protection from noxious stimuli. Hyperglycaemia also decreases resistance to infection.

Diabetic foot problems can be grouped into two main categories, neuropathic and ischaemic, although these often co-exist in the same patient (Edmonds, 1986). The neuropathic foot is deprived of pain sensation. The adjustment of posture or position in response to even minor discomfort is absent and, consequently, trauma occurs. This may be due to excessive weight pressure or sheer pressure from ill-fitting shoes. Foot deformities such as hammer toes and hallux valgus predispose to abnormal pressure areas and neuropathic ulceration.

The typical punched out lesion is usually found on the plantar surface of the foot, most commonly under the head of the first or other metatarsals. Neuropathic ulcers also occur on the heel, dorsal surface and tips of the toes. The ulcer is surrounded by a thick layer of callus and may penetrate so deeply that bone is visible at the base. The ulcer is generally painless and chronic. The neuropathic process may involve the intrinsic muscles of the foot causing weakness and further deformity. Occasionally, disorganization of the ankle occurs and gross deformity results (Charcot's joint).

In contrast, the ischaemic foot is painful. The patient often relates a typical history of claudication. This may progress to rest pain which is worse at night. The ischaemic ulcer shows little sign of healing and has a dead gangrenous edge in contrast to the profuse callus of the neuropathic ulcer. Other sites in the foot may show evidence of ischaemia and peripheral pulses are absent.

Screening for diabetic foot disease. Screening for diabetic foot disease involves taking a careful history and examining the patient. Whilst examining the legs and feet, it is valuable to educate the diabetic patient about the potential problems. Education is a good preventative measure.

Patients with a history of claudication and/or poor peripheral pulses should have an ankle/arm Doppler pressure ratio measured. A value less than one confirms the presence of significant vascular impairment. Angiography and surgery should be considered in these patients.

Careful inspection of the feet will identify deformities, areas of callus and infection and toe nails in need of attention. Measuring vibration perception thresholds and a neurological examination will detect evidence of neuropathy. A pedobarograph is a useful method of identifying high pressure areas.

Management of diabetic foot disease. Diabetics with areas of callus or foot deformity should be seen by the chiropodist for treatment and assessment of footwear. Simple appliances can be made to fit in the shoe to reduce areas of high pressure. In more difficult cases, special footwear will be required.

Foot ulceration in a diabetic patient is an emergency. It is important to educate patients to inspect their feet regularly. If an ulcer is found or they notice pain or a skin colour change, attention should be sought immediately. This service is often best provided by the chiropodist in close liaison with a diabetologist. The ulcer must be thoroughly debrided with removal of all dead skin and callus. A swab should be sent for culture and antibiotics prescribed if infection is suspected. Rest is essential and weight-bearing forbidden. Daily dressings are usually required. Acute infection, poor diabetic control and the need for surgical intervention are all indications for hospital admission.

Amputations as an end result of diabetic foot disease represent a failure in patient education and medical treatment. Patients in whom an ulcer has healed require careful education, footwear assessment and fitting. Generally, long-term chiropody follow-up is necessary.

The organization of diabetic care

The modern management of diabetes centres on attempting to maintain the health of the patient (Hill, 1987). It is clear that many of the complications of diabetes are asymptomatic in the early phases and yet detection is important so that treatment can be initiated. In addition, it is possible to identify certain risk factors which, if corrected, may alter the natural history of the disease. In the past, the main aim of treatment was to control the blood glucose level so that the patient was asymptomatic. Screening for complications was not beneficial since generally there was no effective treatment available. The typical hospital diabetic clinic was established during this era and its organization is generally not suited to the screening now required. Many lack the basic facilities required (Royal College of Physicians and BDA, 1984).

The management of diabetes may now be divided into two distinct categories: first, the supervision of diabetic control which includes controlling blood glucose levels, educating the patient and altering diet and treatment accordingly; and second, the detection of complications and risk factors and their management. The latter is probably best performed during a periodic review examination. This could be performed at annual intervals and it is clear that a specific clinic or longer appointment time would be needed to complete the entire screen (see Table 6). Supervision of diabetic control would need to be at more frequent intervals. Perhaps, the best solution in the hospital setting would be to devote a special review clinic to the annual screening and use the general diabetic clinic for routine diabetic supervision.

The diabetologist should not make such recommendations without considering the workload implications. Recent recommendations suggest that there should be one physician with a special interest in diabetes in each health district in the UK (Spathis, 1986). It was suggested that there should be five out-patient consultant sessions per week for a catchment population of 250 000 and this should be matched by 5.5 out-patient sessions from junior medical staff and clinical assistants. As Table 7 shows, these staffing levels are insufficient to cover the basic requirements of a routine diabetic clinic and annual review clinic if all the diabetics in the area are to be supervised. It also makes no allowance for the other out-patient duties of a diabetologist e.g. the joint eye clinic suggested for retinopathy patients.

Clearly, the hospital service cannot supervise all the diabetics in the area unless manpower is dramatically increased. Financial constraints have made this impossible in many districts. Other schemes have been proposed,

Table 6. Annual review of diabetic patient.

1. *Full history and assessment of glycaemic control*
    home monitoring
    weight loss/gain
    change in eyesight
    chest pain—angina, myocardial infarction
    breathlessness due to heart failure
    neurological symptoms—transient (TIA), stroke, neuropathy
    claudication, rest pain
    genitourinary—impotence
    smoking
    other medication

2. *Examination*
    weight, height
    visual acuity, pupillary dilatation and fundoscopy
    blood pressure lying and standing
    signs of heart failure
    peripheral pulses
    neurological examination including vibration threshold
    foot examination

3. *Investigations*
    urine—Albustix, albumin/creatinine ratio
    MSU—C & S
    blood glucose (fasting or timed postprandial)
    HbA_{1c}
    serum creatinine
    fasting lipids
    resting ECG with beat to beat variation

Table 7. The diabetic workload in an average health district in the United Kingdom.

Catchment population	250 000
Diabetes mellitus (1.01%)*	2525
NIDDM (75%)	1894

Annual review clinic (each diabetic seen × 1/year)
Based on 6 patients per doctor session and 45 clinic sessions per year.
9.4 doctor sessions
per week

Routine diabetic clinic (each diabetic seen × 2/year)
Based on 12 patients per doctor session and 45 clinic sessions per year.
4.7 doctor sessions
per week

*Gatling et al, 1985

e.g. GP mini clinics (Thorn and Russell, 1973) and shared diabetic care with GPs (Hill, 1987). However, shared care schemes are not without their dangers and problems. Hayes reported an increased mortality and morbidity in a group of patients looked after by their family doctors when compared with a matched control group managed in a hospital diabetic clinic (Hayes and Harries, 1984).

There is no single solution to the problem of organizing diabetic care. Whatever scheme operates, there should be a system of audit to ensure that all diabetics are being regularly reviewed and screened for complications. This will involve the maintenance of an accurate register of all diabetics in the area with regular updating of clinical information. A task with major administrative implications.

SUMMARY

The long term management of non-insulin-dependent diabetes falls into two categories: first, the supervision of glycaemic control; and second, the detection of complications, risk factors and their management. To aid the former, home/self monitoring is essential. Patients need to record their results so that they can be reviewed by their physician. At the same time, treatment including diet can be modified to improve control and education about diabetes can be continued. An annual screen is requried to detect the long term complications of diabetes: retinopathy; nephropathy; macrovascular disease; neuropathy; and diabetic foot disease. The early detection of these complications is important to gain maximal benefit from available treatment. The care of non-insulin-dependent diabetics requires skillful organization and in most health districts represents a considerable workload.

REFERENCES

Bloom S, Till S, Sonksen P & Smith S (1984) Use of biothesiometer to measure individual vibration thresholds and their variation in 519 non-diabetic subjects. *British Medical Journal* **288**: 1793–1795.

Boulton AJM, Drury J, Clarke B & Ward JD (1982) Continuous subcutaneous insulin infusion in the management of painful neuropathy. *Diabetes Care* **5**: 386–390.

British Multicentre Study Group (1977) Proliferative diabetic retinopathy: treatment with xenon-arc photocoagulation. Interim report of multicentre randomised controlled clinical trial. *British Medical Journal* **274**: 739–742.

British Multicentre Study Group (1983) Photocoagulation for diabetic maculopathy. A randomised controlled clinical trial using the Xenon arc. *Diabetes* **32**: 1010–1016.

Burns-Cox CJ & Dean Hart JC (1985) Screening diabetics for retinopathy by ophthalmic opticians. *British Medical Journal* **290**: 1052–1054.

Caird FI, Burditt AF & Draper GJ (1968) Diabetic Retinopathy. A further study of prognosis for vision. *Diabetes* **17**: 121–123.

Clark RS, English M, McNeill GP & Newton RW (1985) Effect of intravenous infusion of insulin in diabetics with acute myocardial infarction. *British Medical Journal* **291**: 303–305.

Dahl-Jorgensen K, Brinchmann-Hansen O, Hanssen KF et al (1986) Effect of near normo-glycaemia for two years on progression of early diabetic retinopathy, nephropathy, and neuropathy: The Oslo study. *British Medical Journal* **293**: 1195–1199.

Edmonds M (1986) The diabetic foot: pathophysiology and treatment. *Clinics in Endocrinology and Metabolism* **15(4)**: 889–916.

Ewing DJ & Clarke BF (1986) Autonomic Neuropathy: its diagnosis and prognosis. *Clinics in Endocrinology and Metabolism* **15(4)**: 855–888.

Feldt-Rasmussen B, Mathiesen ER & Deckert T (1986) Effect of two years of strict metabolic control on progression of incipient nephropathy in insulin-dependent diabetes. *Lancet* **ii**: 1300–1304.

Fuller JH, Shipley MJ, Rose G, Jarrett RJ & Keen H (1983) Mortality from coronary heart disease and stroke in relation to degree of glycaemia: the Whitehall Study. *British Medical Journal* **287**: 867–870.

Gatling W, Houston AC & Hill RD (1985) The prevalence of diabetes mellitus in a typical English community. *Journal of the Royal College of Physicians of London* **19**: 248–250.

Gatling W, Knight C, Mullee MA & Hill RD (1988a) Microalbuminuria in diabetes: a population study of the prevalence and an assessment of three screening tests. *Diabetic Medicine* **5**: 343–347.

Gatling W, Mullee MA, Knight C & Hill RD (1988b) Microalbuminuria in diabetes: relationships between urinary albumin excretion and selected variables. *Diabetic Medicine* **5**: 348.

Hayes TM & Harries J (1984) Randomised controlled trial of routine hospital clinic care versus routine general practice care for type II diabetics. *British Medical Journal* **289**: 728–730.

Hill RD (1981) Primary health care screening programme for diabetic eye disease. *Diabetologia* **20**: 670.

Hill RD (1987) *Diabetes Health Care*. London: Chapman and Hall.

Hommel E, Parving HH, Mathiesen E, Edsberg B, Nielsen MD & Giese J (1986) Effect of captopril on kidney function in insulin dependent diabetic patients with nephropathy. *British Medical Journal* **293**: 467–470.

Ireland JT, Viberti GC & Watkins PJ (1982) The kidney and renal tract. In Keen H & Jarrett J (eds) *Complications of Diabetes*, pp 137–178 (second edition). London: Edward Arnold.

Jarrett RJ, Viberti GC, Argyropoulos A, Hill RD, Mahmud U & Murrells TJ (1984) Microalbuminuria predicts mortality in non-insulin dependent diabetes. *Diabetic Medicine* **1**: 17–19.

Jones RH, Hayakawa M, MacKay JD, Parsons V & Watkins PJ (1979) Progression of diabetic nephropathy. *Lancet* **i**: 1105–1106.

Kohner EM, McLeod D & Marshall J (1982) Diabetic eye disease. In Keen H & Jarrett J (eds) *Complications of Diabetes*, pp 19–108 (second edition). London: Edward Arnold.

Mathiesen ER, Oxenboll B, Johansen K, Svendsen PA & Deckert T (1984) Incipient nephropathy in type I (insulin dependent) diabetes. *Diabetologia* **26**: 406–410.

Mogensen CE (1982) Long-term antihypertensive treatment inhibiting progression of diabetic nephropathy. *British Medical Journal* **285:** 685–688.

Mogensen CE (1984) Microalbuminuria predicts clinical proteinuria and early mortality in maturity onset diabetes. *New England Journal of Medicine* **310:** 356–360.

Mohamed A, Wilkin T, Leatherdale BA & Rowe D (1984) Response of urinary albumin to submaximal exercise in newly diagnosed non-insulin dependent diabetics. *British Medical Journal* **288:** 1342–1343.

Pirart J (1978) Diabetes mellitus and its degenerative complications: a prospective study of 4400 patients observed between 1947 and 1973. *Diabetes Care* **1:** 168–188, 252–263.

Royal College of Physicians of London and British Diabetic Association (1984) *The provision of medical care for adult diabetic patients*. London: BDA.

Ryder REJ, Young S, Vora JP, Atiea JA, Owens DR & Hayes TM (1985) Screening for diabetic retinopathy using polariod retinal photography though undilated pupils. *Practical Diabetes* **2:** 34–39.

Shenfield GM, Elton RA, Bhalla IP & Duncan LJP (1979) Diabetic mortality in Edinburgh. *Diabete et Metabolisme* **5:** 149–158.

Sorsby A (1972) The incidence and causes of blindness in England and Wales 1963–1968. *Reports on Public Health and Medical Subjects* **No 28** pp 33, 51. London: Her Majesty's Stationery Office.

Spathis GS (1986) Facilities in diabetic clinics in the UK: shortcomings and recommendations. *Diabetic Medicine* **3:** 131–136.

Thorn PA & Russell RG (1973) Diabetic clinics today and tomorrow: mini clinis in general practice. *British Medical Journal* **267:** 534–536.

Viberti GC, Wiseman M & Redmond S (1984) Microalbuminuria: its history and potential for prevention of clinical nephropathy in diabetes mellitus. *Diabetic Nephropathy* **3:** 79–82.

Waugh NR, Ellingford A & Scott SD (1986) Screening for diabetic retinopathy: options and cost effectiveness. *Practical Diabetes* **3:** 30–31.

WHO Expert Committee on Diabetes Mellitus (1980) *Second Report WHO Technical Report Services* **No 646**. Geneva: WHO.

WHO Multinational Study of Vascular Disease in Diabetes (1985) Prevalence of small vessel and large vessel disease in diabetic patients from 14 centres. *Diabetologia* **28:** 615–640.

Yudkin JS, Boucher BJ, Schopflin KE et al (1980) The quality of diabetic care in a London health district. *Journal of Epidemiology and Community Health* **34:** 277–280.

Index

Note: Page numbers of article titles are in **bold** type.